# DELIBERATE PRACTICE IN
# **PSYCHODYNAMIC**
# **PSYCHOTHERAPY**

# Essentials of Deliberate Practice Series
*Tony Rousmaniere and Alexandre Vaz, Series Editors*

*Deliberate Practice in Child and Adolescent Psychotherapy*
Jordan Bate, Tracy A. Prout, Tony Rousmaniere, and
Alexandre Vaz

*Deliberate Practice in Cognitive Behavioral Therapy*
James F. Boswell and Michael J. Constantino

*Deliberate Practice in Dialectical Behavior Therapy*
Tali Boritz, Shelley McMain, Alexandre Vaz, and
Tony Rousmaniere

*Deliberate Practice in Emotion-Focused Therapy*
Rhonda N. Goldman, Alexandre Vaz, and Tony Rousmaniere

*Deliberate Practice in Motivational Interviewing*
Jennifer K. Manuel, Denise Ernst, Alexandre Vaz, and
Tony Rousmaniere

*Deliberate Practice in Psychodynamic Psychotherapy*
Hanna Levenson, Volney Gay, and Jeffrey L. Binder

*Deliberate Practice in Rational Emotive Behavior Therapy*
Mark D. Terjesen, Kristene A. Doyle, Raymond A. DiGiuseppe,
Alexandre Vaz, and Tony Rousmaniere

*Deliberate Practice in Schema Therapy*
Wendy T. Behary, Joan M. Farrell, Alexandre Vaz, and
Tony Rousmaniere

*Deliberate Practice in Systemic Family Therapy*
Adrian J. Blow, Ryan B. Seedall, Debra L. Miller,
Tony Rousmaniere, and Alexandre Vaz

ESSENTIALS OF DELIBERATE PRACTICE SERIES

TONY ROUSMANIERE AND ALEXANDRE VAZ, SERIES EDITORS

# DELIBERATE PRACTICE IN
# PSYCHODYNAMIC PSYCHOTHERAPY

HANNA LEVENSON

VOLNEY GAY

JEFFREY L. BINDER

**AMERICAN PSYCHOLOGICAL ASSOCIATION**

Published by
American Psychological Association
750 First Street, NE
Washington, DC 20002
https://www.apa.org

Order Department
https://www.apa.org/pubs/books
order@apa.org

Typeset in Cera Pro by Circle Graphics, Inc., Reisterstown, MD

Printer: Gasch Printing, Odenton, MD
Cover Designer: Mark Karis

**Library of Congress Cataloging-in-Publication Data**

Names: Levenson, Hanna, 1945- author. | Gay, Volney P. (Volney Patrick),
    1948- author. | Binder, Jeffrey L., author.
Title: Deliberate practice in psychodynamic psychotherapy / Hanna Levenson,
    Volney Gay, and Jeffrey L. Binder.
Description: Washington, DC : American Psychological Association, [2023] |
    Series: Essentials of deliberate practice | Includes bibliographical
    references and index.
Identifiers: LCCN 2022054589 (print) | LCCN 2022054590 (ebook) |
    ISBN 9781433836732 (paperback) | ISBN 9781433841033 (ebook)
Subjects: LCSH: Psychodynamic psychotherapy. | Psychotherapists--Training of. |
    BISAC: PSYCHOLOGY / Education & Training | PSYCHOLOGY / Movements /
    Psychoanalysis
Classification: LCC RC489.P72 L483 2023 (print) | LCC RC489.P72 (ebook) |
    DDC 616.89/14--dc23/eng/20230320
LC record available at https://lccn.loc.gov/2022054589
LC ebook record available at https://lccn.loc.gov/2022054590

https://doi.org/10.1037/0000351-000

Printed in the United States of America

10 9 8 7 6 5 4 3 2

For Nathan, Evelyn Daisy, Bruin, & Callan

—Your Bonus Grandmother, H. L.

For Florence Gay Clark

—V. G.

For Dr. Cecilia Phillips-Binder, whose memory sustains me

—J. L. B.

# Contents

# Series Preface

*Tony Rousmaniere and Alexandre Vaz*

We are pleased to introduce the Essentials of Deliberate Practice series of training books. We are developing this book series to address a specific need that we see in many psychology training programs. The issue can be illustrated by the training experiences of Mary, a hypothetical second-year graduate school trainee. Mary has learned a lot about mental health theory, research, and psychotherapy techniques. Mary is a dedicated student; she has read dozens of textbooks, has written excellent papers about psychotherapy, and receives near-perfect scores on her course exams. However, when Mary sits with her clients at her practicum site, she often has trouble performing the therapy skills that she can write and talk about so clearly. Furthermore, Mary has noticed herself getting anxious when her clients express strong reactions, such as getting very emotional, hopeless, or skeptical about therapy. Sometimes this anxiety is strong enough to make Mary freeze at key moments, limiting her ability to help those clients.

During her weekly individual and group supervision, Mary's supervisor gives her advice informed by empirically supported therapies and common factor methods. The supervisor often supplements that advice by leading Mary through role-plays, recommending additional reading, or providing examples from her own work with clients. Mary, a dedicated supervisee who shares tapes of her sessions with her supervisor, is open about her challenges, carefully writes down her supervisor's advice, and reads the suggested readings. However, when Mary sits back down with her clients, she often finds that her new knowledge seems to have flown out of her head, and she is unable to enact her supervisor's advice. Mary finds this problem to be particularly acute with the clients who are emotionally evocative.

Mary's supervisor, who has received formal training in supervision, uses supervisory best practices, including the use of video to review supervisees' work. She would rate Mary's overall competence level as consistent with expectations for a trainee at Mary's developmental level. But even though Mary's overall progress is positive, she experiences some recurring problems in her work. This is true even though the supervisor is confident that she and Mary have identified the changes that Mary should make in her work.

The problem with which Mary and her supervisor are wrestling—the disconnect between her knowledge about psychotherapy and her ability to reliably perform psychotherapy—is the focus of this book series. We started this series because most therapists experience this disconnect, to one degree or another, whether they are beginning trainees or highly experienced clinicians. In truth, we are all Mary.

To address this problem, we are focusing this series on the use of deliberate practice, a method of training specifically designed for improving reliable performance of complex skills in challenging work environments (Rousmaniere, 2016, 2019; Rousmaniere et al., 2017). Deliberate practice entails experiential, repeated training with a particular skill until it becomes automatic. In the context of psychotherapy, this involves two trainees role-playing as a client and a therapist, switching roles every so often, under the guidance of a supervisor. The trainee playing the therapist reacts to client statements, ranging in difficulty from beginner to intermediate to advanced, with improvised responses that reflect fundamental therapeutic skills.

To create these books, we approached leading trainers and researchers of major therapy models with these simple instructions: Identify 10 to 12 essential skills for your therapy model where trainees often experience a disconnect between cognitive knowledge and performance ability—in other words, skills that trainees could write a good paper about but often have challenges performing, especially with challenging clients. We then collaborated with the authors to create deliberate practice exercises specifically designed to improve reliable performance of these skills and overall responsive treatment (Hatcher, 2015; Stiles et al., 1998; Stiles & Horvath, 2017). Finally, we rigorously tested these exercises with trainees and trainers at multiple sites around the world and refined them based on extensive feedback.

Each book in this series focuses on a specific therapy model, but readers will notice that most exercises in these books touch on common factor variables and facilitative interpersonal skills that researchers have identified as having the most impact on client outcome, such as empathy, verbal fluency, emotional expression, persuasiveness, and problem focus (e.g., Anderson et al., 2009; Norcross et al., 2019). Thus, the exercises in every book should help with a broad range of clients. Despite the specific theoretical model(s) from which therapists work, most therapists place a strong emphasis on pantheoretical elements of the therapeutic relationship, many of which have robust empirical support as correlates or mechanisms of client improvement (e.g., Norcross et al., 2019). We also recognize that therapy models have already-established training programs with rich histories, so we present deliberate practice not as a replacement but as an adaptable, transtheoretical training method that can be integrated into these existing programs to improve skill retention and help ensure basic competency.

## About This Book

Within the series, this book is a guide for incorporating deliberate practice into the training of psychodynamic trainees and clinicians. To begin, it is important to state that there is no one psychodynamic psychotherapy. Contemporary psychodynamic psychotherapy comprises a diverse family of treatment approaches. This aspect has made writing this book somewhat difficult. The authors needed to come to a more-or-less common understanding of the concepts, ways of formulating, and interventions of psychodynamic psychotherapy that they were going to focus on as a basis for their deliberate practice exercises. Fortunately, there are core common elements that the various psychodynamic approaches share (e.g., importance of conflict, early childhood development, unconscious processes). The psychodynamic therapy (PDT) deliberate practice skills that they have chosen for this book all pertain to these common elements (see Chapter 1 for more details). Consequently, practicing these skills should enhance the development of proficiency in any form of psychodynamic treatment, including both long-term and short-term therapies. In addition, in deriving the skills for this book, they have relied on an attachment-based, relational-psychodynamic treatment that incorporates all the common PDT elements—time-limited dynamic psychotherapy (Binder, 2004; Binder & Betan, 2013, 2022; Levenson, 2017).

By following the 12 skill exercises in this book, trainees can apply these PDT interventions with real patients more rapidly and smoothly than has been the case with traditional training methods, characterized by an awkward jump from classroom to actual therapy settings. Deliberate practice can help therapists integrate core PDT skills into their repertoire and into their own unique style. Deliberate practice as espoused in this book is intended as an enriching addition to PDT traditional training comprising course work, supervised therapy with real patients, and the therapist's own therapy. The PDT skills set forth in this book are not intended to comprehensively cover all relevant therapeutic skills. They have been chosen from a wide range of skills that capable PDT therapists must learn to offer psychodynamic treatments that are responsive to their patients' needs, contexts, and backgrounds.

The authors find this an exciting time to be doing PDT. Psychodynamic ways of thinking have now become so adopted into mainstream society that we hardly can appreciate how revolutionary they were when Freud and his colleagues conceived of them. Freud was a neurologist who hoped to create a neuroscience-based explanation of how the mind worked. His 1895 *Project for a Scientific Psychology* was, as they say, way ahead of its time (Freud, 1950/1895). Freud had to abandon this project because the understanding of the brain/mind during his lifetime was so rudimentary. We have had to wait until modern times to have sophisticated methodologies and noninvasive neuroimaging techniques to begin to explore the neurological correlates of some of the basic ideas behind psychodynamic practice. Today we are discovering that many of the central tenets of contemporary psychodynamic theory and practice (unconscious processes, defenses, transference, the centrality of conflict, representations of self and others, a relational mind, the importance of early development, psychological causality, corrective emotional experiences, and memory) may have neurological correlates. Recent developments in the cognitive neurosciences, neuropsychoanalysis, and developmental psychology have fostered a renewed interest in empirical foundations of psychodynamic forms of psychotherapy with their implications for practice (e.g., Cosolino, 2012; Damasio, 2012; Roffman & Gerber, 2009; Solms & Turnbull, 2011). As opined by Siegel (2017), "Freud is smiling from his grave." Modern science is beginning to support some of what he proposed, albeit in a very contemporary form. In addition, the authors agree with neuroscientist Eric Kandel (1999), who won the Nobel Prize in Medicine in 2000, that psychoanalytically oriented ways of conceptualizing and intervening "still represent the most coherent and intellectually satisfying view of the mind" (p. 505).

One last, prefatory word—the methods of precise rehearsal required of deliberate practice may appear out of place or even off-putting to teachers and supervisors who are training students to work in a field that cherishes awe, reverie, and unplanned "moments of meeting" (Lord, 2017; McWilliams, 1999; Stern, 2004). Nonetheless, the authors invite those with a skeptical attitude and critical eye to try this book, assess the reactions of the trainees and their patients, and then evaluate its usefulness for themselves.

Thank you for including us in your journey toward psychotherapy expertise. Enjoy your learning, enjoy the process! Now let's go practice!

# References

Anderson, T., Ogles, B. M., Patterson, C. L., Lambert, M. J., & Vermeersch, D. A. (2009). Therapist effects: Facilitative interpersonal skills as a predictor of therapist success. *Journal of Clinical Psychology, 65*(7), 755–768. https://doi.org/10.1002/jclp.20583

Binder, J. L. (2004). *Key competencies in brief dynamic psychotherapy. Clinical practice beyond the manual.* Guilford Press.

Binder, J. L., & Betan, E. J. (2013). *Core competencies in brief dynamic psychotherapy. Becoming a highly effective and competent brief dynamic psychotherapist.* Routledge. https://doi.org/10.4324/9780203837412

Binder, J. L., & Betan, E. J. (2022). The cyclical maladaptive pattern. In T. D. Eells (Ed.), *Handbook of psychotherapy case formulation* (3rd ed., pp. 113–143). Guilford Press.

Cosolino, L. (2012). *The neuroscience of human relationships: Attachment and the developing social brain* (2nd ed.). W. W. Norton & Company.

Damasio, A. (2012). Neuroscience and psychoanalysis: A natural alliance. *Psychoanalytic Review, 99*(4), 591–594. https://doi.org/10.1521/prev.2012.99.4.591

Freud, S. (1950). Project for a scientific psychology. In *The standard edition of the complete psychological works of Sigmund Freud* (Vol. 1, pp. 281–291). Imago. (Original work published 1895)

Hatcher, R. L. (2015). Interpersonal competencies: Responsiveness, technique, and training in psychotherapy. *American Psychologist, 70*(8), 747–757. https://doi.org/10.1037/a0039803

Kandel, E. R. (1999). Biology and the future of psychoanalysis: A new intellectual framework for psychiatry revisited. *American Journal of Psychiatry, 156*(4), 505–524. https://doi.org/10.1176/ajp.156.4.505

Levenson, H. (2017). *Brief dynamic therapy* (2nd ed.). American Psychological Association. https://doi.org/10.1037/0000043-000

Lord, S. (Ed.). (2017). *Moments of meeting in psychoanalysis: Interaction and change in the therapeutic encounter.* Routledge. https://doi.org/10.4324/9781315389967

McWilliams, N. (1999). *Psychoanalytic case formulation.* Guilford Press.

Norcross, J. C., Lambert, M. J., & Wampold, B. E. (2019). *Psychotherapy relationships that work* (3rd ed.). Oxford University Press.

Roffman, J. L., & Gerber, A. J. (2009). Neural models of psychodynamic concepts and treatments: Implications for psychodynamic psychotherapy. In R. A. Levy & J. S. Ablon (Eds.), *Handbook of evidence-based psychodynamic psychotherapy* (pp. 305–338). Humana Press. https://doi.org/10.1007/978-1-59745-444-5_13

Rousmaniere, T. G. (2016). *Deliberate practice for psychotherapists: A guide to improving clinical effectiveness.* Routledge Press. https://doi.org/10.4324/9781315472256

Rousmaniere, T. G. (2019). *Mastering the inner skills of psychotherapy: A deliberate practice manual.* Gold Lantern Press.

Rousmaniere, T. G., Goodyear, R., Miller, S. D., & Wampold, B. E. (Eds.). (2017). *The cycle of excellence: Using deliberate practice to improve supervision and training.* Wiley Publishers. https://doi.org/10.1002/9781119165590

Siegel, P. (2017, September 25). The psychodynamic brain: Emotion systems in the brain can run into conflict. *Psychology Today.* https://www.psychologytoday.com/us/blog/freud-lives/201709/the-psychodynamic-brain

Solms, M., & Turnbull, O. H. (2011). What is neuropsychoanalysis? *Neuro-psychoanalysis, 13*(2), 133–145. https://doi.org/10.1080/15294145.2011.10773670

Stern, D. N. (2004). *The present moment in psychotherapy and everyday life.* W. W. Norton & Co.

Stiles, W. B., Honos-Webb, L., & Surko, M. (1998). Responsiveness in psychotherapy. *Clinical Psychology: Science and Practice, 5*(4), 439–458. https://doi.org/10.1111/j.1468-2850.1998.tb00166.x

Stiles, W. B., & Horvath, A. O. (2017). Appropriate responsiveness as a contribution to therapist effects. In L. G. Castonguay & C. E. Hill (Eds.), *How and why are some therapists better than others? Understanding therapist effects* (pp. 71–84). American Psychological Association. https://doi.org/10.1037/0000034-005

# Acknowledgments

First and foremost, we thank our students who inspired this book—our past students, who embraced, struggled, and were courageous as part of their learning psychodynamic psychotherapy, and our present students who over the past 3 years have provided helpful and innovative comments as we tried out various exercises, many of which appear in this book. In particular, H. L. would like to acknowledge the feedback from her Case Conference students (2019–2022) at the Wright Institute, who formed the initial "lab" for testing out our exercises and participating in research about deliberate practice as a training method.

This book would not have come into being without the invitation, expert advice, and good humor of the editors of this series, Tony Rousmaniere and Alexandre Vaz. Their ongoing support was invaluable and enriching.

We are sincerely grateful to Richard Lane, Jacqueline Persons, and Joan Sarnat for their insightful consultations during critical phases of the book. We also extend our thanks to Sarina Volari, who helped get our drafts into proper form; Sarah Zemelman, who did videos of trainees doing example exercises; and Narayan Singh who added a sophisticated student's perspective to the exercises in various stages of development.

We acknowledge Rodney Goodyear for his significant contribution to starting and organizing this book series. We are grateful to Susan Reynolds, David Becker, Elizabeth Budd, Joe Albrecht, and Emily Ekle at American Psychological Association (APA) Books for providing expert guidance and insightful editing that has significantly improved the quality and accessibility of this book.

We are deeply indebted to K. Anders Ericsson, the inventor of the concept of deliberate practice; John D. Bransford, who introduced cutting-edge instructional methods and technologies; and Hans H. Strupp, whose work in time-limited dynamic psychotherapy was inspirational.

Finally, the writing of any book takes time—namely, time away from family, friends, and other endeavors. To our partners, colleagues, children, and grandchildren, thank you for your forbearance and encouragement. To our four-legged members of the family, your constant companionship during otherwise solitary hours at the computer was much appreciated.

The exercises in this book underwent extensive testing at many different training programs. For the following pilot site leaders and trainees who volunteered to "test run" this work and provided critically important feedback throughout the exercise refinement and writing process, we cannot thank you enough:

- Matthew R. Baity, Douglas Court, Hannah Greeley, Kayla Kaiser, Heidy Marcos, Nicole McClure, Sophia Miller, Jessa Mohaddess, El Phillip, Laura Pluckhan, Brian Raines, Traci Schrader, Megan Tedrow, Cherelle Young, Damien Brunt, Marina Chi, Jim McVeigh, Casey Rasmussen, Thomas Roche, Alex Miguel, Cassie Wells, Anna Feinman, Courtney Lodin, Jennifer Zhang, Kade Martineau, Ryan Shickman, and Jolene Spellman, Alliant International University, Sacramento, CA, United States

- Matt Blanchard, Walid Ali, Jonathan Applebaum, Maya Chandy, Yijia Dai, Mae Jones, Anita Sun, Roheena Moosa, William Ndama, Andrea Oberhauser Mendez, Nathra Palepu, Isadora Rodrigues, Catherine Coats, Jannatun Ferdowsi, Danielle Gurfinkel, Christian Marrero, Jimenez Rodriguez, Maria Angela, Chengwei Xu, Jessica Tsang, Nirj Mistry, and Charlette Yan, New York University Student Health Counseling and Wellness, New York, NY, United States

- Stephanie Chen, Richard Rubio, and Petra Janopaul, Counseling Program, Wright Institute, Berkeley, CA, United States

- Sallie G. DeGolia, Debra L. Safer, Maria Ocampo, Monica Allen, Aliza Goldberg, Jason Tucciarone, Alexandra Liu, Desiree Li, Bailey Shoenberger, Jason Tinero, Aimee Zhang, Meena Denduluri, Patricia Pop, Marissa Sia, Rebecca Cook, Sarah Joelson, Omar Bravo, Maggie Wang, Danielle Esses, Nekhya Fox, Emily Fox, Rosy Karna, Rachel Weiler, Monica Allen, Benjamin Goldwasser, Amanda Chang, Elizabeth Michael, Alix Simonson, Alex Macy, and Jennifer Stephens, Stanford University, Stanford, CA, United States

- Robert Hatcher, Victoria Martin, Dave Cazeau, Elisa Cameron, Tema Watstein, Julius Robins, Shruthi Jayashqankar, Kendell Doyle, Molly Finkel, Shiyun Chen, and Tingyun Tseng, Wellness Center, Graduate Center/City University of New York, New York, NY, United States

- Mark Hilsenroth, Taylor Groth, Natassia Johnson, Kate McMillen, Bianca Cersosimo, Lylli Cain, and Michael Katz, Adelphi University, Garden City, NY, United States

- Joel Jin, Narayan Singh, Emi Ichimura, and Melissa-Ann Lagunas, Seattle Pacific University, Seattle, WA, United States

- Richard D. Lane, Karen Weihs, Scott Salamone, Nick Ahrendt, Amanda Freitas, Vivian Le, Jen Bao, Allison Peet, Ramsha Rao, Marisa Fernandez, Prabh Singh, Michael Duerden, Mehrban Pour Parsi, Tyler Shiflett, Diana Crocker, Johannes Kieding, Ole Thiehaus, Beth Bernstein, and Amy Hu, University of Arizona, Tucson, AZ, United States

- Hanna Levenson, Rachel Coopersmith, Sydney Emerson, Rikki Feurstein, Jeremy Graves, Danya Lebell, Jason Leigh, Tessa Van der Meer, Madrone Love, Olga Gerasimenko, Mia Semelman, Kelsey Shogren, Sarina Volari, Madeleine Welte, and Joy Yamazaki-Jones, Wright Institute, Berkeley, CA, United States

- Michelle J. Montagno, Carisse Cronquist, Katherine Karimian, Cristian Lemus, Everardo Leon, Madeleine Marcus, Priscilla Phan, Brittani DeCloedt, Juliene Fresnedi, Natalia Giles, Megan McCarthy, and Jolene Spelman, University of San Francisco, San Francisco, CA, United States

- Teresa Ann Ostler, Paula Amat Norma, Marissa Benecke, Ellen Elghammer, Erin Galen, Julia Gold, Gayle Levin, Kaleb Pollum, Shaheli Seth, and Nathaniel Whitfield, University of Illinois at Urbana-Champaign, Champaign, IL, United States

- Jacqueline Persons and Garret G. Zieve, Oakland Cognitive Behavioral Therapy Center, Oakland, CA, United States

- Alexandre Vaz and Inês Amaro, Psinove, Lisbon, Portugal

We are also deeply grateful to the following colleagues and graduate students who graciously provided their valuable perspectives:

- Jordan Bate and Katie Aafjes-van Doorn, Ferkauf Graduate School of Psychology, Yeshiva University, New York, NY, United States
- Richard D. Lane, University of Arizona, Tucson, AZ, United States
- Jacqueline Persons, Oakland Cognitive Behavioral Therapy Center, Oakland, CA, United States
- Tracy A. Prout, IMPACT Psychological Services, Mamaroneck and Beacon, NY, United States
- Teri Quatman, Santa Clara University, Santa Clara, CA, United States
- Joan Sarnat, Psychoanalytic Institute of Northern California, Independent Practice, Oakland, CA, United States
- Thomas E. Schacht, East Tennessee State University, Johnson City, TN, United States
- Narayan Singh, Seattle Pacific University, Seattle, WA, United States
- Hans Welling, Integra, Lisbon, Portugal
- Garret G. Zieve, University of California, Berkeley, CA, United States

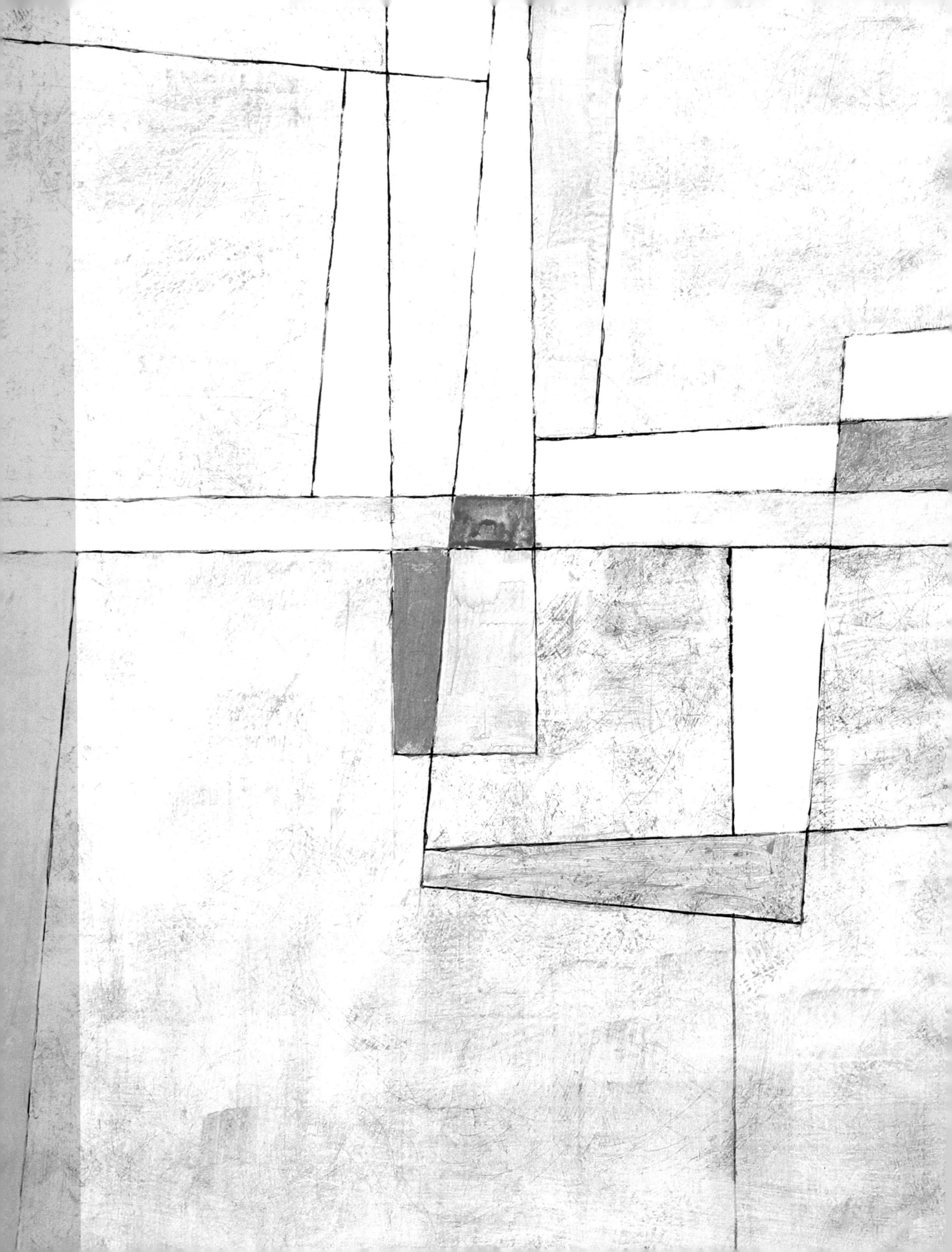

# Overview and Instructions

In Part I, we provide an overview of deliberate practice, including how it can be integrated into psychodynamic clinical training programs and instructions for performing the deliberate practice exercises in Part II. **We encourage both trainers and trainees to read both Chapters 1 and 2 before performing the deliberate practice exercises for the first time.**

Chapter 1 provides a foundation for the rest of the book by introducing important concepts related to deliberate practice and its role in psychotherapy training more broadly and psychodynamic therapy (PDT) training more specifically. Because so many models of PDT have evolved over time, we decided to focus on those features that all psychodynamic therapies hold in common. In addition, we provide background on the PDT conceptual framework including how it applies to psychopathology and psychotherapy. We also individually review the 12 PDT skill exercises.

Chapter 2 lays out the basic, most essential instructions for performing the PDT deliberate practice exercises in Part II. They are designed to be quick and simple and provide you with just enough information to get started without being overwhelmed by too much information. Chapter 3 in Part III provides more in-depth guidance, which we encourage you to read once you are comfortable with the basic instructions in Chapter 2.

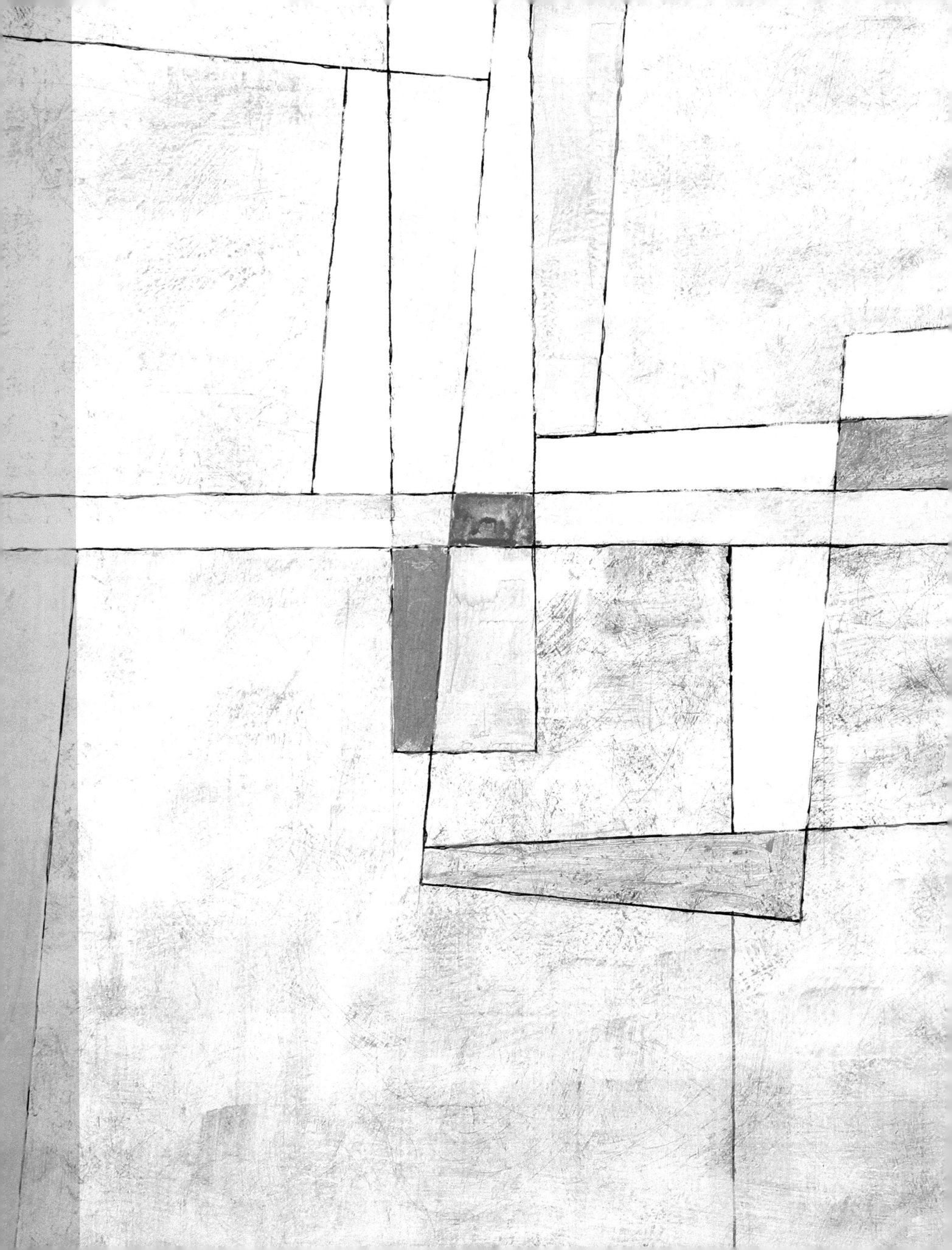

# Introduction and Overview of Deliberate Practice and Psychodynamic Therapy

It's almost 10 a.m. on a Sunday morning in the San Francisco Bay area. I've finished reading the front-page section of *The New York Times* along with my cup of Peet's coffee, and I'm setting up my computer on the kitchen table to get on Zoom to connect with Jeff Binder and Volney Gay, who are in Nashville, Tennessee. We have been meeting like this for 2 years now—almost overlapping entirely with COVID's sheltering-in-place protocols. I've known Jeff for more than 40 years since my early days at the San Francisco VA Medical Center, which was my first real-time job after I became a clinical psychologist. There I was responsible for training students and doing outpatient therapy mainly with Vietnam-era veterans. As part of my training responsibilities, I was heading up a Brief Psychodynamic Therapy Program for psychology predoctoral interns and third-year psychiatric residents. As part of this program, each trainee was assigned to work with one patient in a time-limited therapy (maximum 20 sessions). All sessions had to be videotaped, and trainees engaged in a group supervision every week where they would share portions of their videotaped sessions for that week. I would stop these tapes at critical junctures and ask the group members what they would say or do now and why. I would routinely call on the students to share their thoughts, feelings, and behavioral inclinations about their patients and about their colleagues' patients (what I called their *interactive countertransference*). We would often use those reactions to hypothesize how down the road they might "get hooked" (Kiesler, 1988) into reenacting some dysfunctional dynamic with the patient. There was a lot of focus on learning microskills, the absence of which became starkly clear during the drama of actual sessions.

It was during this time, in the early 1980s, that I heard about a National Institute of Mental Health (NIMH) study that was being conducted at Vanderbilt University in Nashville (which came to be nicknamed "Vandy II"). And that's how I met Jeff Binder. I invited myself to Nashville to see what was happening. Jeff was conducting the NIMH study with Hans Strupp, already a giant in the field of psychodynamic research and scholarly writing; they were in the process of supervising experienced therapists in how to do a relational form of time-limited dynamic psychotherapy (TLDP) that was designed to help therapists manage their countertransference reactions when seeing "difficult patients."

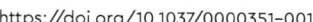

https://doi.org/10.1037/0000351-001
*Deliberate Practice in Psychodynamic Psychotherapy*, by H. Levenson, V. Gay, and J. L. Binder

It had been noted in "Vandy I" (a study done some years earlier) that certain patients (especially those who were outwardly hostile, demeaning, or otherwise unpleasantly provocative) were very adept at undermining their therapists' competent use of clinical skills. Therapists facing these difficult patients found that they were so preoccupied with managing their own emotional reactivity to their patients' demeaning or hostile stances, that they lost their therapeutic perspective and became enmeshed in their patients' *mishigas* (a Yiddish expression loosely translated as "their own neurotic stuff"). Jeff went on to write the now-classic book with Hans, *Psychotherapy in a New Key: A Guide to Time-Limited Dynamic Psychotherapy* (Strupp & Binder, 1984), that explicated this model of modern psychodynamic–interpersonal therapy designed to help therapists formulate and intervene without becoming unwitting accomplices to their patients' dysfunctional pushes and pulls in the therapeutic relationship.

So when Tony Rousmaniere approached me to write a manual for beginners to learn psychodynamic skills through deliberate practice, I immediately thought of Jeff as a coauthor. Jeff had by this time written his own papers and books on how to teach clinical competencies, and I admired how his mind worked. Just as personal computers were becoming available to the public, Jeff wrote about using hyperlinks to teach psychotherapy skills. I knew I had met an exceptional thinker when he suggested that "common sense" could be a very helpful therapeutic tool.

When I contacted Jeff to tantalize him into working on this endeavor with me, he immediately replied that we needed to involve a third person, Volney Gay, in the project. He described Volney as a Renaissance therapist's therapist who had held professorships in psychology, religious studies, and anthropology, as well as being a training and supervising analyst. The minute Volney showed us a video of how to learn to ride a bicycle step by step (hint: the first step doesn't involve pedaling), I knew we had found our third musketeer—a training analyst, who while seeing the infinite complexities of connecting with another human mind, could also envision clinical learning as incorporating discrete microskills.

Back to me at my kitchen table Zooming in to meet with Jeff and Volney for our regularly scheduled 2-hour Sunday meeting to discuss the skill we were working on that month for this book. There would be laughter, discussions of philosophies of human nature, and pedagogical methods, interspersed with working on the conception, composition, and testing of scores of exercises—12 of which made it into this manual. There were times we were daunted by what we were trying to do, and then there would be flashes of encouragement and relief as we watched videos of trainees trying out our exercises and exclaiming, "Hey, we're beginning to get it!"

Adding up the years the three of us have been teaching, supervising, and doing clinical work, the number is around 150! When we started out in this profession, our hair was darker and there was more of it. But as we came together to write this book, we were still just as excited and eager to venture into uncharted territories as when we began our careers. We are pleased to introduce this enlivening way to learn in a field that we promise will never be tedious or monotonous, but rather continuously challenging and enriching.

## Overview of the Deliberate Practice Exercises

This book focuses on 14 exercises that have been thoroughly tested and modified based on feedback from psychodynamic therapy (PDT) trainers and trainees. Each of the first 12 exercises each represent an essential psychodynamic skill. Table 1.1

**TABLE 1.1. The 12 Psychodynamic Skills Presented in the Deliberate Practice Exercises**

| Intermediate Skills | Advanced Skills |
| --- | --- |
| 1. Engaging in a therapeutic inquiry | 7. Making transference interpretations |
| 2. Being aware of countertransference reactions | 8. Using metaphors |
| 3. Deepening emotional experience | 9. Exploring fantasy |
| 4. Making process comments | 10. Case formulation: gathering data for the cyclical maladaptive pattern |
| 5. Pointing out defenses and inquiring about underlying fear | 11. Using supervision to recognize reenactments |
| 6. Introducing the rationale for treatment | 12. Providing a corrective emotional experience |

presents the 12 skills that are covered in these exercises. The last two exercises are more comprehensive, consisting of an annotated psychodynamic-relational transcript of an actual case (Exercise 13) and improvised mock therapy sessions (Exercise 14). Together they teach students how to integrate these 12 skills into more expansive clinical scenarios.

In these exercises, trainees work in pairs under the guidance of a teacher and role-play as a patient and a therapist, switching back and forth between the two roles. Each of the 12 skill-focused exercises consists of 15 patient statements grouped by difficulty—beginner, intermediate, and advanced—that calls for a specific skill. For each skill, trainees are asked to read through the description of the skill, its criteria, and some examples of it. The trainee playing the patient then reads the statements, which present possible symptoms, problems, and emotional states. The trainee playing the therapist then improvises a response that meets the criteria that define that particular skill. The one exception to this format is Exercise 11, where the role-plays are between a trainee playing the supervisor and a trainee playing the therapist.

After each patient statement and therapist response couplet is practiced several times, the trainees will stop to receive feedback from their teacher. Guided by the teacher, the trainees will be instructed to try statement–response couplets several times, working their way down the list. In consultation with their teacher, trainees will go through the exercises, starting with the least challenging and moving to more advanced levels. The triad (teacher–patient–therapist) will have the opportunity to discuss whether exercises were too hard or too easy and adjust them accordingly.

In consultation with teachers, trainees can decide which skills they wish to work on and for how long. On the basis of our testing experience, we have found practice sessions should last about an hour for maximum benefit. Anything longer can cause trainee fatigue and reduce learning efficiency.

We envision these exercises being done during an hour of class time or as homework assignments. We found that using the internet (e.g., Zoom calls) provided an easy way to partner with another classmate and provided a simple way to record the sessions for later review or viewing by the teacher. We understand that in the pragmatics of teaching many students at once, the teacher or supervisor may not be available for students while they are practicing. In that case, the exercise will be the therapist–patient dyad alone. Anticipating this adjustment, at the end of all exercises, we provide a few plausible therapist responses so students can judge whether they have met the skill criteria. It is best for the role-playing therapist to improvise responses before consulting the possible responses provided, staying true to the tenets of deliberate practice.

Ideally, learners of psychodynamic–interpersonal theory and practice will both gain confidence and achieve competence through practicing these exercises. *Competence* is defined here as the ability to perform a psychodynamic skill in a manner that is flexible and responsive to the patient. We have chosen skills we view as essential to PDT and that beginning practitioners often find challenging to implement.

The skills identified in this book are not comprehensive. They do not represent everything one needs to learn to become a competent psychodynamic clinician. Far from it! A short history of psychodynamic–interpersonal approaches and a brief description of the deliberate practice methodology will be provided to explain how we have arrived at the union between them.

## The Goals of This Book

We have three primary goals: (a) to familiarize trainees with the format of deliberate practice so that they can draw on deliberate practice throughout their professional careers, (b) to help trainees achieve competence in core psychodynamic–interpersonal skills, and (c) to introduce the background and function of deliberate practice to teachers/supervisors and thereby encourage its use.

In addition, these deliberate practice exercises are designed to achieve the following:

1. Help therapists-in-training develop their ability to apply the skills in a range of clinical situations.

2. Move these skills into procedural memory (Squire, 2004) so therapists can access them even when they are tired, stressed, overwhelmed, or discouraged.

3. Provide therapists-in-training with an opportunity to exercise a particular skill using a style and language that is congruent with who they are.

4. Provide the opportunity to use these skills in response to varying patient statements, presenting problems, and affects. We designed them to build confidence to adopt skills in a broad range of circumstances within different patient contexts.

5. Provide therapists-in-training with many opportunities to fail and then correct their failed response on the basis of feedback. This helps build confidence and persistence.

6. Finally, this book aims to help trainees discover their personal learning style so they can continue their professional development long after their formal training is concluded.

## Who Can Benefit From This Book?

This book can be used in multiple contexts, including in graduate-level courses, supervision, postgraduate training, and continuing education programs. We assume the following:

1. The trainer is knowledgeable about and competent in PDT.

2. The trainer can demonstrate how to use PDT skills across a range of therapeutic situations, via role-play and/or video. There are numerous accessible American Psychological Association (APA) videos illustrating psychodynamic strategies and techniques that can be used for this purpose (e.g., Levenson, 1999; Levenson & Carlson, 2008,

2010; McCullough & Carlson, 2005; McWilliams & Carlson, 2008; Safran & Carlson, 2008, 2009; Wachtel & Carlson, 2007).

3. The trainer can provide feedback to students regarding how to craft and improve their application of PDT skills.

4. Trainees will have accompanying readings, such as books and articles, that explain the theory, research, and rationale of PDT and each particular skill. Recommended reading for each skill is provided in the sample syllabus (Appendix C).

The exercises covered in this book were piloted many times in various training sites. This book pertains to trainers and trainees from different cultural backgrounds worldwide. For guidance on how to improve one's skills in dealing with multicultural issues, see the forthcoming book *Deliberate Practice in Multicultural Therapy* (Harris et al., in press).

We wrote this book for those in all stages of formal training (from never having seen a patient to postdoctoral settings). However, it will be of interest to seasoned therapists as well. Experienced therapists know that to do clinical work competently, one needs to pursue lifelong learning approach. All exercises feature guidance for assessing and adjusting the difficulty to precisely target the needs of each individual learner. The term *trainee* in this book is used broadly, referring to anyone in the field of professional mental health seeking to acquire PDT skills.

## Deliberate Practice in Psychotherapy Training

How does one become an expert in a professional field? What is trainable and what is simply beyond one's reach, due to innate or uncontrollable factors? Questions such as these touch on our fascination with expert performers and their development. A mixture of awe, admiration, and even confusion surround people such as Mozart, Leonardo da Vinci, or more contemporary top performers such as basketball legend Michael Jordan and chess virtuoso Garry Kasparov. What accounts for their consistently superior professional results? Evidence suggests that the time spent on a particular type of practice is essential to developing expertise in virtually all domains (Ericsson & Pool, 2016). "Deliberate practice" is an evidence-based method that can improve performance in an effective and reliable manner.

The concept of deliberate practice originated in a classic study by K. Anders Ericsson and colleagues (1993). They found that the amount of time practicing a skill and the quality of the time spent doing so predicted mastery and acquisition. They identified five key activities in learning and mastering skills: (a) observing one's own work, (b) getting expert feedback, (c) setting small incremental learning goals just beyond the performer's ability, (d) engaging in repetitive behavioral rehearsal of specific skills, and (e) continuously assessing performance. Ericsson and his colleagues termed this process *deliberate practice*, a cyclical process that is illustrated in Figure 1.1.

Lengthy engagement in deliberate practice is associated with expert performance across various professional fields, such as medicine, sports, music, chess, computer programming, and mathematics (Ericsson et al., 2018). People may associate deliberate practice with the widely known "10,000-hour rule" popularized by Malcolm Gladwell in his 2008 book, *Outliers*, although the actual number of hours required for expertise varies by field and by individual (Ericsson & Pool, 2016). This "rule," however, perpetuated two errors. The first is that the number of deliberate practice hours needed to

**FIGURE 1.1. Cycle of Deliberate Practice**

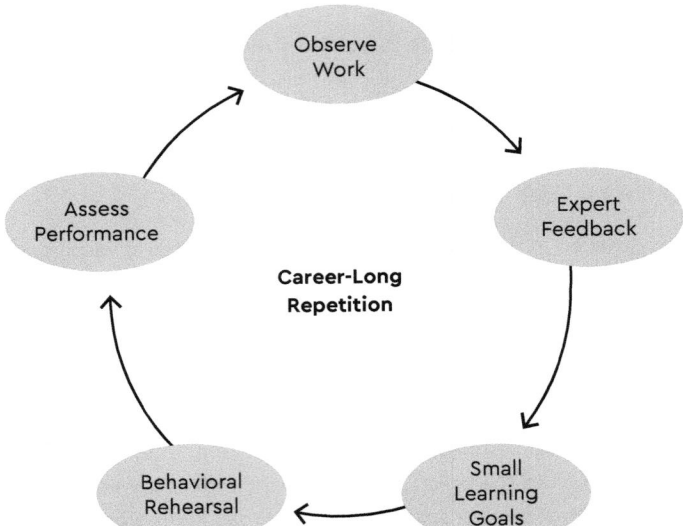

*Note.* From *Deliberate Practice in Emotion-Focused Therapy* (p. 7), by R. N. Goldman, A. Vaz, and T. Rousmaniere, 2021, American Psychological Association (https://doi.org/10.1037/0000227-000). Copyright 2021 by the American Psychological Association.

attain expertise is fixed. On the contrary, there is considerable variability in how many hours are required in different domains.

The second error is asserting that engagement in 10,000 hours of work performance will generate expertise in that domain. This error applies to psychotherapy, where the number of hours of clinical work has traditionally been used as a measure of proficiency (Rousmaniere, 2016). However, research suggests that the number of hours of experience does not predict therapist effectiveness (Goldberg, Babins-Wagner, et al., 2016; Goldberg, Rousmaniere, et al., 2016). It seems more likely that the presence or absence of deliberate practice is a key factor.

Recognizing the value of deliberate practice in other fields, psychotherapy scholars have incorporated deliberate practice into training for mental health professionals (e.g., Bailey & Ogles, 2019; Binder & Betan, 2013; Hill et al., 2020; Rousmaniere et al., 2017; Taylor & Neimeyer, 2017; Tracey et al., 2015). There are good reasons to question analogies made between psychotherapy and other professional fields, like sports or music. In comparison, psychotherapy is complex and free-form. Sports have clearly defined goals, and classical music follows a written score. In contrast, the goals of psychotherapy shift with the unique presentation of each patient in each session. Therapists do not have the luxury of following a score.

Instead, good psychotherapy is more like improvisational jazz (Noa Kageyama, cited in Rousmaniere, 2016). In jazz improvisations, a complex mixture of group collaboration, creativity, and interaction are coconstructed among band members. Like psychotherapy sessions, no two jazz improvisations are identical. However, improvisations are not a random collection of notes. They are grounded in a comprehensive conceptual understanding and technical proficiency that is developed only through continuous deliberate practice. For example, prominent jazz instructor Jerry Coker (1990) listed 18 skill areas that students must master, each of which has multiple discrete skills including tone quality, intervals, chord arpeggios, scales, patterns, and licks. In this sense, more creative and artful improvisations reflect previous commitments to repetitive skill practice and acquisition. As legendary jazz musician Miles Davis put it, "Sometimes you have to play a long time to be able to play like yourself" (Cook, 2005, p. 34).

We want our book on deliberate practice to help PDT therapists become themselves. The goal is to acquire skills so that you have them on hand when you need them. Practice the skills to make them your own. Incorporate aspects that feel right for you. Ongoing and effortful deliberate practice does not impede flexibility and creativity. It enhances both. Effective PDT therapists integrate previously acquired skills with properly attuned flexibility. The core PDT responses we provide as examples are meant as templates or possibilities, rather than "answers." Please interpret and apply them as you see fit, in a way that makes sense to you. We encourage flexible and improvisational play!

## Simulation-Based Mastery Learning

Deliberate practice uses simulation-based mastery learning (Ericsson, 2004; McGaghie et al., 2014). That is, the stimulus material for training consists of "contrived social situations that mimic problems, events, or conditions that arise in professional encounters" (McGaghie et al., 2014, p. 375). In other words, stimuli used in training are sufficiently like real-world experiences that they provoke similar reactions. This facilitates *state-dependent learning*. Using deliberate practice, students acquire skills in an environment that evokes emotions and cognitive challenges evoked in real-life contexts (R. P. Fisher & Craik, 1977; Smith, 1979). For example, pilots train with flight simulators that present mechanical failures and dangerous weather conditions, and surgeons practice with surgical simulators that present medical complications. Training in simulations with challenging stimuli increases professionals' capacity to perform effectively under stress. In this book, the "simulators" are typical patient statements that might be presented in the course of therapy sessions and call on the same skill needed in that context. The fact that the learning is interpersonal (e.g., role-plays with peers) rather than individual, adds to the stressful environment, simulating the tension that occurs when working with actual patients.

## Declarative Versus Procedural Knowledge

*Declarative knowledge* is what a person can understand, write, or speak about. It often refers to information that can be consciously recalled through memory and is often acquired relatively quickly. In contrast, procedural learning is implicit in memory and "usually requires *repetition of an activity*, and associated learning is demonstrated through *improved task performance*" (Koziol & Budding, 2012, p. 2694, emphasis added). *Procedural knowledge* is what a person can perform, especially under stress (Squire, 2004). There may be a wide difference between demonstrations of declarative versus procedural knowledge. For example, an "armchair quarterback" is a person who criticizes an athletic performance but would have trouble performing it at a level commensurate with their critique. Likewise, most dance, music, or theater critics can write eloquently about their subjects but would be flummoxed if asked to perform them.

In PDT training, the gap between declarative and procedural knowledge appears, for example, when a trainee or therapist can recognize and appreciate a metaphor that lands adeptly on the edge of the patient's awareness, pushing the patient forward to new insights ever so subtly. The same student struggles to provide similar metaphors with real patients. **The sweet spot for deliberate practice is the gap between**

**declarative and procedural knowledge.** In other words, effortful practice should target those skills that the trainee could write a good paper about but would have trouble performing with an actual patient. We start with declarative knowledge, learning skills theoretically, and observing others perform them. Once students can do that, we seek to foster procedural learning using deliberate practice exercises. Our goal is to give therapists "automatic" access to these 12 skills so they can use them easily when necessary. Following in-class training with simulated patients, supervisors can help students further refine their skills with actual patients (Binder, 1999, 2004; Levenson, 2017).

Let us turn to some background on PDT to help contextualize these 12 skills and locate them in contemporary, psychodynamic theory and practice.

## Psychodynamic–Interpersonal Therapy

### Common Features

The terms *psychoanalytic therapy* and *psychodynamic therapy* for the most part can be considered synonymous. Both terms refer to a "family" of therapies that can have different views of human functioning and malfunctioning and may have variations in language, but share certain features. We base our book on a contemporary, attachment-based, relational–interpersonal approach used by a wide range of psychodynamic practitioners. More specifically, we use a model of TLDP (Levenson, 1995; Strupp & Binder, 1984). TLDP incorporates elements relevant to many psychodynamic approaches. It provides a teachable way of formulating and intervening, has a research base, and the availability of additional materials (e.g., books, videos). TLDP is compatible with short- and long-term applications, and is well-known to the authors of this manual.

What features do PDTs have in common? There are several informative sources. Blagys and Hilsenroth (2000) reviewed publications that consistently and significantly differentiated psychodynamic–interpersonal therapy from cognitive behavior therapy (CBT) in at least two studies, in at least two different research labs. These investigators delineated seven activities or focal areas that distinguished short-term, manualized psychodynamic-interpersonal therapy from CBT (see Exhibit 1.1).

---

**EXHIBIT 1.1. Summary of Distinctive Features of Psychodynamic–Interpersonal Psychotherapy**

1. Focus on affect and the expression of patients' emotion
2. Exploration of patients' attempts to avoid topics or engage in activities that hinder the progress of therapy
3. The identification of patterns in patients' actions, thoughts, feelings, experiences, and relationships
4. Emphasis on past experiences
5. Focus on patients' interpersonal experiences
6. Emphasis on the therapeutic relationship
7. Exploration of patients' wishes, dreams, or fantasies

*Note.* From "Distinctive Features of Short-Term Psychodynamic-Interpersonal Psychotherapy: A Review of the Comparative Psychotherapy Process Literature," by M. D. Blagys and M. J. Hilsenroth, 2000, *Clinical Psychology: Science and Practice, 7*(2), p. 185 (https://doi.org/10.1093/clipsy.7.2.167). Copyright 2000 by the American Psychological Association.

Shedler (2022) has described stereotyped, outmoded, and misunderstood aspects of psychodynamic practice and theory that have little resemblance to modern PDT. In a paper, provocatively titled "That Was Then, This Is Now: Psychoanalytic Psychotherapy for the Rest of Us," he explicates how psychodynamic theory and practice have developed over time. He asked, "If psychoanalysis is not a theory about the id, ego and superego, or fixations, or repressed memories, what *is* it about?" (p. 406). He then goes on to name and describe the following distinctive features of contemporary psychodynamic technique: an emphasis on unconscious mental life, the mind in conflict, the past affecting the present, transference in the therapeutic relationship, defensive processes, and psychological causation.

Similarly, when therapists representing three theoretical approaches identified essential processes for their approach (Boterhoven De Haan & Lee, 2014), distinct differences emerged. Essential features for PDT were a focus on the patient's feelings; insight; therapy relationship; recurrent themes; nonjudgmental acceptance; discussion of scheduling, fees, and interruptions in treatment; therapeutic process; interpersonal relationships; and interpretation of unconscious wishes, feelings, and ideas.

These lists from three perspectives (examination of publications, tracking development over time, and therapists' self-reports) overlap to a considerable degree. Using these research findings, we formed our operational definition of PDT. In this book, we discuss skills exemplifying these characteristic features: (a) focus on unconscious processes; (b) focus on affect and expressions of emotion; (c) identification of patterns of actions, thoughts, feelings, fantasies, and interpersonal relationships; (d) focus on defenses (i.e., coping strategies to avoid uncomfortable topics and unwittingly hinder therapeutic progress); (e) emphasis on how past experiences influence current thinking and behavior; and (f) focus on transference and countertransference (i.e., identifying how the patient's problematic patterns are manifested in the therapeutic relationship). For convenience, in this book we use the term *psychodynamic therapy*, or PDT.

## Research in PDT

Regarding treatment research findings, we would like to address a widespread misconception among both psychodynamic clinicians and practitioners representing other treatment orientations. It is commonly assumed that, in contrast to CBT, which has been extensively studied and is considered evidence-based, psychodynamic therapies are not supported by empirical evidence and are therefore an inferior form of treatment. In fact, as of 2021, there had been at least 243 randomized controlled trials (RCTs) comparing the efficacy of both long- and short-term psychodynamic therapies to control groups representing no treatment, treatment as usual, or other gold standard therapies, such as CBT. RCTs and meta-analyses consistently have found psychodynamic therapies to be significantly more effective than control groups and, compared with other therapy approaches, equally effective in treating mood, anxiety, and personality disorders (Barber et al., 2021).

## Conceptual Framework

To take full advantage of the skill exercises in this book, the reader should possess compatible models of personality, psychopathology, and therapeutic processes. A psychodynamic therapist must have a cognitive map or "working model" of the immediate therapeutic situation, including just enough theory to comprehend the problem context and design intervention strategies, but not so much as to get in the way of attunement to the patient and spontaneous reactions to the changing context. Such a mental model will provide readers who use the exercises a conceptual framework within which to see the therapeutic role that each skill plays in furthering therapeutic progress.

### A Theory of Personality

*Personality Structure.*   The building blocks of personality can be viewed as *interaction structures* that contain self-representations associated with a sense of individual identity (Beebe et al., 1997; Sandler & Sandler, 1978). These interaction structures are composed of self-representations and object-representations that are inextricably linked together by transactional scenarios characterized by particular affective tones (Mitchell, 1988). Psychological structures are not stable, impermeable edifices. Rather, they are ingrained patterns of mental activity that reflect adaptations to one's internal and external environments; they are slow to form and slow to change. Interaction structures occupy the foreground of personality, whereas cognitive and perceptual processes are conceived as occupying the background of personality. In that capacity, they function as information processors of the content contained in the interaction structures.

The interaction structures that characterize each personality are the product of the unique physiologic and genetic makeup of the person plus that person's internalization of relationships with others. From the moment of birth on, transactions with others, particularly those on whom the individual relies for protection and physical and emotional sustenance (i.e., "significant others"), are internalized. They shape the organization and content of the emerging personality structure.

The interaction structures that comprise the foundation of personality are composites of multiple, discrete internalized experiences that share common narrative elements. Although we use the word *structures*, we do not mean a static template but a dynamic process leading to action. If you took videos depicting a child interacting with parents, friends, and teachers in which the child is rejected, for example, that set of videos would be a visible, public record of the child's private, interpersonal schema. Typically, these schemas are not directly accessible to the child's conscious awareness. Many of these memory traces were laid down before the infant could comprehend speech; they are embodied. Indeed, they are procedural memories. However, they contain the rules of approved behavior, and so they dominate all later interactions. And, as learned procedures, they implicitly and silently guide one's expectations and patterns of behavior with others. In the language of cognitive psychology, they represent procedural interpersonal knowledge (Binder, 2004). While operating behind the scenes, these structures contribute to self- and object-relational units that are maintained in conscious awareness (Horowitz, 1998).

In any interpersonal encounter, an individual follows a cognitive map or *internal working model* of the situation (Bowlby, 1988). An adaptive working model is flexible and can be modified by immediate feedback as the interaction unfolds, even though it is the product of combining schematic themes and direct observations of the current situation in which the person is engaged (Horowitz, 1998). The salient themes that characterize a person's internal working models are reflected in the distinguishing features of their personality and interpersonal style. An individual's characteristic pattern of interacting with others tends to evoke a circumscribed, reciprocal range of reactions from others. These reactions, in turn, tend to reinforce the likelihood that the original interpersonal actions will be repeated because they tend to fulfill the expectations of the instigator of the original actions. Through such complementary transactions, an interpersonal style—for good or ill—tends to become self-perpetuating (Binder, 2004; Strupp & Binder, 1984). Wachtel (1993) termed such a reciprocally reinforcing system *cyclical psychodynamics*.

*Motivation and Development.* Classic psychoanalytic theory of motivation posited the reduction of sexual and aggressive tensions through the discharge of biologically based "drives." Beginning in the mid-20th century, British object relations theorists began to replace the drive theory of motivation with theories that viewed human beings as innately *object-seeking* (Fairbairn, 1952). The American interpersonal psychiatrist, H. S. Sullivan (1954) proposed that the fundamental human motivation was a sense of security produced by harmonious interpersonal interactions. By far the most influential motivation theorist was John Bowlby (1969/1982). Using attachment theory, he took an evolutionary perspective in which he postulated the existence of biologically ingrained behavioral systems whose purpose is to achieve and maintain physical proximity to caretakers to ensure protection from predators and other dangers.

Bowlby's attachment theory emphasizes the human motivation to seek connected-ness with other humans. Blatt (beginning in 1974 and culminating in his 2008 book, *Polarities of Experience*), added a seemingly opposing but complementary motive, which is to seek autonomy, mastery, self-sufficiency, and self-definition. Examining the fields of personality development, psychopathology, and therapeutic process, Blatt (2008) described the dialectic tension that exists between the motives for meaningful inter-personal relatedness and the motives for a coherent and integrated self-definition. He stated, "Development in the sense of the self leads to increasingly mature levels of inter-personal relatedness that, in turn, facilitate further differentiation and integration of the development of the self" (pp. 3–4). This same sentiment is evidenced in the work of Safran and Muran (2000) on negotiating therapeutic alliances and originally in Bowlby's (1988) view of attachment. They suggest that taking independent action in the world is possible only if one is sure that a *secure base* of interpersonal intimacy awaits one's return.

## A Theory of Psychopathology

Corresponding with the move of contemporary psychoanalytic theories away from Freudian structural theory (e.g., ego, id, superego) and drive theory (e.g., libido, aggres-sion), has come a deemphasis on concepts of inner conflict, defense, and compromise formation. Instead, contemporary psychoanalytic theories of psychopathology share an emphasis on parental empathic failures in attuning to an infant's and child's devel-opmental needs and individual temperament.

The long period in which human infants and children need adult parental figures to care for and protect them gives parental figures vast influence on the child's personality development. If the child is not under significant physiological or interpersonal stress, the child will develop representations of relational experiences that are adaptive and realistic. However, if a child endures extended stress, the child will develop impaired cognitive and perceptual functions, resulting in maladaptive person schemas. Another contribution to the development of maladaptive person schemas occurs when the parenting figures pressure the child to assume certain personality characteristics and behaviors and to avoid or disavow others. When infants or children feel compelled to shape themselves in a particular way to maintain emotional bonds with their parenting figures, their resultant person schemas will be rigidly maintained and will be interpersonally circumscribed.

A person's self-representations and expectations of others developed while coping with early relations with parenting figures are rigidly clung to and do not adequately consider current interpersonal realities. In other words, the adult is burdened with early modes of relating that at one time were adaptive but are now maladaptive (Eagle, 2011). Or as more poetically put by William Faulkner (1951) in his novel *Requiem for a Nun*, "The past is never dead. It's not even past."

Consequently, in all its manifestations psychopathology essentially represents personality characterized by internal person schemas or working models that are rigidly adhered to and delimit the repertoire of corresponding modes of relating available to the person (Binder, 2004). Persons with impaired working models will inevitably show impairments to their cognitive and perceptual functions. Severe warping of narrative structures, synonymous with *personality disorders*, often is associated with difficulties managing emotions (i.e., overcontrol or dysregulation) and self-soothing (e.g., self-esteem problems). When insults to cognitive and perceptual functions distort reality-testing, psychotic symptoms such as delusions and hallucinations appear. These sorts of personality malformations and maladaptations are invariably associated with symptoms of anxiety and depression.

## A Theory of Psychotherapy

Congruent with contemporary PDT's theories of personality and psychopathology, the primary PDT in-session or process goal is to identify salient, maladaptive interaction structures and corresponding maladaptive patterns of interpersonal relating. The primary *outcome goal* is to modify these maladaptive internal representations and interpersonal patterns and replace them with new, more adaptive and satisfying ways of experiencing and relating to self and to others. The ultimate therapeutic aim is to help patients remove impediments to their ability to make choices that will, at least, provide an opportunity for increased satisfaction and happiness (Binder, 2004; Eagle, 2011; Levenson, 2017).

Contemporary psychodynamic therapists seek to engage actively with their patients and display a more overtly emotional connection, characterized by empathy and nonjudgmental acceptance. The therapist actively listens to the patient. This interpersonal stance on the therapist's part is often a novel experience for the patient. It contributes to *corrective emotional experiences* in which the therapist's attitudes and behavior disconfirm the patient's maladaptive and negative interpersonal expectations. Another powerful "corrective" experience occurs when therapists realize they have been unwittingly recruited by the patient into playing a role in the patient's maladaptive scenario and begin to disembed themselves (Kiesler, 1988; Levenson, 2017; Muran & Barber, 2010; Safran & Muran, 2000; Strupp & Binder, 1984). These interactions disconfirm the patient's negative expectations and so weaken the maladaptive interaction structures producing them (Alexander & French, 1946; Eagle, 2011). These corrective emotional experiences, which may be a function of memory reconsolidation, are considered to be a primary change agent (Levenson et al., 2020).

In addition to experiential learning, another primary change agent is *insight*, or increased awareness of one's idiosyncratic views of self and others, as well as one's own motivations, expectations, assumptions, feelings, and behavior (Binder, 2004; Levenson, 2017). There is now solid empirical support for the association of increased insight and positive outcome in PDT (Barber et al., 2021). Related to increased insight are changes for the better in measures of internal interaction structures or *quality of object relations*, less reliance on immature defenses, and increase in *mentalization* (i.e., increases in the capacities for self-reflection and for empathizing with others), the ability to comprehend one's own and other's mental states, and to use that information to explain and guide interpersonal behavior (Barber et al., 2021; Fonagy & Bateman, 2006).

From empirical and clinical points of view, the change agent most consistently predictive of positive treatment outcomes is the *therapeutic alliance*. Contemporary psychodynamic approaches differ regarding how they conceptualize the therapeutic alliance. One view is that a positive alliance is a necessary interpersonal context for the therapist's technical strategies to be effective; another view is that a strong, positive alliance is necessary and sufficient to produce therapeutic progress. Safran and Muran (2000) proposed another way in which the therapeutic alliance is associated with therapeutic progress. They posited that during any psychotherapy, ruptures to the alliance will inevitably occur and the therapist's identifying and resolving these ruptures is essential for a positive therapy outcome.

Therapeutic alliance ruptures are, to a great degree, synonymous with transference-countertransference enactments (Safran & Muran, 2000). As previously mentioned, a primary distinguishing feature of psychoanalytic therapies is their focus on analyzing transference patterns. Originally, transference was conceptualized as the projection of the interpersonal manifestation of the patient's core unconscious conflicts onto the "blank screen" of the therapist. A contemporary conceptualization of transference appreciates the ubiquitous nature of that process and how the person of the therapist inevitably cocreates enactments. From the same vantage point, the therapist's countertransference can be viewed as a combination of one's own personal issues (classic countertransference) and an understandable reaction to the patient's evocative transferential behavior (interactive countertransference; Binder, 2004; Levenson, 1995; Safran & Muran, 2000; Strupp & Binder, 1984). Hence, transference and countertransference are inextricably entwined.

The classic technical strategy for initiating a therapy discourse is "free association"—directing patients to verbalize unedited whatever comes into their mind. The theoretical rationale was that because drives sought discharge, unedited verbalizations would contain drive derivatives that would serve as clues to important unconscious conflicts. Contemporary PDT bases its technical strategy for initiating discourse on findings of cognitive science research; most cognitive activity, particularly problem solving, goes on outside of conscious awareness. Therefore, encouraging the patient to lead the therapeutic discourse as spontaneously as possible serves to evoke underlying affective and interpersonal themes. The therapist's overriding technical aim is to further the therapeutic dialogue, providing the ground on which change processes such as insight, corrective emotional experiences, and enhanced mentalization can occur.

By now you can appreciate how much a psychodynamic therapist must do during the course of a psychotherapy session; everything from interpersonal pattern recognition, to self-monitoring one's own personal reactions, to deciding which specific types of interventions are going to evoke the most productive responses from the patient. Psychotherapy researchers used to be enthusiastic about searching for "the best techniques" leading to improved outcomes. Today they recognize that a potentially more fruitful research strategy is to study what personal and professional characteristics make for an effective therapist (Wampold & Owen, 2021). Furthermore, more researchers and psychotherapy trainers are realizing that many of the traits that make for an expert psychotherapist are shared by experts in other complex performance domains, such as sports, music, and medicine (Ericsson et al., 2018).

The skills that you will practice and ideally acquire from this text are foundational parts of the psychodynamic therapist's competent and then expert performance. Mastering these skills is not easy, and the effort is not always pleasant, but we guarantee you will appreciate the outcome.

## Psychodynamic–Interpersonal Skills in Deliberate Practice

Drawing on the central features of contemporary PDT enumerated earlier, we have chosen to include exercises on facilitating the goals of insight and corrective emotional experiences; deepening feelings and emotions; pointing out defenses and the therapeutic process, focusing on transference and countertransference; making interpretations, using fantasy and speaking directly to the unconscious, and gathering data on recurrent interpersonal and intrapsychic patterns.

Following recommendations from the editors of this deliberate practice series, Drs. Rousmaniere and Vaz, we picked skills that trainees commonly have trouble using in actual clinical sessions, based on our experience as teachers and supervisors. For example, we have been surprised how often trainees avoid following up on what the patient is saying out of a misguided assumption that they should know what the patient is talking about and need to fake such knowledge. It still amazes us to see how "polite" our trainees feel they need to be, waiting indefinitely for patients to raise a topic "in their own time." They do not (yet) know how straightforward inquiries can not only help therapists understand patients better but, just as important, help patients learn and understand more about themselves—their unstated expectations, unacknowledged longings, and unexpressed feelings. Therefore, we have developed skill training focused on asking simple questions.

Another set of skills emanates from our clinical experience and the results of empirical studies—namely, how a little negative interpersonal process between therapist and patient goes a long way to undermining therapeutic progress (Binder & Henry, 2010; Henry et al., 1986). Therefore, several of the skills in this book speak to averting or repairing therapeutic ruptures. We focus on skills that facilitate therapist emotional awareness, especially using supervision to manage the supervisee's vulnerability to be pushed and pulled into reenactments of dysfunctional patterns of engagement with difficult patients. Also, we present skills that help the therapist speak to the patient's unconscious processes and thereby lessen resistance. And finally, we include skills that foster empathy for the patient, so that the therapist's tendencies toward being frustrated, angry, or even hostile toward patients are lessened.

In choosing the skills in this book, we have privileged those skills with an empirical basis. We recognize how the field of psychotherapy has been advanced incrementally by scientific scrutiny. For many years, most psychodynamic practitioners believed that the practice of PDT was not researchable. PDT was considered an art as much as anything else. However, through empirical work in child development, neuroscience, and therapeutic process, PDT now has a large research base.

In writing this book, we did encounter an issue that speaks to how PDT differs from many other therapeutic approaches. When the series editors gave us templates for the skills, we understood that they wanted us to compose a client statement to which the trainee role-playing the therapist would give a response that met the criteria for that skill. The implication was that there would be an appropriate intervention that the trainee could practice with a variety of client statements. However, in PDT there is rarely a one-size-fits-all intervention. In other words, in most cases, there could be no generic client statement that would receive a "good-enough," generic therapist response. What a psychodynamic therapist would say to one patient who said "X" would not be the same as what would be said to a different patient who said the same thing. To decide on a useful intervention, clinicians need to know the dynamics of the case—who is this person, what is their life experience, what is their attachment style, what is their internal working model, and what is the tone of the therapeutic alliance, for example. To construct PDT-relevant exercises, we needed to provide the therapist-in-training with enough of a patient's backstory to make the task more realistic (albeit, more demanding)—what would one say to this patient, at this time, in this way? To provide a variety of cases, we sorted through patient profiles with unique personality styles corresponding to their placement on an interpersonal circumplex model built around the two orthogonal dimensions of control (dominance, power) and affiliation (friendliness, warmth; Wiggins & Broughton, 1985. As one moves around the circle, each octant reflects a blend of the two axial dimensions, permitting a mixture of agreeableness and dominance. In this manner, we were successful in presenting a range of patient dynamics. In addition, we focused on three patients in particular in our more advanced exercises, so that trainees could have the experience of incrementally gathering information sufficient to formulate a patient's dynamics.

Before turning to the specifics of the 12 skills, we wish to discuss our decision to use the word *patient* throughout the book instead of *client*. As Shedler (2006) pointed out, "in truth, both words are problematic, but *patient* seems to me the lesser of evils" (p. 10). The Latin root of patient is "one who is suffering," and it seems to us that the work of the therapist is to ease suffering and restore robustness. In addition, we believe that the doctor–patient relationship implies more responsibility than the more business-like relationship between people offering services and their clients. In PDT, we do not provide clients with a range of professional services, leaving it up to them to choose those they prefer, like a manicurist asking their client to pick out a color of nail polish. As therapists, we have a responsibility to determine what might be causing the pain and then to choose appropriate methods and interventions that would minimize distress and promote health and healing, while taking into account the patient's preferences and cultural identities (broadly defined). Because we see so much of the cause of a person's suffering is out of their awareness, trusting them to choose a remedy does not make sense. In fact, most people come into therapy because they are avoiding feeling and doing the very things that would be ameliorative. In addition, our society, laws, and mores place a great deal of power in the hands of a therapist. With this enhanced power comes greater responsibility. Our whole therapeutic endeavor demands trust— trust that we will put the needs of our patients before our own.

However, by using the term *patient*, we are not implying a hierarchical power relationship where "doctors" perform procedures on passive patients. The psychodynamic model we are presenting demands a deeply interpersonal and intertwined collaboration. Nonetheless, if the term *patient* is aversive to you because it implies sickness, helplessness, or some other negative connotation, please replace it with whatever term you prefer.

## The Psychodynamic–Interpersonal Skills Presented in Exercises 1–12

Other books in the APA deliberate practice series have divided the skills into three difficulty levels—beginner, intermediate, and advanced. However, it struck the editors of this series that because interventions in PDT needed to consider certain patient and relationship factors as a matter of course (i.e., demanding therapist responsiveness from the get-go), there would only be two levels of skills—intermediate and advanced.

### Intermediate Skills

*Skill 1: Engaging in a Therapeutic Inquiry.* In PDT, one of the therapists most useful skills is asking good questions. Deceptively, this looks like an easy skill. This exercise combines three inquiry skills so that the therapist learns to ask the patient questions designed to "help me see it as you see it," "help me understand it as you understand it," and "help me see the implications of it as you do."

*Skill 2: Being Aware of Countertransference Reactions.* This skill is considered fundamental when conducting PDT because patients can exert strong emotional and interpersonal pulls and pushes on the therapist, and yet the therapist needs to maintain responsive equanimity. The therapist must track not only the patient's thoughts, feelings, and behaviors but also their own thoughts, feelings, and behaviors that the patient may have triggered. In PDT, the therapist's internal and external reactions can provide information about the patient. Although therapist awareness is placed as the second skill in this book, trainees should realize that this is a complex skill because it involves being mindful of one's own experience while simultaneously listening to the experience of the patient. As Safran (2012), an analyst, researcher, and leader in the field of the contemporary relational movement, stated,

> Over time I have come to believe that one of the most important skills for therapists to develop is an *internal skill, rather than a technical one.* This internal skill involves attending to our own emotions when working with clients and cultivating the ability to tolerate and process painful or disturbing feelings in a nondefensive fashion. (p. 111, emphasis added)

Safran reasoned that by processing and managing the powerful feelings evoked in us by patients (*containment*), we can help regulate our patients much as parents do with an overwhelmed child. Exercise 11 builds on this skill by allowing trainees to practice how they might share their countertransference experiences with supervisors.

*Skill 3: Deepening Emotional Experience.* The psychodynamic therapist must be an emotional detective/midwife/catalyst—capable of evoking and deepening emotion so that the patient's nascent emotions can be recognized, named, and processed. There are several strategies for intensifying the patient's most poignant feelings, and this skill will allow the trainee to try out four of them.

*Skill 4: Making Process Comments.* Beginning therapists often get caught up in the content of what the patient is saying. But in an interpersonal PDT, the therapist privileges attending to the process of what is going on between therapist and patient. Paying attention to the process of such transactions is a window into the patient's implicit internal working model. *Commenting on the here and now, in the here and now* is an invaluable skill for the therapist and one that will be called forth in many more complex skills, such as those in Exercises 5 and 7.

*Skill 5: Pointing Out Defenses and Inquiring About Underlying Fear.* Defense mechanisms are self-protective acts; they are used to avoid experiences that were linked to danger at an earlier developmental level. Unfortunately, these idiosyncratic avoidance processes begin to feel like a part of one's personality. That makes it difficult for people to change, even when it comes at a cost to their authenticity. Recognizing and pointing out such defenses are fundamental skills in a therapist's armamentarium.

*Skill 6: Introducing the Rationale for Treatment.* Therapists can use this skill unprompted or in response to patient inquiries about how PDT works and what will happen in the sessions. You may wonder why explaining the treatment rationale is Skill 6 rather than Skill 1. Here is our reason: Patients enter therapy for myriad reasons—most are nervous and unsure about what they are getting themselves into. To begin therapy takes courage, and for many it is still (unfortunately) associated with stigma, failure, or downright terror of being found crazy. To explain something as complicated as PDT in a few sentences is difficult enough, but to explain it to a person who is having intense feelings and who might be dealing with them by being defensive (e.g., placating, challenging, self-recriminating) is a daunting task. And of course, explaining a treatment rationale is not a one-time-only event; rather, it should be used as needed, especially when a patient expresses confusion about or doubt in some aspect of PDT. We suggest learning this skill midway in the book but also repeating it after completing all 12 skill-based exercises. It is one of those skills that serves many purposes, such as facilitating repairs of relational ruptures.

### Advanced Skills

*Skill 7: Making Transference Interpretations.* Transference as a process is ubiquitous—people see others through a lens that is largely determined by their preexisting, significant-other representations. There has been a great deal of controversy, however, about therapists' interpreting transference when they suspect it. Present research evidence suggests that low to moderate levels of transference interpretations are highly effective. Nonetheless, learning this skill will help you become aware of the transference dynamics that occur in-session. That knowledge is invaluable for understanding who you represent to the patient at any point in time, regardless if you interpret it or not.

*Skill 8: Using Metaphors.* Metaphors are deceptively simple. Because emotion so often infiltrates metaphors and because of their power to capture how the speaker feels viscerally, exploring metaphors in PDT is invaluable. Furthermore, metaphors can often effectively paint a powerful picture when ordinary phrasing with words is inadequate to convey a sense of what is happening, what is hoped for, and what is feared. In therapy, metaphors used by both the patient and the therapist greatly enhance the depth of the communication. This exercise will give trainees three ways of practicing using metaphors: staying within the patient's metaphor, stating an implicit message behind the metaphor, and creating metaphors as powerful ways to engage patients.

*Skill 9: Exploring Fantasy.* Fantasies can provide, like dreams, a "royal road" (Freud, 1900/1997) to understanding the unconscious activities of the mind. Some psychoanalytic therapists view fantasies as a way of getting a relatively uncensored window into the patient's wants, desires, and needs that often do not get expressed in rationale discourse. Fantasies (along with wishes and dreams) are one of the seven ways Blagys and Hilsenroth (2000) distinguished what psychodynamic therapists focus on versus clinicians who use other treatment models. There are many ways of working with fantasies in therapy at various levels of manifest (on the surface) and latent (hidden) content. Exercise 9 provides one way of making use of daydreams that come up in sessions.

*Skill 10: Case Formulation: Gathering Data for the Cyclical Maladaptive Pattern.* Over time PDTs have developed a variety of theories about what makes people tick, each focusing on different phenomena (e.g., instinctual urges, failures in empathic responsiveness, self–object representations). Because PDT is a multimodel theoretical system, there are multiple ways to formulate a case, and there is an expansive literature devoted to the different methods for formulating cases, each with its own sources of data. For example, Pine (1990) specified four of them (drive, ego, object relations, and self-experience), each with its own "complex, in-depth view of the mind" (p. 3). Messer and Warren (1995) differentiated between those models that focus on conflict and those that are relational. What is common among all of these, and what we have based our formulation exercise on, is the process of looking for recurrent themes that occur in the patient's current, past, and present relationships, including those with the therapist.

*Skill 11: Using Supervision to Recognize Reenactments.*   Exercise 2 focuses on helping trainees become aware of their countertransferences as an inner skill. Exercise 11 builds on that skill. Here we are using the vehicle of talking to one's supervisor about one's overwhelming or interfering feelings that are evoked in sessions. Unfortunately, many trainees do not speak to supervisors about their difficult feelings. This exercise was designed to accomplish three goals: (a) have trainees become more aware of feelings that get evoked and provoked by patients, (b) see supervision as a way to metabolize such feelings, and (c) be encouraged to approach their supervisors to have what might be difficult (yet rewarding) discussions about difficult feelings.

*Skill 12: Providing a Corrective Emotional Experience.*   The last exercise in the skill series involves one of the main curative change agents in psychotherapy. Although much has been written and discussed about the importance of insight in PDT, here we give the corrective emotional experience its due. Alexander and French (1946) defined the *corrective emotional experience,* almost poetically, as "reexperiencing the old, unsettled conflict but with a new ending." Bowlby (1985) perhaps said it best:

> Our [therapists'] role is in sanctioning the patient to think thoughts that his parents have discouraged or forbidden him to think, to experience feelings his parents have discouraged or forbidden him to experience, and to consider actions that his parents have forbidden him to contemplate. (p. 198)

Over the years and from various theoretical vantage points an impressive body of research (e.g., Castonguay & Hill, 2012) has supported the importance of this in-session "new ending." Now we are beginning to understand the neuroprocesses (i.e., memory reconsolidation) that may scaffold such mutative change (Levenson et al., 2020).

## A Note About Vocal Tone, Facial Expression, and Body Posture

PDT clinicians attend carefully to the nonverbal and paralinguistic cues expressed by both patient and therapist. Silence is also valued and used strategically. Among the overarching aims of this book is the hope that learners will develop the ability to apply skills in a range of clinical situations and use this as an opportunity to exercise the skills using a style and language that are congruent with who they are. Just as we encourage those who are role-playing the patient to adjust the difficulty of the stimuli (e.g., their tone and the intensity of affect), we also encourage those role-playing the therapists to adjust and experiment with their vocal tone, facial expressions, and body postures. We do know that one of the ways PDT has changed over time is that there is less importance placed on maintaining a neutral tone and posture. Especially with relationally focused PDT, the therapist's emotional expression and tone of voice can be used to speak volumes. Research has indicated that therapist's emotional expression is positively associated with treatment outcome (e.g., Peluso & Freund, 2018). There are also helpful articles with extensive patient–therapist transcripts illustrating how to incorporate more emotionally focused interventions into PDT (e.g., Levenson, 2020). Because so much cannot be conveyed by the written word, PDT learners will find it useful to watch recorded examples of experts performing therapy (e.g., APA's clinical training video series) so that they can observe these key principles in action, as well as to record their sessions, so that they can watch them privately, and/or show them in supervision.

## Overview of the Book's Structure

This book is organized into three parts. Part I contains this chapter and Chapter 2, which provides basic instructions on how to perform these exercises. We found through testing that providing too many instructions up front overwhelmed trainers and trainees. Therefore, we kept these instructions as simple as possible. Further guidelines for getting the most out of deliberate practice are provided in Chapter 3, and additional instructions for monitoring and adjusting the difficulty of the exercises are provided in Appendix A. **Do not skip the instructions in Chapter 2, and be sure to read the additional guidelines and instructions in Chapter 3 and Appendix A once you are comfortable with the basic instructions.**

Part II contains the 12 skill-focused intermediate and advanced exercises (see Table 1.1). Each contains an overview of the exercise, example patient–therapist interactions to help guide trainees, step-by-step instructions for conducting that exercise, and a list of criteria for mastering the relevant skill. We present patient statements and sample therapist responses organized by difficulty (beginner, intermediate, and advanced). The statements and responses are presented separately. This gives the trainee playing the therapist more freedom to improvise responses without being influenced by the sample responses. Exercises 4, 9, 10, and 12 present recurring patients—Mr. Hiram Johnson, Ms. Ann Lee, and Dr. Nevell Ingram[1]—so that trainees can see how cases develop over time in PDT. The case of Mr. Johnson has been presented in four chapters (Levenson, 1995) and there is a commercially available video with an actor playing Mr. Johnson (Levenson, 1999). Ms. Lee's six-session therapy and case formulation have previously been discussed (Levenson, 2017), and a commercially available video of the entire therapy with the actual patient is available through APA (Levenson, 2010). In addition, Ms. Lee's therapy has been the subject of several empirical investigations (Friedlander et al., 2018, 2020; Levenson, 2020; Levenson et al., 2020; Luo et al., 2022). These additional resources can supplement the exercises in this book, along with the APA video of the first author discussing the skills-based approach and illustrating it with video examples (Levenson & Friedlander, in production). The final two exercises in Part II provide opportunities to practice the 12 skills within simulated psychotherapy sessions. Exercise 13 provides two sample psychotherapy session transcripts (of the case of Ms. Lee) in which the PDT skills are used and clearly labeled, demonstrating how they might flow together in an actual therapy session. PDT trainees are invited to run through the

---

1.  The patients' identities have been disguised to protect confidentiality.

sample transcripts with one playing the therapist and the other playing the patient to get a feel for how a session might unfold. Exercise 14 provides suggestions for undertaking mock sessions, as well as patient profiles ordered by difficulty (beginner, intermediate, and advanced) that trainees can use for improvised role-plays.

Part III contains Chapter 3, which provides additional guidance for trainers and trainees. Chapter 2 is more procedural, whereas Chapter 3 covers big-picture issues. It highlights seven ways to get the most out of deliberate practice. In it, we discuss the importance of appropriate responsiveness, attending to trainee well-being and respecting privacy, and trainer self-evaluation, among other topics.

Three appendixes conclude this book. Appendix A provides instructions for monitoring and adjusting the difficulty of each exercise as needed. It provides a Deliberate Practice Reaction Form for the trainee playing the therapist to complete to indicate whether the exercise is too easy or too difficult. Appendix B includes a Deliberate Practice Diary Form that can be used to during a training session's final evaluation to process the trainees' experiences. However, its primary purpose is to give trainees a format to explore and record their experiences while engaging in additional, between-session deliberate practice activities without the supervisor. Appendix C presents a sample syllabus demonstrating how the 12 deliberate practice exercises and other support material can be integrated into a wider PDT training course. Instructors may choose to modify the syllabus or pick elements from it to integrate into their own courses.

Downloadable versions of this book's appendixes, including a color version of the Deliberate Practice Reaction Form, can be found in the "Clinician and Practitioner Resources" tab online (https://www.apa.org/pubs/books/deliberate-practice-psychodynamic-psychotherapy).

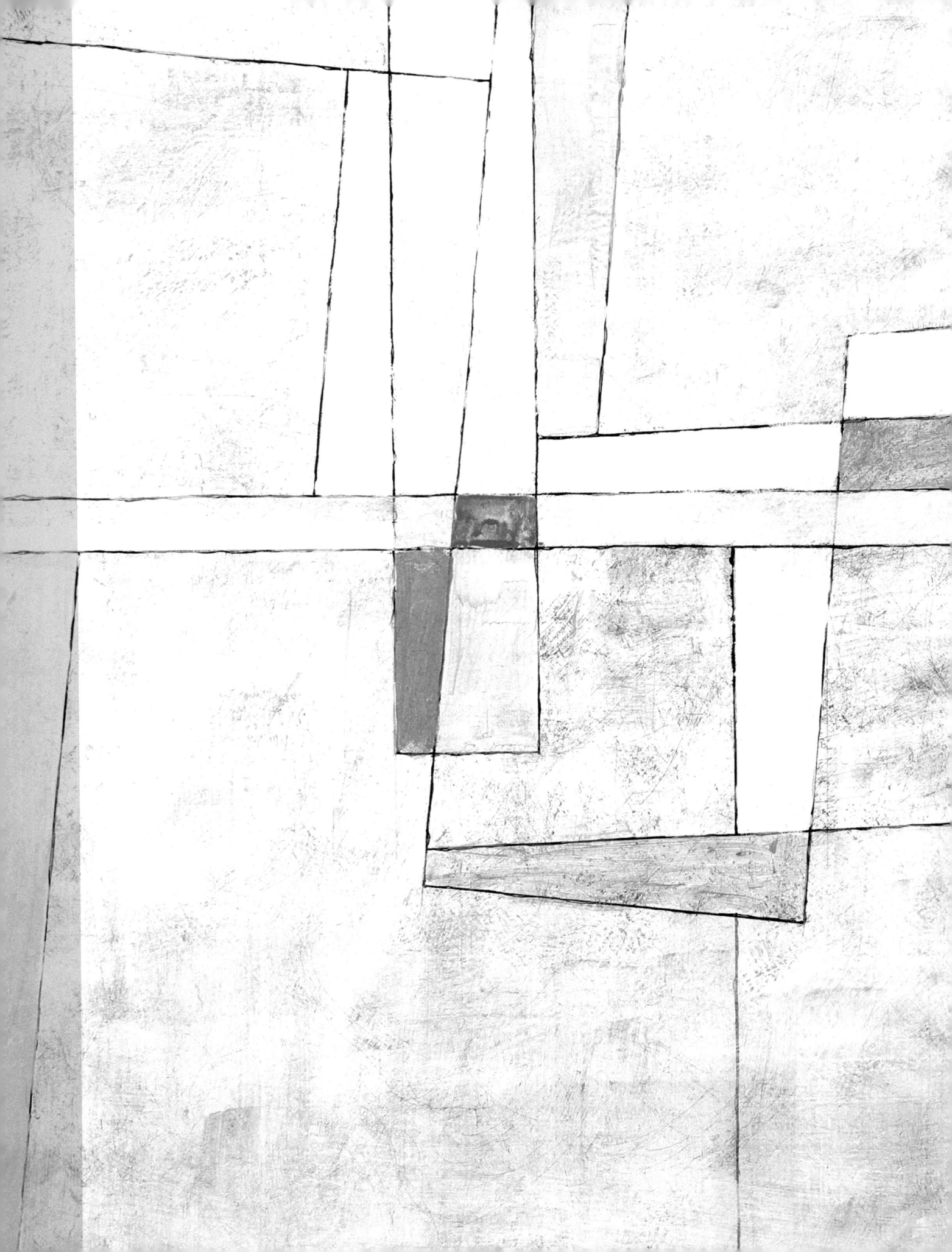

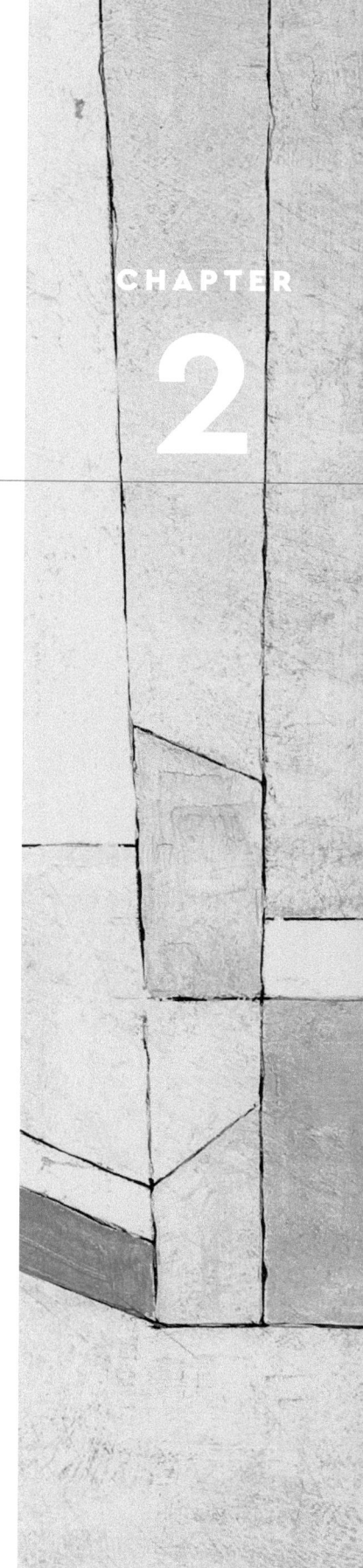

# Instructions for the Psychodynamic Therapy Deliberate Practice Exercises

This chapter provides basic instructions that are common to all the exercises in this book. More specific instructions are provided in each exercise. Chapter 3 also provides important guidance for trainees and trainers that will help them get the most out of deliberate practice. Appendix A offers additional instructions for monitoring and adjusting the difficulty of the exercises as needed after getting through all then patient statements in a single difficulty level, including a Deliberate Practice Reaction Form the trainee playing the therapist can complete to indicate whether they found the statements too easy or too difficult. **Difficulty assessment is an important part of the deliberate practice process and should not be skipped.**

## Overview

The deliberate practice psychodynamic therapy (PDT) exercises in this book involve role-plays of hypothetical situations in therapy. The role-play involves three people: One trainee role-plays the therapist, another trainee role-plays the patient, and a trainer (professor or supervisor) observes and provides feedback. Alternately, a peer (e.g., the trainee who role-plays the patient) can observe and provide feedback.

This book provides a script for each role-play, each with a patient statement and an example therapist response. The patient statements are graded in difficulty from beginner to advanced, although these difficulty grades are only estimates. The actual perceived difficulty of patient statements is subjective and varies widely by trainee. For example, some trainees may experience a stimulus of a patient's being angry as easy to respond to, whereas another trainee may experience it as very difficult. Thus, it is important for trainees to provide difficulty assessments and adjustments to ensure that they are practicing at the right difficulty level: neither too easy nor too hard.

https://doi.org/10.1037/0000351-002

*Deliberate Practice in Psychodynamic Psychotherapy*, by H. Levenson, V. Gay, and J. L. Binder

## Time Frame

We recommend a 70-minute time block for every exercise (although other time frames can be used), structured roughly as follows:

- First 20 minutes: Orientation—the trainer explains the PDT skill and demonstrates the exercise procedure with a volunteer trainee, using example scripts provided for each exercise.

- Middle 30 minutes: Trainees perform the exercise in pairs. The trainer or a peer provides feedback throughout this process and monitors or adjusts the exercise's difficulty as needed after each set of statements (see Appendix A for more information about difficulty assessment).

- Final 20 minutes: Review, feedback, and discussion.

## Preparation

1. Every trainee will need their own copy of this book.

2. Each exercise requires the trainer to fill out a Deliberate Practice Reaction Form after completing all the statements from a single difficulty level. This form is available in the "Clinician and Practitioner Resources" tab at https://www.apa.org/pubs/books/deliberate-practice-psychodynamic-psychotherapy and in Appendix A.

3. Trainees are grouped into pairs. One volunteers to role-play the therapist and one to role-play the patient (they will switch roles after 15 minutes of practice). As noted previously, an observer who might be either the trainer or a peer trainee will work with each pair.

## The Role of the Trainer

The primary responsibilities of the trainer are to

1. provide corrective feedback, which includes both information about how well the trainees' response met expected criteria and any necessary guidance about how to improve the response, and

2. remind trainees to do difficulty assessments and adjustments after each level of patient statements is completed (beginner, intermediate, and advanced).

## How to Practice

Each exercise includes its own step-by-step instructions. Trainees should follow these instructions carefully, as every step is important.

## Skill Criteria

Each of the first 12 exercises focuses on one essential PDT skill with two to five skill criteria that describe the important components or principles for that skill.

**The goal of the role-play is for trainees to practice improvising responses to the patient statement in a manner that (a) is attuned to the patient, (b) meets skill criteria as much as possible, and (c) feels authentic for the trainee.** Trainees are provided scripts with example therapist responses to give them a sense of how to incorporate the skill criteria into a response. **It is important, however, that trainees do not read the example responses verbatim in the role-plays!** Therapy is highly personal and improvisational; the goal of deliberate practice is to develop trainees' ability to improvise within a consistent framework. Memorizing scripted responses would be counterproductive for helping trainees learn to perform therapy that is responsive, authentic, and attuned to each individual patient.

The three authors of this text wrote the scripted example responses. However, trainees' personal style of therapy may differ slightly or greatly from that in the example scripts. It is essential that, over time, trainees develop their own style and voice, while simultaneously being able to intervene according to the model's principles and strategies. To facilitate this, the exercises in this book were designed to maximize opportunities for improvisational responses informed by the skill criteria and ongoing feedback. Trainees will note that some of the scripted responses do not meet all the skill criteria. These responses are provided as examples of flexible application of PDT skills in a manner that prioritizes attunement with the patient.

## Review, Feedback, and Discussion

The review and feedback sequence after each role-play has these two elements:

- First, the trainee who played the patient **briefly** shares how it felt to be on the receiving end of the therapist response. This can help assess how well trainees are attuning with the patient.

- Second, the trainer provides **brief** feedback (less than 1 minute) based on the skill criteria for each exercise. Keep feedback specific, behavioral, and brief to preserve time for skill rehearsal. If one trainer is teaching multiple pairs of trainees, the trainer walks around room, observing the pairs and offering brief feedback. When the trainer is not available, the trainee playing the patient gives peer feedback to the therapist, based on the skill criteria and how it felt to be on the receiving end of the intervention. Alternatively, a third trainee can observe and provide feedback.

Trainers (or peers) should remember to keep all feedback specific and brief and not to veer into discussions of theory. There are many other settings for extended discussion of PDT theory and research. In deliberate practice, it is of utmost importance to maximize time for continuous behavioral rehearsal via role-plays.

## Final Evaluation

After both trainees have role-played the client and the therapist, the trainer provides an evaluation. Participants should engage in a short group discussion based on this evaluation. This discussion can provide ideas for where to focus homework and future deliberate practice sessions. To this end, Appendix B presents a Deliberate Practice Diary Form, which can also be downloaded from the "Clinician and Practitioner Resources" tab online (https://www.apa.org/pubs/books/deliberate-practice-psychodynamic-psychotherapy). This form can be used as part of the final evaluation to help trainees process their experiences from that session with the supervisor. However, it is designed primarily to be used by trainees as a template for exploring and recording their thoughts and experiences between sessions, particularly when pursuing additional deliberate practice activities without the supervisor, such as rehearsing responses alone or if two or more trainees want to practice the exercises together—perhaps with another trainee filling the supervisor's role. Then, if they want, the trainees can discuss these experiences with the supervisor at the beginning of the next training session.

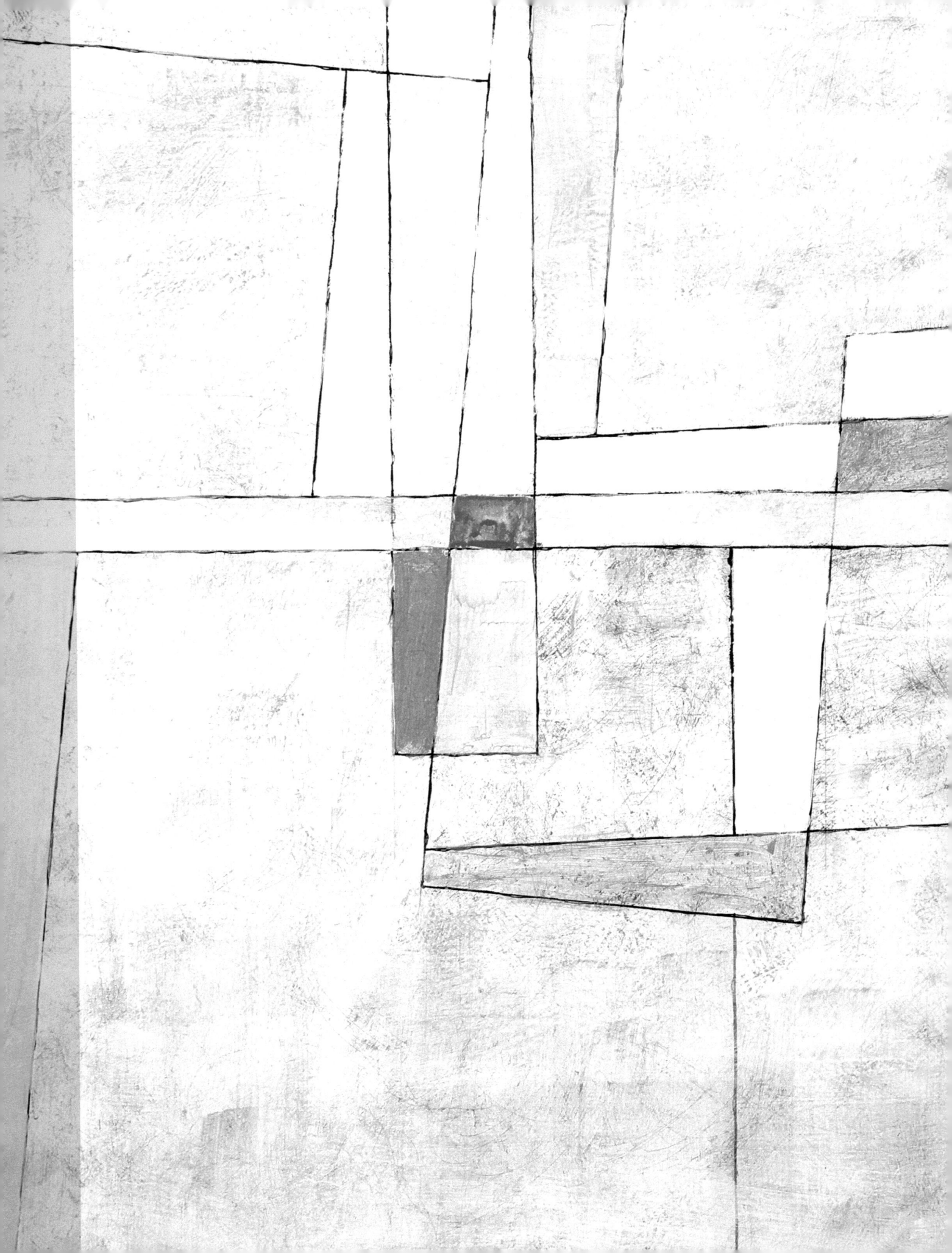

# Deliberate Practice Exercises for Psychodynamic Therapy Skills

This section of the book provides 12 deliberate practice exercises for essential psycho-dynamic therapy (PDT) skills. These exercises are organized in a developmental sequence, from those that are more appropriate to someone just beginning PDT training to those for practitioners who have progressed to a more advanced level. Although we anticipate that most trainers would use these exercises in the order we have suggested, some may find it more appropriate to their training circumstances to use a different order. We also provide two comprehensive exercises that bring together the PDT skills using annotated PDT session transcripts and mock PDT sessions.

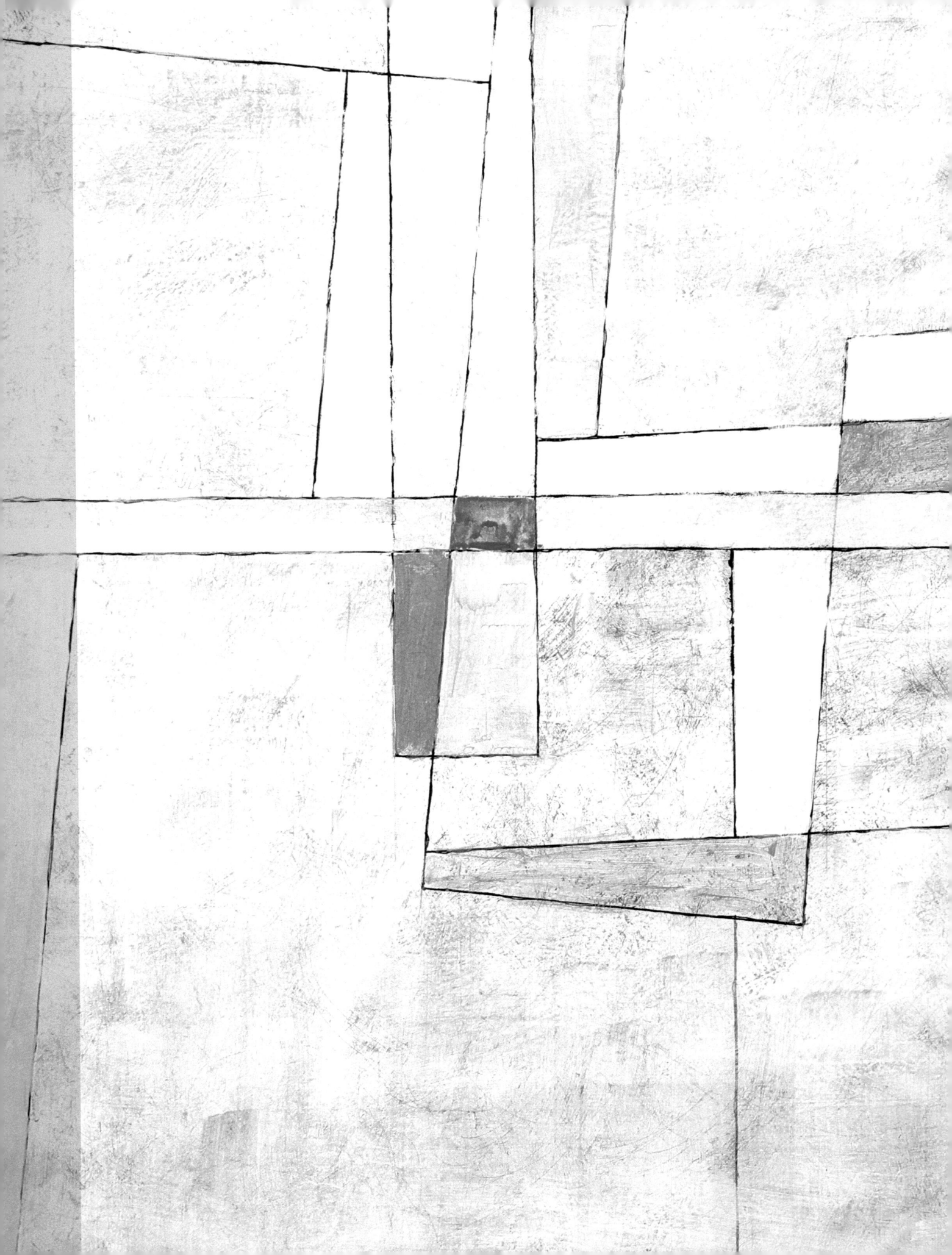

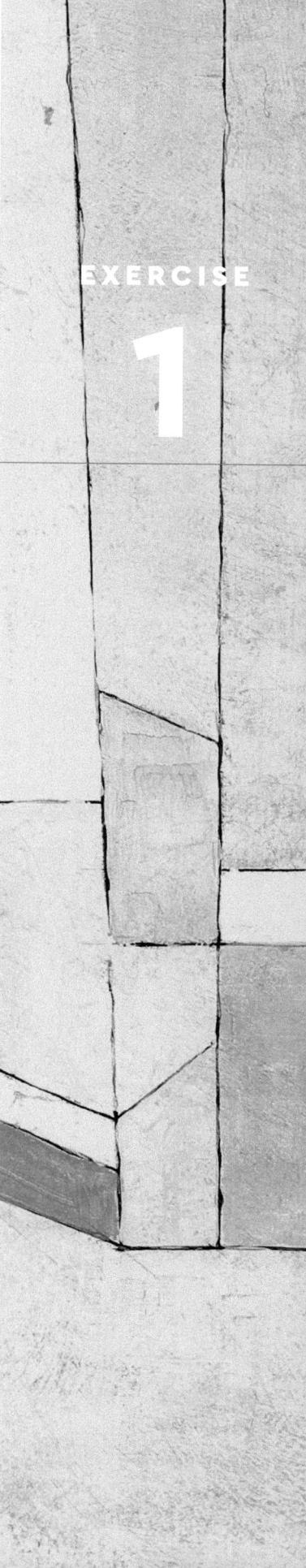

# Engaging in a Therapeutic Inquiry

## Preparations for Exercise 1

1. Read the instructions in Chapter 2.

2. Download the Deliberate Practice Reaction Form and the Deliberate Practice Diary Form at https://www.apa.org/pubs/books/deliberate-practice-psychodynamic-psychotherapy (see the "Clinician and Practitioner Resources" tab; also available in Appendixes A and B, respectively).

## Skill Description

### Skill Difficulty Level: Intermediate

In psychodynamic–interpersonal therapy, inquiry encourages a patient to tell their *personal story*. This story will include plausible reasons for the patient's difficulties, including the origins of these difficulties and current factors that they believe cause their difficulties. Dynamic therapists assume that some of those beliefs cause suffering and that the patient cannot understand how this occurs. This unfortunate situation occurs partly because the patient lacks awareness of sufficient details to understand why they are trapped in this particular story—or, sometimes, even that there is a story—so they continue to participate in it. In addition to helping the patient fill out their narrative, further benefits of doing a detailed inquiry are that the therapist achieves a thorough understanding of the patient's experience and the patient appreciates this earnest effort by the therapist. That, in turn, strengthens the alliance between patient and therapist.

To obtain these details, you must help the patient elaborate a spontaneous version of their personal story into a narrative that allows you both to construct a rich and vivid picture of life seen through the patient's eyes. This process requires you to minimize your assumptions about what specifically the patient is referring to and what their words mean as you listen to the narrative. It also requires you to maintain an attitude of intense curiosity

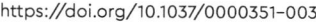

https://doi.org/10.1037/0000351-003
*Deliberate Practice in Psychodynamic Psychotherapy*, by H. Levenson, V. Gay, and J. L. Binder

and to compare the patient's version of the story to your commonsense comprehension of whatever is being described. Finally, your most useful tool is asking good questions. This is an undervalued skill; asking good questions often requires much know-how because in retrospect, the questions often seem so obvious. With these skills on hand, you are ready to conduct a detailed examination of the patient's narrative.

We will focus on three inquiry strategies that facilitate the elaboration of the patient's personal, often unarticulated story. The trainee should improvise a response to each patient description using the following skill criteria.

1. **For the beginner patient statements:** Ask about **missing details** in the narrative or to clarify a vague or confusing part of the narrative. Use this inquiry strategy when a part of the mental picture that you have constructed from the patient's ongoing narrative is either missing or too vague to see clearly. Therefore, you ask the patient to fill in the missing detail or more clearly describe or explain a particular detail. "Help me see it as you see it."

2. **For the intermediate patient statements:** Ask about how the patient **comprehends** or understands a part of the narrative. Use this inquiry strategy when you want to obtain a clearer or richer understanding of what a part of the narrative means to the patient. "Help me understand it as you understand it."

3. **For the advanced patient statements:** Ask about the **implications** the narrative has for the future. Use this strategy when you want to discover how the patient imagines a part of the narrative will unfold going forward. Often one is not aware of implications for the future of a particular scenario. "Help me see it as you anticipate it."

---

**SKILL CRITERIA FOR EXERCISE 1**

1. For the beginner patient statements: Ask about missing details in the narrative or clarify a vague or confusing part of the narrative.
2. For the intermediate patient statements: Ask about how the patient comprehends or understands a part of the narrative.
3. For the advanced patient statements: Ask about the implications of the narrative for the future.

---

## Examples of Therapists Engaging in a Therapeutic Inquiry

### Example 1: Asking for Details or Clarification

PATIENT: [*sad*] There is no one in my life that I can count on.

THERAPIST: When you said that, were you thinking of someone in particular?

### Example 2: Asking About Comprehension

PATIENT: [*irritated*] My sister was the athlete in the family.

THERAPIST: Does that hold some particular meaning for you as the other child in the family?

### Example 3: Asking About Implications

PATIENT: [*suspicious*] I don't hate therapy. I've just not found therapists very helpful.

THERAPIST: Do you expect that I will not be very helpful either?

| INSTRUCTIONS FOR EXERCISE 1 |
|---|

**Step 1: Role-Play and Feedback**

- The patient says the first beginner patient statement. The therapist **improvises** a response based on the skill criteria.
- The trainer (or, if not available, the patient) provides **brief** feedback based on the skill criteria.
- The patient then repeats the same statement, and the therapist again improvises a response. The trainer (or patient) again provides brief feedback.

**Step 2: Repeat**

- Repeat Step 1 for all the statements **in the current difficulty level** (beginner, intermediate, or advanced).

**Step 3: Assess and Adjust Difficulty**

- The therapist completes the Deliberate Practice Reaction Form (see Appendix A) and decides whether to make the exercise easier or harder or to repeat the same difficulty level.

**Step 4: Repeat for Approximately 15 Minutes**

- Repeat Steps 1 to 3 for at least 15 minutes.
- The trainees then switch therapist and patient roles and start over.

**Now it's your turn! Follow Steps 1 and 2 from the instructions.**

*Remember:* The goal of the role-play is for trainees to practice improvising responses to the patient statements in a manner that (a) uses the skill criteria and (b) feels authentic for the trainee. **Example therapist responses for each patient statement are provided at the end of this exercise. Trainees should attempt to improvise their own responses before reading the example responses.**

| BEGINNER-LEVEL PATIENT STATEMENTS FOR EXERCISE 1: ASKING FOR DETAILS OR CLARIFICATION |
| --- |
| *Beginner Patient Statement 1* |
| [Anxious] My significant other said they didn't want a "clingy" partner, so I'm afraid to complain about how little time they spend with me. |
| *Beginner Patient Statement 2* |
| [Sad] Later in life, when my spouse, who drank a lot, threatened to leave me, I was hospitalized with depression for the first time. |
| *Beginner Patient Statement 3* |
| [Timid] At family dinners, I could barely talk because I was afraid of my father, who could be violent when he drank. |
| *Beginner Patient Statement 4* |
| [Frustrated] I find the colleagues in my department at the university insufferable at times. |
| *Beginner Patient Statement 5* |
| [Sad] My two older siblings are the favorites in the family. I think my parents were exhausted by the time they had me. |

**Assess and adjust the difficulty before moving to the next difficulty level (see Step 3 in the exercise instructions).**

| INTERMEDIATE-LEVEL PATIENT STATEMENTS FOR EXERCISE 1: ASKING ABOUT COMPREHENSION |
| --- |
| *Intermediate Patient Statement 1* |
| **[Sad]** When I'm feeling down, I go work out in the gym. |
| *Intermediate Patient Statement 2* |
| **[Irritated]** My parents say I'm the "bookish" one in the family. |
| *Intermediate Patient Statement 3* |
| **[Ashamed]** You know, I was the only one in my family not to graduate college. |
| *Intermediate Patient Statement 4* |
| **[Proud]** My father is a great dentist. He's committed to his patients above everyone else. |
| *Intermediate Patient Statement 5* |
| **[Boastful]** I will be the youngest tenured professor in the history of my department. |

**Assess and adjust the difficulty before moving to the next difficulty level (see Step 3 in the exercise instructions).**

| ADVANCED-LEVEL PATIENT STATEMENTS FOR EXERCISE 1: ASKING ABOUT IMPLICATIONS |
| --- |
| *Advanced Patient Statement 1* |
| **[Anxious]** My significant other doesn't want a "clingy" partner, so I'm afraid to complain about how little time they spend with me. |
| *Advanced Patient Statement 2* |
| **[Embarrassed]** When I don't know what to do, my daughter steps in to tell me what I should do. |
| *Advanced Patient Statement 3* |
| **[Coldly]** To be honest, I'm disappointed that you're not a real psychoanalyst. |
| *Advanced Patient Statement 4* |
| **[Nervous]** I know I'm allowed only 20 sessions. I'm worried about what happens when I run out of sessions. |
| *Advanced Patient Statement 5* |
| **[Exasperated sigh]** I am really frustrated! You haven't told me anything about me that I didn't already know. |

🤚 **Assess and adjust the difficulty here (see Step 3 in the exercise instructions). If appropriate, follow the instructions to make the exercise even more challenging (see Appendix A).**

## Example Therapist Responses: Engaging in a Therapeutic Inquiry

*Remember:* Trainees should attempt to improvise their own responses before reading the example responses. **Do not read the following responses verbatim unless you are having trouble coming up with your own responses!**

| EXAMPLE RESPONSES TO BEGINNER-LEVEL PATIENT STATEMENTS FOR EXERCISE 1: ASKING FOR DETAILS OR CLARIFICATION |
| --- |
| *Example Response to Beginner Patient Statement 1* |
| Can you tell me more about what you mean when you say "afraid"? |
| *Example Response to Beginner Patient Statement 2* |
| Can you describe how you experienced your "depression"? |
| *Example Response to Beginner Patient Statement 3* |
| What did your father do when he drank and became violent? |
| *Example Response to Beginner Patient Statement 4* |
| Can you say more about what you find insufferable about your colleagues? |
| *Example Response to Beginner Patient Statement 5* |
| What did your parents do that made you think they were exhausted? |

| EXAMPLE RESPONSES TO INTERMEDIATE-LEVEL PATIENT STATEMENTS FOR EXERCISE 1: ASKING ABOUT COMPREHENSION |
| --- |
| *Example Response to Intermediate Patient Statement 1* |
| Can you explain how working out helps when you are feeling "down"? |
| *Example Response to Intermediate Patient Statement 2* |
| Calling you "bookish," what does that mean to you? |
| *Example Response to Intermediate Patient Statement 3* |
| Help me understand what being the only one not to graduate college means to you. |
| *Example Response to Intermediate Patient Statement 4* |
| How do you feel knowing that your father's patients come first? |
| *Example Response to Intermediate Patient Statement 5* |
| Help me understand what being the youngest tenured professor in your department's history means for you. |

| EXAMPLE RESPONSES TO ADVANCED-LEVEL PATIENT STATEMENTS FOR EXERCISE 1: ASKING ABOUT IMPLICATIONS |
| --- |
| *Example Response to Advanced Patient Statement 1* |
| What do you imagine would happen if you did complain about how little time your significant other spends with you? |
| *Example Response to Advanced Patient Statement 2* |
| What do you imagine would happen if she didn't tell you what you should do? |
| *Example Response to Advanced Patient Statement 3* |
| How do you imagine our work together might be different if I were a psychoanalyst? |
| *Example Response to Advanced Patient Statement 4* |
| How do you imagine you will feel when the 20 sessions are done? |
| *Example Response to Advanced Patient Statement 5* |
| I can see you're really frustrated with me. What do you imagine my reaction is to how you're feeling and what you just told me? |

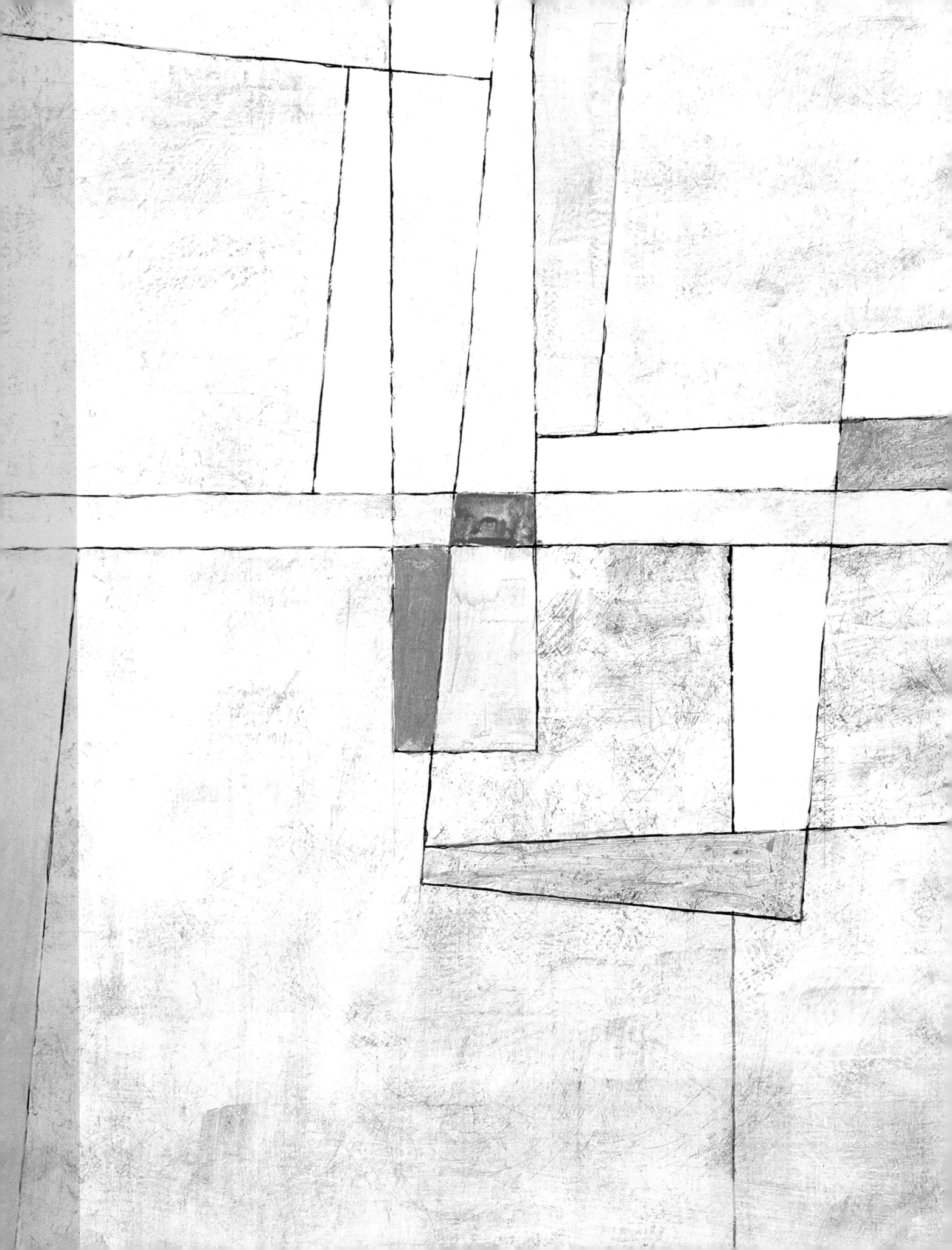

# Being Aware of Countertransference Reactions

## Preparations for Exercise 2

1. Read the instructions in Chapter 2.

2. Download the Deliberate Practice Reaction Form and the Deliberate Practice Diary Form at https://www.apa.org/pubs/books/deliberate-practice-psychodynamic-psychotherapy (see the "Clinician and Practitioner Resources" tab; also available in Appendixes A and B, respectively).

## Skill Description

### Skill Difficulty Level: Intermediate

In many ways, this exercise is the most basic and essential underlying skill in psychodynamic psychotherapy. It involves being aware of one's bodily sensations, feelings, thoughts, and behavioral urges as one is doing or reflecting on the therapy. At first glance, this skill may appear deceptively simple. In fact, it is quite complex because it involves being mindful of one's own experience while simultaneously listening to the patient's experience, both at several levels.

This exercise helps trainees practice becoming aware of their reactions to patients—their countertransferences. This term was originally used by Freud (1910/1957) to refer to therapists' unconscious reactions to patients derived from their own unresolved issues stemming from their unique pasts. If unrecognized, this type of personal or *classical countertransference* is not helpful to the treatment and might even be harmful to it, such as when a therapist unknowingly uses a patient to meet the therapist's personal psychological needs. However, the therapist's *awareness of their countertransference* can facilitate the therapeutic process (Hill, 2020). Therefore, the therapist's own therapy and supervision are extremely important for learning about such vulnerabilities (MacDevitt, 1987).

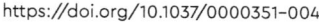

https://doi.org/10.1037/0000351-004

*Deliberate Practice in Psychodynamic Psychotherapy*, by H. Levenson, V. Gay, and J. L. Binder

There is another type of countertransference, however, that is viewed as an "inevitable aspect of psychotherapy that could have positive or negative effects depending upon how the therapist dealt with it" (Hayes et al., 2018, p. 497). This type is called *complementary countertransference*. Relational psychodynamic therapists focus on how therapists react to the patient's in-session behavior in a fashion that complements the patients' relational style (Kiesler et al., 1997). For example, a patient's aggressive behavior usually evokes a complementary urge in the therapist to be aggressive or submissive, whereas another patient's friendly demeanor usually pulls for a friendly response. In this way, the therapist becomes "hooked" (Kiesler, 1988) into acting out the complementary response to the patient and reacts to the patient in ways that other people similarly feel pulled to react. The therapist, therefore, has a firsthand, gut-level experience of what it is like for others interacting with the patient, creating a potentially useful source of information. In this way, the therapist's own reactions can help them understand the type and effect of a patient's maladaptive interpersonal pattern, begin to have an idea of what needs to change (i.e., treatment goals), and devise informed interventions. From this perspective, if properly used, countertransference facilitates rather than hinders a treatment.

Unfortunately, trainees often have this idealized model of the "good therapist" as one who only has positive feelings about every patient. This image is stultifying because it requires the therapist to shut off awareness of a whole range of potentially unpleasant, but informative, feelings. The therapist is inclined to label these feelings as "negative" rather than see them as helpful for understanding why the patient is having difficulty in their interpersonal relationships. Therefore, the therapist's becoming aware of their reactions to patients, both from a classical and complementary point of view, is of paramount importance.

This exercise is different from the other exercises in this book because trainees are not practicing what to say out loud to patients in real therapy sessions. Rather, trainees practice self-awareness by observing and labeling their internal processes (bodily reactions, feelings, thoughts, and behavioral inclinations), to develop a skilled inner voice when sitting with a real patient. One of the later exercises of this book (Exercise 11) will invite you to practice talking about your countertransference in supervision. Making this material available in supervision will allow your supervisor to help you navigate the complex use of self-awareness in psychodynamic formulation and intervention.

## Special Instructions

One trainee will role-play a patient who talks about a potentially emotionally arousing topic. The other trainee will not role-play; instead, their task is to monitor their internal thoughts, feelings, and bodily felt responses as they are listening to the patient and to disclose only those internal experiences that they feel comfortable sharing. A trainer (professor or peer role-playing the "patient") observes and provides feedback. In this task, the therapist does not respond to the patient but instead describes their experience out loud. The therapist should try not to think about the appropriate clinical interventions or responses to the patient's words. Instead, the focus is fully on heightening the therapist's awareness of their own internal processes.

The patient reads the first patient statement to the therapist. The therapist monitors their own internal experience and reactions (thoughts, feelings, bodily reactions, and urges) while listening to the patient. When the patient is finished reading, the therapist describes out loud any feelings or bodily felt experiences that they feel comfortable disclosing. For example, the therapist could say, "As I hear this, I feel disgusted, and I am aware I don't want to see this patient in therapy," "I feel warmth in my chest," "I feel excited at the prospect of working with this person," "I feel intimidated as I listen to how they are talking," or "I feel very compassionate for the patient and have an urge to hug them."

The Deliberate Practice Reaction Form (Appendix A) provides common responses, but you may notice your own bodily felt responses that are not listed on this form. Try to notice and describe at least one aspect of your experience. It may be a feeling like sadness or anger, or a thought or memory, or an urge to act or react. It may be a sensation you are aware of internally, such as a pit in your stomach or a closing of your throat. It may also involve an externally apparent experience, such as flushing of your face or a smile coming across your lips. The goal is to continually scan for inner experiences, although at first you may have trouble identifying any experience at all. Only describe responses that you feel comfortable disclosing. It is important that trainees have the right not to reveal responses they wish to keep private.

The trainee should improvise a response to each patient description following these skill criteria:

1. **Observe and track your own thoughts, feelings, wishes, physical sensations, and urges while simultaneously listening to the patient.** In this exercise, you will probably be affected by both types of countertransference—the classical type, where your own dynamics, influenced by your unique, past history, and present situations (e.g., as a therapist-in-training), will affect how you feel about the patient, and the complementary type, where the patient's dynamics "pull you" to react in ways similar to other people who interact with this patient. At this point, you need not be concerned with what type of countertransference is giving rise to your internal reactions. Just try to track them.

2. **Disclose reactions that you feel comfortable sharing.** Protect your own privacy and boundaries by not disclosing reactions that feel too personal. (The trainer should ask if therapist is able to do this.) Remember, you are not saying these things to the patient but just saying them aloud to help you practice being aware of them. (Self-disclosure or revealing one's countertransference to patients can be a powerful technique that should be used carefully and only in certain situations, as indicated by a supervisor.)

3. **If you have reactions in the "too hard" category, ask the trainer to make the role-play easier.** Remember, that deliberate practice works best if you stay in the Goldilocks zone of not too easy, not too hard.

---

### SKILL CRITERIA FOR EXERCISE 2

1. Observe and track your own thoughts, feelings, wishes, physical sensations, and urges while simultaneously listening to the patient.
2. Disclose reactions that you feel comfortable sharing.
3. If you have reactions in the "too hard" category, ask the trainer to make the role-play easier.

## INSTRUCTIONS FOR EXERCISE 2

### Step 1: Role-Play and Feedback

- The patient either says the first beginner patient statement or uses it as an improvisation prompt (i.e., there is no need to repeat every word, but the patient needs to convey the general content and tone of the statement).
- The therapist does not respond to the patient but instead describes their experience out loud, sharing whatever thoughts, feelings, or bodily experiences they feel comfortable sharing.
- The trainer (or, if not available, the patient) provides **brief** feedback.

### Step 2: Repeat

- Repeat Step 1 for all the statements **in the current difficulty level** (beginner, intermediate, or advanced).

### Step 3: Assess and Adjust Difficulty

- The therapist completes the Deliberate Practice Reaction Form (see Appendix A) and decides whether to make the exercise easier or harder or to repeat the same difficulty level.

### Step 4: Repeat for Approximately 15 Minutes

- Repeat Steps 1 to 3 for at least 15 minutes.
- The trainees then switch therapist and patient roles and start over.

### Now it's your turn! Follow Steps 1 and 2 from the instructions.

*Remember:* We do not provide sample therapist responses to the patient statements because, unlike the other exercises, this one does not focus on developing the most appropriate response to the patient. Instead, the main goal of this exercise is for trainees to explore and communicate their own genuine internal reactions.

| BEGINNER-LEVEL PATIENT STATEMENTS FOR EXERCISE 2 |
| --- |

*Beginner Patient Statement 1*

[Cheerfully] I am in graduate school to study to be a therapist like you. I also work at a bank part-time and have a long-distance relationship with my boyfriend. I thought I would start therapy to see what it was like. I'm a pretty go-go person. And I come from a devoted family. My sister is a fantastic volleyball player and just won an athletic scholarship at a really good university. I am living at home right now to take care of my mother. She drinks a bit too much, and I just like keeping an eye on her as dad is busy coaching my sister, and next year she'll be away at school. I'm really looking forward to being in therapy.

*Beginner Patient Statement 2*

[Upbeat] I got transferred to you because my last therapist finished their training rotation. They were really wonderful. Right off the bat, they just seemed to know who I was and what I needed. My therapist was very insightful and gave me some good advice about how to solve the problems I brought into therapy. I asked for someone similar. I hope you can help me.

*Beginner Patient Statement 3*

[Thoughtfully] I lost my spouse last year. In fact, just about a year ago next week. I'm realizing that I am having some kind of anniversary reaction. Seems like I'm missing them more now than in the previous 6 months. I've started dreaming about them. I think it would help me to talk about my grief with someone who wasn't a friend. I have a lot of friends and they mean well, but when they tell me that I'll feel better with time, it really doesn't help. I'd just like to be able to talk to someone who will listen to me. Does that sound OK to you?

*Beginner Patient Statement 4*

[Sarcastically] So you're the new therapist? Well, you should know that over the years I've seen a lot of therapists while I've been coming to the counseling center, and some helped. But then they all leave. I've wondered about the therapists that I've had. Did I ever matter to them? Will I matter to you? Will you leave also?

*Beginner Patient Statement 5*

[Friendly] I've really had a rough couple of years. I am having trouble finding a job I like and meeting someone I like. Maybe I haven't been trying hard enough. But, you know, it isn't that easy to find work that matches my skills, and finding a person who excites me as a partner isn't easy either. But maybe I finally got some good luck with you as my therapist.

 **Assess and adjust the difficulty before moving to the next difficulty level (see Step 3 in the exercise instructions).**

## INTERMEDIATE-LEVEL PATIENT STATEMENTS FOR EXERCISE 2

### Intermediate Patient Statement 1

[Serious] Before we start therapy, I'd like to ask you some questions about yourself. If you are gay or bisexual or even gender fluid, I'd appreciate your letting me know. Have you had any experience working with gay people? Have you had gay patients? I am asking because sometimes therapists I've seen don't get me or where I'm coming from at all. My last therapist got really self-conscious talking about sexual identity. If I'm really going to be honest with someone, I want to know they will understand where I'm coming from. And I want them to be honest with me, so I will know where they are coming from. Can you be that kind of therapist with me?

### Intermediate Patient Statement 2

[Boastful] My parents have been trying to fix me ever since I was born. My teeth were a little crooked, so they got me braces. They were concerned about my weight. Did I tell you my dad is a diet doctor and my mother is petite? So they made me keep track of every single thing that went into my mouth. I didn't like that very much. They would still be trying to fix me to this day if I let them. I'm pretty complex. You are looking at me like I'm from the moon or something. Why don't we meet two or three times a week so you can figure me out and tell me what I need to do to move forward in my life.

### Intermediate Patient Statement 3

[With a trembling voice] Well, uh, it started when we were evicted from our apartment. I should have found another place that would have kept us all together, but I got so nervous and confused. And then I started to drink. Uh, right now I feel like I need to get some food in me. I have diabetes and I'm feeling pretty lightheaded. I feel like I could pass out. I skipped breakfast this morning to rush over here. Is there a place where I could get a tomato juice or something?

### Intermediate Patient Statement 4

[Casual] Some people think I have an anger problem. I don't think so. I've never hit anyone, although one time, I tossed a glass of water at someone who was pissing me off. And sometimes I swear at bad car drivers, but who doesn't? Otherwise I'm pretty easygoing. My friend is concerned that my anger will get me into trouble someday and suggested I come to therapy. So here I am. What do you think?

### Intermediate Patient Statement 5

[Monotone] I usually keep other people at arm's length. I don't dislike them or anything, but oftentimes people are not trustworthy. If I don't protect me, who will? My grown children have each other, and so they don't need me so much. And my relatives gossip, and I don't care for that very much. So I keep to myself a lot. This is probably the most I've ever talked to anyone. Hopefully I'll be able to give you what you need in this therapy for your psychology degree or psychotherapy training or whatever.

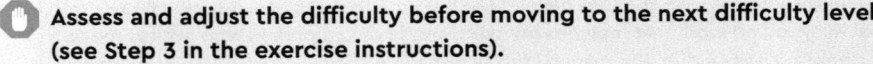 **Assess and adjust the difficulty before moving to the next difficulty level (see Step 3 in the exercise instructions).**

## ADVANCED-LEVEL PATIENT STATEMENTS FOR EXERCISE 2

### Advanced Patient Statement 1

[Irritated] You are spending way too much time asking about my childhood. I know that's how you therapists work, but I think that's just a bunch of Freudian crap. You need to get to know me, to understand who I am right now. My problems are now, not back then. It is really hard for me to come and see you, and my situation is so difficult—I really can't afford to waste any time talking about the past. I need help now!

### Advanced Patient Statement 2

[With authority] My doctor sent me here because he thought it might help with my high blood pressure. But I get stressed for real reasons. It mainly comes from needing to work under people who are not very good at their jobs—either they are not that bright or they are not that committed. People tend to be intimidated by me because of my accomplishments. I got almost perfect SATs and graduated from college in 3 years with honors. I have to tell you, I have my doubts about seeing a trainee. Do you have enough experience to really be of help to me?

### Advanced Patient Statement 3

[Seductively] My ex is a really good person but just really couldn't relate to me on a deep level. You seem like the kind of person I could really have deep conversations with. When I look closely at your face and listen to the sound of your voice, I can intuit that you are a caring person—really warm and engaging. And I can see in your eyes that you can see those qualities in me as well. You seem like the kind of person I could really have a meaningful relationship with. I know you can't tell me that you are attracted to me, but I am getting the feeling that maybe you are.

### Advanced Patient Statement 4

[Monotone and slow] I've been depressed for as long as I can remember. I've been hospitalized twice, had shock treatments twice, and have taken every antidepressant known to man, [pause] but although they help at first, I always return to wondering what the purpose of my life is. I don't have work I enjoy; I don't have real friends. I go from therapy to therapy, hoping each time it will be different. But it never is. I don't think I can really keep doing this much longer.[1]

### Advanced Patient Statement 5

[Irritated] All right, I know what you are going to say. I shouldn't have been drinking and driving. But I just had a couple of glasses of wine with dinner. I don't go out much, so I was just letting off a little steam. I've earned the right to do that. I'm sure you are going to give me a lecture about the dangers of being on the road after drinking—but seriously, it was just a couple of glasses of wine. It's so hard for people to really understand the pressures I'm under and how the alcohol just takes the edge off my anxiety. And it wasn't like I was driving bad. I didn't even get pulled over for weaving or anything like that—just an out-of-date registration sticker. I mean really. And then the cop gives me a ticket for a DUI.

 **Assess and adjust the difficulty here (see Step 3 in the exercise instructions). If appropriate, follow the instructions to make the exercise even more challenging (see Appendix A).**

---

1. Expressions such as "I don't think I can really keep doing this much longer" may reflect an expression of a feeling and not an intent to harm oneself. Nevertheless, therapists need to use a multitude of contextual patient indicators to determine suicidal intent. Trainees should seek close supervision for patients who may be at risk of self-harm or suicide.

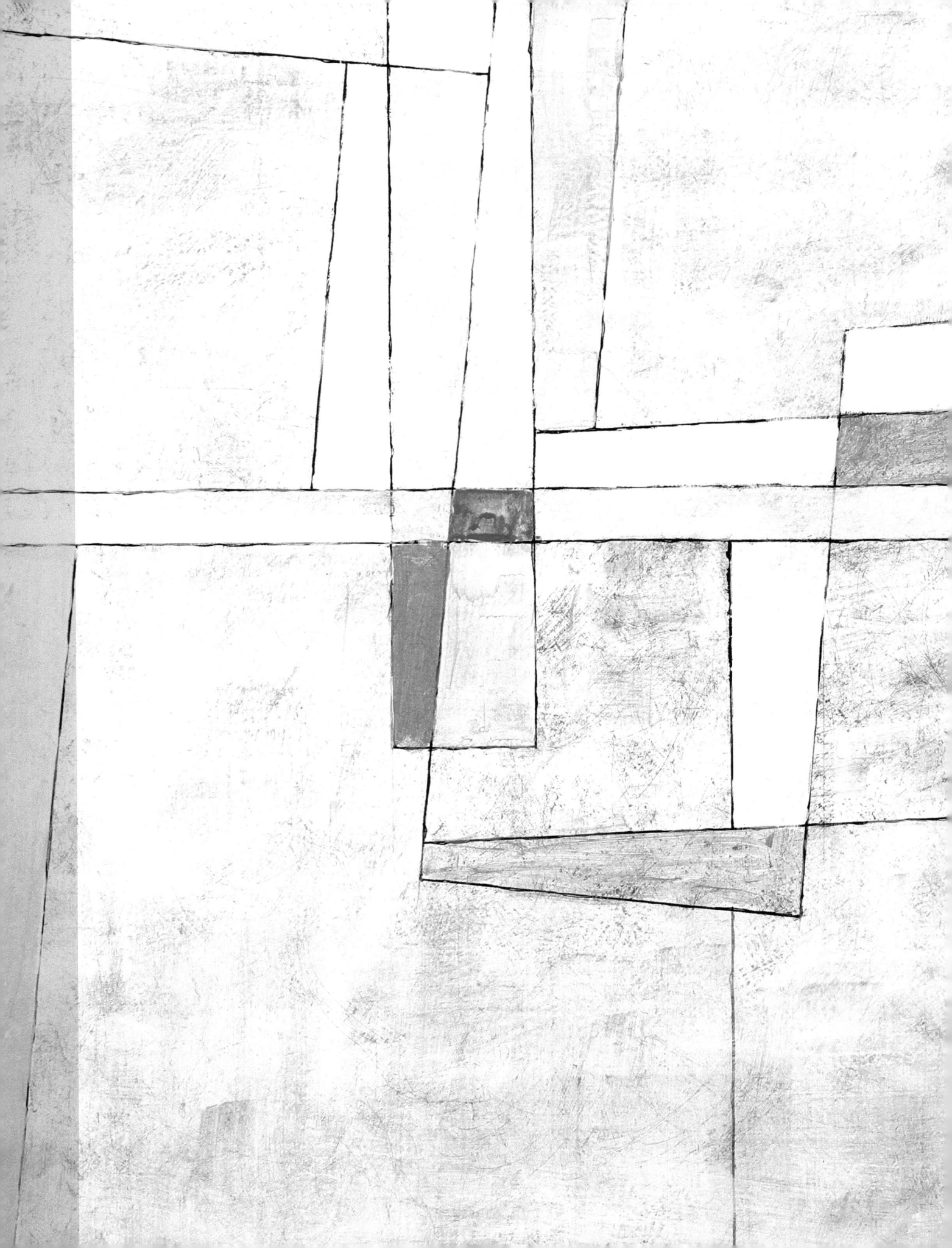

# Deepening Emotional Experience

## Preparations for Exercise 3

1. Read the instructions in Chapter 2.

2. Download the Deliberate Practice Reaction Form and the Deliberate Practice Diary Form at https://www.apa.org/pubs/books/deliberate-practice-psychodynamic-psychotherapy (see the "Clinician and Practitioner Resources" tab; also available in Appendixes A and B, respectively).

## Skill Description

### Skill Difficulty Level: Intermediate

Of the seven strategies that distinguish manualized psychodynamic therapy from manualized cognitive behavior therapy, the first one mentioned is the analyst's focus on affect and expression of emotion (Blagys & Hilsenroth, 2000). Research indicates that the more patients become aware of and experience their emotions in therapy, the more their outcomes are improved (Furrow et al., 2012; Lane et al., 2015). And recent findings indicate that in psychodynamic therapy in particular, helping patients experience their feelings leads to their better functioning (H. Fisher et al., 2016). Therefore, the psychodynamic therapist must be an emotional detective/midwife/catalyst—capable of evoking and deepening emotion so that the patient's nascent emotions can be recognized, named, and understood and become gateways for change.

Empathic evocations are used to "bring experience to life through vivid imagery, elaborate description, analogy, or metaphor" (Goldman et al., 2021, p. 83). They help patients get in touch with the depth of their emotional experience—especially involving emotions that they avoid and that may be at the root of the patient's conflicts. In this way, patients can begin to appreciate the enormous way emotions are implicated in

https://doi.org/10.1037/0000351-005

their sense of self, motivation, values, and capacities for relationships. Quite often therapists will use their voice and intonation to match emotions that are on the verge of awareness or expression (e.g., soft and slow to bring out sadness). Another technique involves therapists speaking as if they were the patient (e.g., using the first person "I"). In knowing which way to proceed, the therapist should be guided by what feels like the most poignant aspect of the patient's message, whether this is conveyed through the patient's words, face, body, or posture.

The trainee should improvise a response to each patient description following one or more of these skill options:

- **Option 1: Use vivid language and match your tone of voice and manner to the patient's underlying emotion.** This helps fan the patient's flickering emotional embers into flames visible to the patient and the therapist.

- **Option 2: Use an "I" statement spoken as if it is from the patient's point of view.** This shows the therapist's willingness to put themselves in the shoes of the patient and dramatically seeds an emotional tone.

- **Option 3: Use a metaphor or analogy.** As in poetic and dramatic speech, metaphors and analogies convey feelings with immediacy.

---

**SKILL OPTIONS FOR EXERCISE 3**

1. Use one or more of the following to intensify the most poignant feeling and meaning embedded within the patient's statement:
   - Option 1: Use vivid language and match your tone of voice and manner to the patient's underlying emotion.
   - Option 2: Use an "I" statement spoken as if it is from the patient's point of view.
   - Option 3: Use a metaphor or analogy.

---

## Examples of the Therapist Deepening Emotional Experience

### Example 1

PATIENT: [*angry*] I would like my mother to listen to me.

THERAPIST: You'd like to grab her by the shoulders and force her to listen! (Option 1)

### Example 2

PATIENT: [*angry*] I would like my mother to listen to me.

THERAPIST: [*intensifying the patient's firm tone*] Mother, I need you to listen to me right now! (Options 1 and 2)

### Example 3

PATIENT: [*angry*] I would like my mother to listen to me.

THERAPIST: Her listening to you would take 50 pounds off your shoulders. (Option 3)

## INSTRUCTIONS FOR EXERCISE 3

### Step 1: Role-Play and Feedback

- The patient says the first beginner patient statement. The therapist **improvises** a response based on the skill option.
- The trainer (or, if not available, the patient) provides **brief** feedback based on the skill option.
- The patient then repeats the same statement, and the therapist again improvises a response. The trainer (or patient) again provides brief feedback.

### Step 2: Repeat

- Repeat Step 1 for all the statements **in the current difficulty level** (beginner, intermediate, or advanced).

### Step 3: Assess and Adjust Difficulty

- The therapist completes the Deliberate Practice Reaction Form (see Appendix A) and decides whether to make the exercise easier or harder or to repeat the same difficulty level.

### Step 4: Repeat for Approximately 15 Minutes

- Repeat Steps 1 to 3 for at least 15 minutes.
- The trainees then switch therapist and patient roles and start over.

> **Now it's your turn! Follow Steps 1 and 2 from the exercise instructions.**

*Remember:* The goal of the role-play is for trainees to practice improvising responses to the patient statements in a manner that (a) uses the skill option and (b) feels authentic for the trainee. **Example therapist responses for each patient statement are provided at the end of this exercise. Trainees should attempt to improvise their own responses before reading the example responses.**

| BEGINNER-LEVEL PATIENT STATEMENTS FOR EXERCISE 3 |
| --- |
| *Beginner Patient Statement 1* |
| [Anxious] My boss called on me in the middle of the meeting, and I got so anxious I couldn't speak and everyone just stared at me. |
| *Beginner Patient Statement 2* |
| [Matter-of-fact] My grown children went away and left me alone, and I've been alone all weekend. So that's all that's been happening. |
| *Beginner Patient Statement 3* |
| [Mournful] And back when I was in school, none of the girls seemed to like me. I don't know why. |
| *Beginner Patient Statement 4* |
| [Angry, clenched jaw] And, in the meeting, no one acknowledged my observations. |
| *Beginner Patient Statement 5* |
| [Exasperated] The other speaker droned on and on, limiting my time to speak. |

> **Assess and adjust the difficulty before moving to the next difficulty level (see Step 3 in the exercise instructions).**

| INTERMEDIATE-LEVEL PATIENT STATEMENTS FOR EXERCISE 3 |
| --- |
| *Intermediate Patient Statement 1* |
| [Ashamed] When I was a kid, my mother told me not to dwell on my sad feelings; I should be thankful for what I have. |
| *Intermediate Patient Statement 2* |
| [Sad] My grown children act like they don't really need me; and that's OK with me because I have plenty of other people in my life. |
| *Intermediate Patient Statement 3* |
| [Confused] I drive for 2 hours to see my partner every weekend. Once in a while, it would be nice for them to come and see me. |
| *Intermediate Patient Statement 4* |
| [Voice quivering] If my daughter were to move away, I don't know what I would do. |
| *Intermediate Patient Statement 5* |
| [Tearful] I just feel so upset; I can't stop crying! |

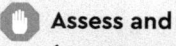 **Assess and adjust the difficulty before moving to the next difficulty level (see Step 3 in the exercise instructions).**

| ADVANCED-LEVEL PATIENT STATEMENTS FOR EXERCISE 3 |
| --- |
| *Advanced Patient Statement 1* |
| [Matter-of-fact] My doctor sent me here because they think I'm depressed. I don't know how they got that idea. Everything in my life is going very well. |
| *Advanced Patient Statement 2* |
| [Flat affect] It's hard to say my stepfather made me have sex, but it came down to that. |
| *Advanced Patient Statement 3* |
| [Indignant] People call me "Professor," not "Mr.," if you don't mind. |
| *Advanced Patient Statement 4* |
| [Tearing up] I'm sorry about having to use so many of your Kleenex today. |
| *Advanced Patient Statement 5* |
| [Irritated] My partner was picking me up from school where I teach. I was talking to some of my students when my partner pulled up and yelled at me to hurry up. |

🖐 **Assess and adjust the difficulty here (see Step 3 in the exercise instructions). If appropriate, follow the instructions to make the exercise even more challenging (see Appendix A).**

# Example Therapist Responses: Deepening Emotional Experience

*Remember:* Trainees should attempt to improvise their own responses before reading the example responses. **Do not read the following responses verbatim unless you are having trouble coming up with your own responses!**

| EXAMPLE RESPONSES TO BEGINNER-LEVEL PATIENT STATEMENTS FOR EXERCISE 3 |
| --- |
| *Example Response to Beginner Patient Statement 1* |
| It's like all of a sudden everyone was looking at me and I just wanted to crawl into a hole. (Options 2 and 3) |
| *Example Response to Beginner Patient Statement 2* |
| So they went away and left you all alone, like you didn't matter. That sounds really painful. (Option 1) |
| *Example Response to Beginner Patient Statement 3* |
| Sounds like that is still sad for you to think about all these years later. (Option 1) |
| *Example Response to Beginner Patient Statement 4* |
| From the look on your face now, you could have spit fire. (Option 3) |
| *Example Response to Beginner Patient Statement 5* |
| It must have felt like torture, waiting for your turn to speak. (Options 1 and 3) |

| EXAMPLE RESPONSES TO INTERMEDIATE-LEVEL PATIENT STATEMENTS FOR EXERCISE 3 |
| --- |
| **Example Response to Intermediate Patient Statement 1** |
| So no matter what you are feeling now as an adult, you hear your mother's voice ringing in your ears, "Don't feel; be thankful!" (Options 1 and 3) |
| **Example Response to Intermediate Patient Statement 2** |
| I hear you say it's OK not to have your children be part of your life, yet your voice sounds quite sad as you say it. (Option 1) |
| **Example Response to Intermediate Patient Statement 3** |
| I drive to see my partner every weekend. Just once I'd like them to make the effort to come see me! (Options 1 and 2) |
| **Example Response to Intermediate Patient Statement 4** |
| That would feel like being set adrift in a small boat in the middle of the ocean. (Option 3) |
| **Example Response to Intermediate Patient Statement 5** |
| If those tears could talk, what would they say? (Options 1 and 3) |

| EXAMPLE RESPONSES TO ADVANCED-LEVEL PATIENT STATEMENTS FOR EXERCISE 3 |
| --- |
| *Example Response to Advanced Patient Statement 1* |
| I really don't know why I am here. My life is going really well. (Option 2) |
| *Example Response to Advanced Patient Statement 2* |
| Oh, my goodness. It's even hard to talk about, let alone have any feelings about! (Option 1) |
| *Example Response to Advanced Patient Statement 3* |
| I don't want to have my status diminished and I won't tolerate that from you. (Option 2) |
| *Example Response to Advanced Patient Statement 4* |
| You feel you need to apologize to me, your therapist, for showing your true feelings? (Option 1) |
| *Example Response to Advanced Patient Statement 5* |
| Did you want to disappear or disappear your partner? (Option 3) |

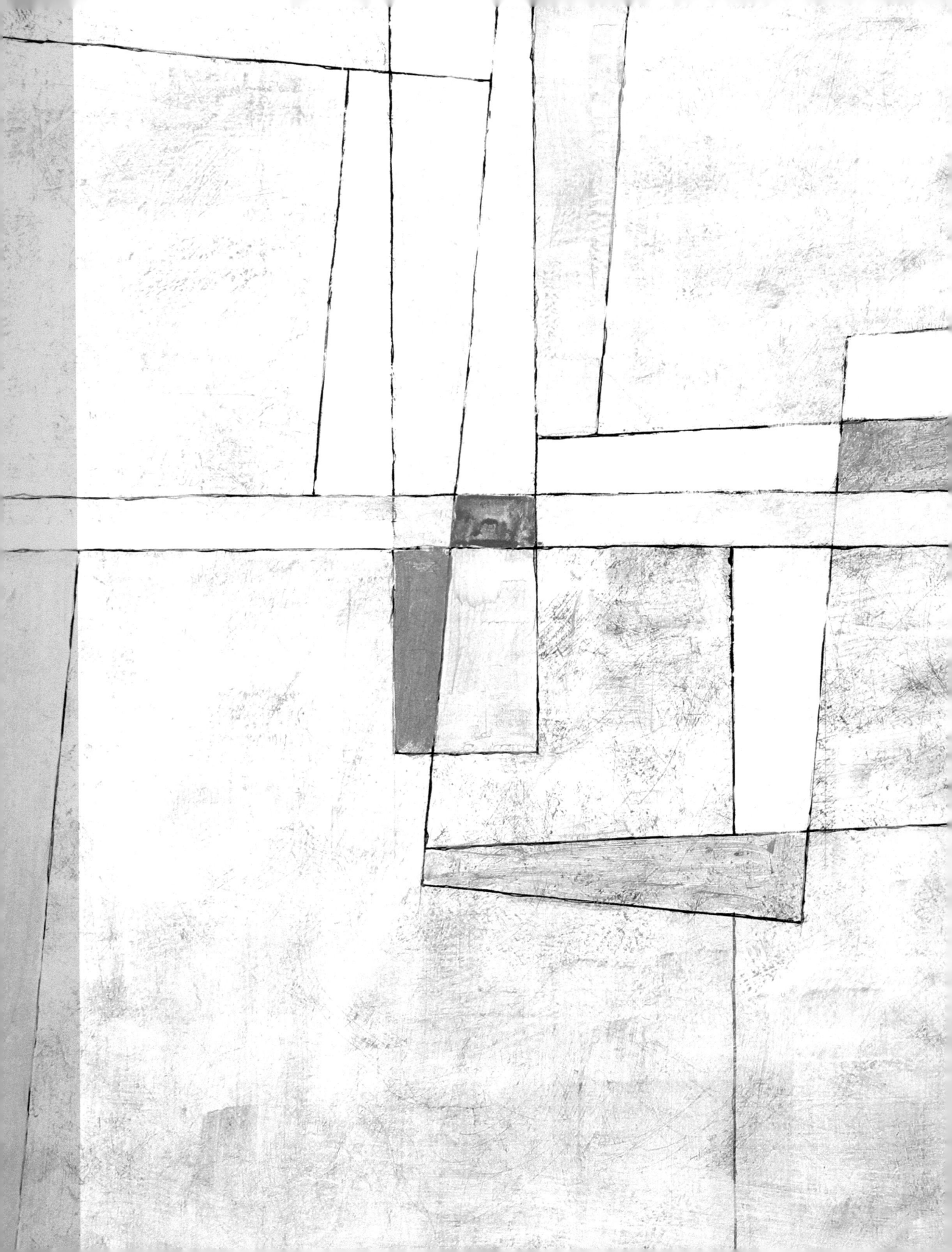

# Making Process Comments

## Preparations for Exercise 4

1. Read the instructions in Chapter 2.

2. Download the Deliberate Practice Reaction Form and the Deliberate Practice Diary Form at https://www.apa.org/pubs/books/deliberate-practice-psychodynamic-psychotherapy (see the "Clinician and Practitioner Resources" tab; also available in Appendixes A and B, respectively).

## Skill Description

### Skill Difficulty Level: Intermediate

Beginning therapists often get caught up in the content of what the patient is saying, which can be quite interesting and relevant to the clinical work. But in an interpersonal psychodynamic therapy, the therapist privileges attending to the process (Kiesler, 1988) of the transactions between therapist and patient because it gives invaluable information as to what is going on relationally and how to intervene productively. Furthermore, significant gains can also be made by helping patients appreciate what is going on in the session in real time.

The relational psychodynamic therapist focuses on the therapeutic relationship as a change mechanism. Here we mean more than the therapeutic alliance. The therapist uses their experience of interacting with the patient to provide information about what it is like to be in relationship with this person, what is the cyclical maladaptive pattern the therapist and patient might end up recreating, and what corrective emotional experiences and insights could be curative.

Irving Yalom (1995, 2002) referred to focusing on the process as talking about the here and now in the here and now, and Greenson (1967), more than 50 years ago, referred to it as working in the moment. At the most surface level, process comments

https://doi.org/10.1037/0000351-006

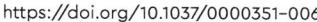

*Deliberate Practice in Psychodynamic Psychotherapy*, by H. Levenson, V. Gay, and J. L. Binder

focus on pointing out behavioral transactions between the patient and therapist: "I notice when I did X, you did Y." Other types of process comments involve a therapist's "inquiring about or disclosing immediate feelings about the client, herself or himself in relation to the client, or the therapeutic relationship" (Hill et al., 2014, p. 299). Sometimes this kind of sharing is called *immediacy* (Hill et al., 2014), *metacommunication* (Kiesler, 1988), or *countertransference disclosures* (Gabbard & Wilkinson, 2000). What all of these have in common is helping patients gain an awareness of their interpersonal patterns and how they get triggered in the session.

In this exercise, you will start off practicing making process comments at the most general level. In future exercises, you will be able to practice commenting on the patient's defenses in the here and now (Exercise 5) and helping patients become aware of similarities between the way they relate in session and outside session (making transference interpretations; Exercise 7).

The identities of all patients have been disguised to protect their confidentiality. Ann is based on a real patient whose case has previously been discussed and published (Levenson, 2017). In addition, there is a video of all six sessions done with Ann that is commercially available (Levenson & Carlson, 2010), as well as a two-session version containing an interview with her therapist (Hanna Levenson) discussing the case from a skills-based point of view, *Psychodynamic Therapy Skills* (Levenson & Friedlander, in production). A transcript of the two sessions can be found in Exercise 13. There have also been four published studies using the video of Ann that can be found in the references (Friedlander et al., 2018, 2020; Levenson, 2020; Levenson et al., 2020). The case of Mr. Johnson (pseudonym) is based on a real patient whose case has previously been discussed and published (Levenson, 1995). There is also a video of Mr. Johnson (using an actor; see Levenson, 1999).

The trainee playing the therapist should then improvise a response to each patient description and statement following these skill criteria:

1. **Ask permission to take a look at what happened right now between the therapist and patient.** Process comments made in the moment can expose interpersonal issues in tangible, emotional ways that talking about interpersonal behaviors in the past cannot.

2. **Name what just transpired between therapist and patient.**

3. **Option 1: Invite the patient to explore their feelings about what transpired.**

   or

   **Option 2: Conjecture (make your best guess) about the patient's feelings about what transpired.** In this way, process comments can help a therapist repair interpersonal ruptures with patients (e.g., "I wonder if when I made that comment, that hurt you, and for that I am deeply sorry").

### SKILL CRITERIA FOR EXERCISE 4

1. Ask permission to take a look at what happened right now between the therapist and patient.
2. Name what just transpired between therapist and patient.
3. Option 1: Invite the patient to explore their feelings about what transpired.

   or

   Option 2: Conjecture about the patient's feelings about what transpired.

## Examples of Therapists Making Process Comments

**Note:** <u>Underlined text</u> before each patient statement should be read aloud to provide context. Take your time in reading this slowly and repeating if necessary.

### Example 1

<u>The patient said, "My family tells me that I need to help myself." The therapist responded, "You are coming here to therapy."</u>

**PATIENT:** [*with an exhausted sigh*] Wow, I'm feeling pretty weak.

**THERAPIST:** Can we pause here for a minute and look at what just transpired? (Criterion 1) I just stated that you were doing something to help yourself by coming to therapy, and then you responded about feeling weak. (Criterion 2) I'm wondering how you are feeling about my saying something positive about you? (Criterion 3, Option 1)

> or

It's almost like you got uncomfortable with my saying something positive about you. (Criterion 3, Option 2)

### Example 2

<u>The therapist asks the patient a challenging question about what the patient was feeling as they were talking about something upsetting.</u>

**PATIENT:** [*monotone*] Are you going to be here next week?

**THERAPIST:** Can we take a look at what just happened? (Criterion 1) I noticed that after I asked you about your feelings, you asked me if I'm going to be here next week. (Criterion 2) I am wondering what was going on for you just then. (Criterion 3, Option 1)

### Example 3

<u>The patient has been talking excitedly about their new book project; the therapist glances at the clock on the wall behind the patient.</u>

**PATIENT:** [*confused*] Well, uh, now I forgot what I was saying. How odd. Anyway, now I feel like kind of hopeless.

**THERAPIST:** Can we take a look at what just happened? (Criterion 1) You were speaking about your new book project, and when I glanced at my clock, you stopped talking. (Criterion 2) I'm wondering what my looking at the clock meant for you. (Criterion 3, Option 1)

> or

Did you think when I looked at my clock, I wasn't interested in what you were saying? (Criterion 3, Option 2)

## INSTRUCTIONS FOR EXERCISE 4

### Step 1: Role-Play and Feedback

- The patient reads the <u>underlined text</u> aloud then says the first beginner patient statement. The therapist **improvises** a response based on the skill criteria.
- The trainer (or, if not available, the patient) provides **brief** feedback based on the skill criteria.
- The patient then repeats the same statement, and the therapist again improvises a response. The trainer (or patient) again provides brief feedback.

### Step 2: Repeat

- Repeat Step 1 for all the statements **in the current difficulty level** (beginner, intermediate, or advanced).

### Step 3: Assess and Adjust Difficulty

- The therapist completes the Deliberate Practice Reaction Form (see Appendix A) and decides whether to make the exercise easier or harder or to repeat the same difficulty level.

### Step 4: Repeat for Approximately 15 Minutes

- Repeat Steps 1 to 3 for at least 15 minutes.
- The trainees then switch therapist and patient roles and start over.

> **Now it's your turn! Follow Steps 1 and 2 from the instructions.**

*Remember:* The goal of the role-play is for trainees to practice improvising responses to the statements in a manner that (a) uses the skill criteria and (b) feels authentic for the trainee. **Example therapist responses for each patient statement are provided at the end of this exercise. Trainees should attempt to improvise their own responses before reading the example response.**

   *Note:* <u>Underlined text</u> before each patient statement should be read aloud to provide context. Take your time in reading this slowly and repeating if necessary.

| BEGINNER-LEVEL PATIENT STATEMENTS FOR EXERCISE 4 |
| --- |
| ***Beginner Patient Statement 1*** |
| <u>Mr. Johnson has been talking dejectedly about being such a loser: "I can't do anything right." The therapist responds supportively by telling him, "You've decided to try therapy and have shown up right on time."</u> <br><br> PATIENT: **[Sad]** Yeah, but I almost didn't make it on time. |
| ***Beginner Patient Statement 2*** |
| <u>The therapist has just asked Mr. Johnson how he felt about his daughter's leaving him alone for the weekend to go on a short trip with some friends. He responds with a sad and trembling voice, saying, "What did you say, doctor?" The therapist repeats the question about his daughter's leaving him alone.</u> <br><br> PATIENT: **[Sad and confused]** I'm sorry, doctor, I still didn't hear you. |
| ***Beginner Patient Statement 3*** |
| <u>Ann Lee comes into the session smiling. The therapist asks her how her weekend visit with her boyfriend went. Ann's facial expression immediately goes from sunny to gloomy, and her eyes well up with tears.</u> |
| ***Beginner Patient Statement 4*** |
| <u>The therapist has arrived at the session 5 minutes late and apologizes briefly to Mr. Johnson. Mr. Johnson sits in silence, which is unusual for him.</u> |
| ***Beginner Patient Statement 5*** |
| <u>The therapist has asked Mr. Johnson, "I'm wondering how you felt when your daughter asked you to loan her some money so she could move out."</u> <br><br> PATIENT: **[Frustrated]** Right now I just feel hungry. I'm having trouble concentrating on what you are saying. I think I need to eat something. |

 **Assess and adjust the difficulty before moving to the next difficulty level (see Step 3 in the exercise instructions).**

| INTERMEDIATE-LEVEL PATIENT STATEMENTS FOR EXERCISE 4 |
| --- |
| **Intermediate Patient Statement 1** |
| Dr. Ingram has been talking about how hard he has been working toward obtaining faculty tenure in his department. Recently his research paper had been returned by a journal for revisions. The therapist asks him how he felt about the manuscript's not being accepted as is.<br><br>PATIENT: [Confused] Oh, excuse me, did you say something? |
| **Intermediate Patient Statement 2** |
| The therapist asks Mr. Johnson a challenging question about what he was feeling as they were talking about something upsetting.<br><br>PATIENT: [Monotone] Are you going to be here next week? |
| **Intermediate Patient Statement 3** |
| Ann begins the session uncustomarily talking very quickly to the point where it is hard to understand what she is saying. |
| **Intermediate Patient Statement 4** |
| Mr. Johnson is sitting in the waiting room alongside a second patient the therapist has erroneously scheduled for the same time. Seeing the error, the therapist invites Mr. Johnson into the therapy office, and then goes back to the waiting room to reschedule the second patient. Upon returning to the office, the therapist says, "I am sorry for the mix-up."<br><br>PATIENT: [Apologetic] Well, uh, did I do something wrong? I know it's probably my fault. |
| **Intermediate Patient Statement 5** |
| Dr. Ingram has been sitting in a clinic waiting room with several other patients who are there to see other therapists.<br><br>PATIENT: [Upset, entering therapy office] It is very difficult for me waiting with such, well, low-class people. |

 **Assess and adjust the difficulty before moving to the next difficulty level (see Step 3 in the exercise instructions).**

## ADVANCED-LEVEL PATIENT STATEMENTS FOR EXERCISE 4

### *Advanced Patient Statement 1*

The therapist questioned Ann about why she stayed in a relationship with a partner who seemed to neglect her and often left her feeling very unhappy.

**PATIENT:** **[Forcefully]** You know, I am taking a psychology course, and the instructor showed us an article from a prestigious journal that stated that about 70% of the people in psychotherapy don't get lasting benefits.

### *Advanced Patient Statement 2*

The therapist has just announced to Mr. Johnson that it's time to end the session.

**PATIENT:** **[Dejectedly]** You know, I have been feeling kind of hopeless lately. Sometimes I feel like there's no point in going on.

### *Advanced Patient Statement 3*

Dr. Ingram enters the room looking down. The therapist greets him with a cheerful "Welcome!"

**PATIENT:** **[Irritated]** You know, it's almost insulting to come here, like a defeated puppy. **[Suddenly shifts his tone to matter-of-fact]** Well, anyway, I'm here.

### *Advanced Patient Statement 4*

Dr. Ingram has been talking excitedly about his new book project; the therapist glances at the desk clock.

**PATIENT:** **[Confused]** Well, uh, now I forgot what I was saying. How odd. Anyway, now I feel like kind of confused.

### *Advanced Patient Statement 5*

The therapist starts off the session by saying to Dr. Ingram, "Toward the end of our last session, you mentioned the topic of sex. Might we start there today?"

**PATIENT:** **[Irritated]** Well, I'm not sure that "I" mentioned sex. I think that you did. Like you are again, today!

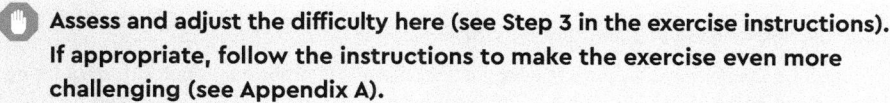 **Assess and adjust the difficulty here (see Step 3 in the exercise instructions). If appropriate, follow the instructions to make the exercise even more challenging (see Appendix A).**

## Example Therapist Responses: Making Process Comments

*Remember:* Trainees should attempt to improvise their own responses before reading the example responses. **Do not read the following responses verbatim unless you are having trouble coming up with your own responses!**

| EXAMPLE RESPONSES TO BEGINNER-LEVEL PATIENT STATEMENTS FOR EXERCISE 4 |
| --- |
| *Example Response to Beginner Patient Statement 1* |
| Can we pause here for a minute and look at what just transpired? (Criterion 1) I just said that you were doing something right to help yourself by coming to therapy on time, and you continued to find fault with yourself, despite what I said. (Criterion 2) I'm wondering how you are feeling about my acknowledging the positive steps you have taken. (Criterion 3, Option 1)<br><br>or<br><br>It's almost like you got uncomfortable with my seeing something positive in your behavior. (Criterion 3, Option 2) |
| *Example Response to Beginner Patient Statement 2* |
| Can we take a look at what just happened? (Criterion 1) It seems that when I asked you how you felt about your daughter's leaving you alone, you had trouble hearing me. (Criterion 2) I wonder what was happening just then. (Criterion 3, Option 1)<br><br>or<br><br>Maybe my question made you uncomfortable and you preferred not to hear it. (Criterion 3, Option 2) |
| *Example Response to Beginner Patient Statement 3* |
| Wow! Something just happened in here. (Criterion 1) It seems when I asked you how your weekend went with your partner, your whole expression changed and you started to cry. (Criterion 2) Looks like my question evoked a lot of sadness for you? (Criterion 3, Option 2) |
| *Example Response to Beginner Patient Statement 4* |
| Would it be OK if we took a look at what just happened? (Criterion 1) I apologized for being late and you were silent; you aren't often silent in here. (Criterion 2) So I'm wondering about your silence. Can you help me understand? (Criterion 3, Option 1)<br><br>or<br><br>I am wondering if perhaps your silence indicates some upset with me for begin late. (Criterion 3, Option 2) |
| *Example Response to Beginner Patient Statement 5* |
| Can we take a look at what just happened? (Criterion 1) I asked you how you felt when your daughter asked you for money, and you suddenly became hungry and needed some food. (Criterion 2) Did you have any feelings about my asking you about your daughter? (Criterion 3, Option 1) |

## EXAMPLE RESPONSES TO INTERMEDIATE-LEVEL PATIENT STATEMENTS FOR EXERCISE 4

### Example Response to Intermediate Patient Statement 1

Can we take a look at what just happened? (Criterion 1) We were talking about something very important to you—a journal returning your manuscript. When I asked you how you felt about it, you suddenly forgot the topic. (Criterion 2) What do you make of that? (Criterion 3, Option 1)

### Example Response to Intermediate Patient Statement 2

Can we take a look at what just happened? (Criterion 1) I noticed that after I asked you about your feelings, you changed the subject and asked me if I'm going to be here next week. (Criterion 2) I am wondering what was going on for you just then. (Criterion 3, Option 1)

### Example Response to Intermediate Patient Statement 3

Sorry to interrupt, but could we take a look at what is occurring right now in session? (Criterion 1) You came into the session, sat down, and started speaking pretty quickly—so quickly that your words were running together. In fact, I am having some trouble following what you are saying. (Criterion 2) Are you aware of why you are talking so quickly today? (Criterion 3, Option 1)

### Example Response to Intermediate Patient Statement 4

Might we look at what just happened between us? (Criterion 1) I made a mistake and scheduled two people for the same time. Yet you blamed yourself. (Criterion 2) I wonder how it is that you came to blame yourself when I was at fault. (Criterion 3, Option 1)

### Example Response to Intermediate Patient Statement 5

Before we begin today, could we pause and look and what you said about the experience you just had my waiting room? (Criterion 1) You said it was difficult waiting with such low-class people. (Criterion 2) I'd be interested in hearing what made it so difficult for you. (Criterion, Option 1)

| EXAMPLE RESPONSES TO ADVANCED-LEVEL PATIENT STATEMENTS FOR EXERCISE 4 |
| --- |
| *Example Response to Advanced Patient Statement 1* |
| Can we take a look at what just happened? (Criterion 1) I asked you about why you tolerated your partner's behavior. And you responded by citing evidence that therapy is not equally helpful to everyone. (Criterion 2) It makes me wonder how you felt about my question? (Criterion 3, Option 1) |
| *Example Response to Advanced Patient Statement 2* |
| Can we take a look at what just happened? (Criterion 1) When I said that our time for today was up, you voiced a feeling of hopelessness and implied that you might have thoughts of hurting yourself. (Criterion 2) Was there something about my saying our time was up that caused some disturbing thoughts or feelings? (Criterion 3, Option 2) |
| *Example Response to Advanced Patient Statement 3* |
| Could we talk about your reaction when I said "Good morning," and you replied that you felt insulted? (Criteria 1 and 2) Perhaps something I said or how I said it was irritating to you? (Criterion 3, Option 2) |
| *Example Response to Advanced Patient Statement 4* |
| Can we take a look at what just happened? (Criterion 1) You were speaking about your new book project and suddenly you stopped. Just before, I had glanced at my clock. (Criterion 2) I'm wondering what my looking at my clock meant for you. (Criterion 3, Option 1) |
| *Example Response to Advanced Patient Statement 5* |
| Could we please look at what just transpired between us? (Criterion 1) I brought up the topic of sex because I remembered it's where we left off, and you had a strong reaction. (Criterion 2) Perhaps my asking about sex today felt out of place. Is that right? (Criterion, Option 2) |

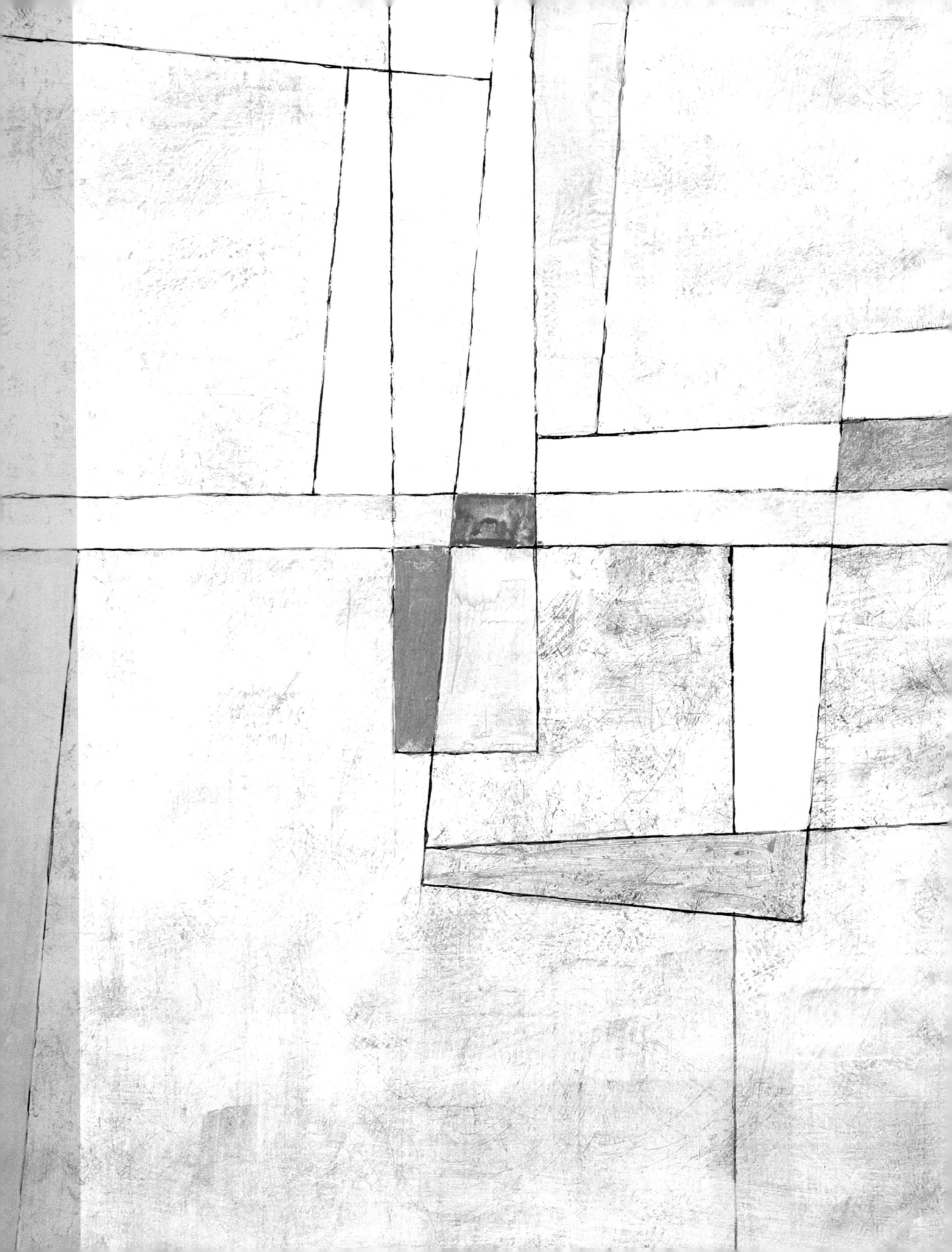

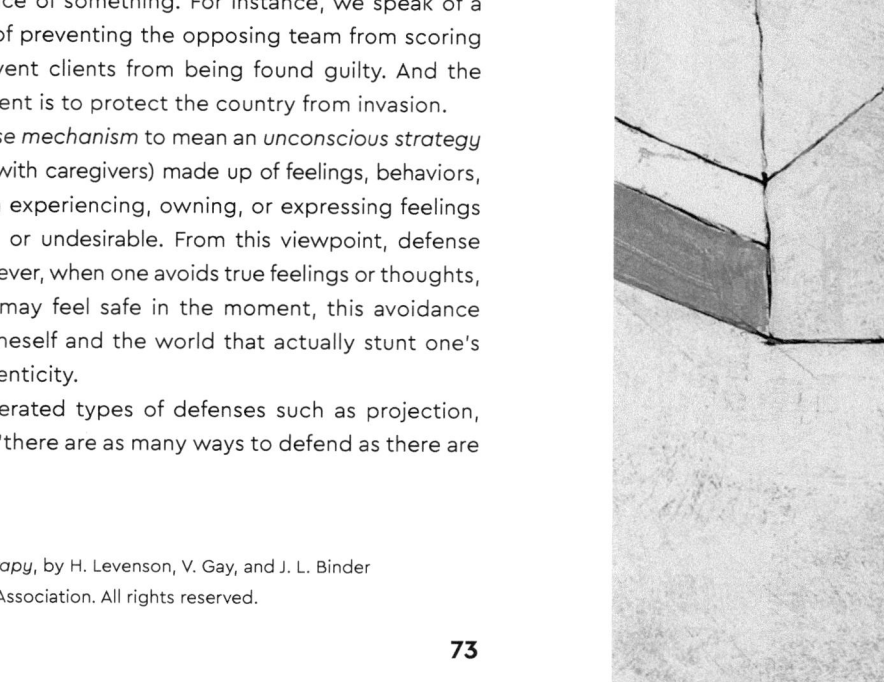

# Pointing Out Defenses and Inquiring About Underlying Fear

## Preparations for Exercise 5

1. Read the instructions in Chapter 2.

2. Download the Deliberate Practice Reaction Form and the Deliberate Practice Diary Form at https://www.apa.org/pubs/books/deliberate-practice-psychodynamic-psychotherapy (see the "Clinician and Practitioner Resources" tab; also available in Appendixes A and B, respectively).

## Skill Description

### Skill Difficulty Level: Intermediate

We use the terms *defense* and *defensive* in everyday conversation. They actually are quite appropriate descriptors because the function of a defense in common parlance is as a protection against or an avoidance of something. For instance, we speak of a defensive maneuver in sports as a way of preventing the opposing team from scoring points. A defense attorney tries to prevent clients from being found guilty. And the purpose of a country's defense department is to protect the country from invasion.

Sigmund Freud coined the term *defense mechanism* to mean an *unconscious strategy* (often learned through early experiences with caregivers) made up of feelings, behaviors, or thoughts that blocks the person from experiencing, owning, or expressing feelings because they are considered dangerous or undesirable. From this viewpoint, defense mechanisms are self-protective acts. However, when one avoids true feelings or thoughts, it comes at a dear cost; although one may feel safe in the moment, this avoidance creates habitual ways of dealing with oneself and the world that actually stunt one's awareness, flexibility, intimacy, and authenticity.

Freud's daughter, Anna Freud, enumerated types of defenses such as projection, repression, and rationalization. Actually, "there are as many ways to defend as there are

https://doi.org/10.1037/0000351-007

*Deliberate Practice in Psychodynamic Psychotherapy*, by H. Levenson, V. Gay, and J. L. Binder

snowflakes or fingerprints" (McCullough & Carlson, 2005) because just about anything can be used as a defense mechanism to avoid thoughts and feelings. Therefore, what is productive in therapy is to help patients discover their idiosyncratic avoidant processes, which can then lead to an understanding of what may be perpetuating their pain and present difficulties.

In this exercise, you will get practice noticing and pointing out the patient's defensive strategies to the patient. These defensive patterns are usually learned so early in life, used so consistently, and incorporated so deeply into a person's interactional repertoire that they often feel like a part of one's personality rather than defensive maneuvers. In such cases, we might even say such patterns are *ego-syntonic*—acceptable (even ideal) to the patient. And of course, like most unconscious habits, until they are pointed out, we do not have a means of changing them.

A patient's increasing awareness of their own defensive patterns can begin to loosen their view of their defenses as a desirable part of themselves; patients may begin to see the damage their defenses have done, making the once unconsciously embraced defensive strategies *ego-dystonic* (unacceptable). Once this occurs, it becomes easier for patients to collaborate with their therapists toward achieving a common goal (getting unstuck). Later you will work with Exercise 12, which is focused on helping patients have new (corrective) emotional experiences when they do not use their customary defenses and therefore do not avoid crucial thoughts and feelings in the session. But for now, you will focus on pointing out the defense—a critical first step. Helpful hint: Before challenging a defense, validate it, conveying that you see its need from the patient's point of view. Remember, defenses start out as self-protective acts.

The trainee should improvise a response to each patient description following these skill criteria:

1. **Point out the defensive strategy to the patient in an empathic and validating manner.** From the perspective of the therapist, a common element indicating a defensive strategy is any thought, feeling, or behavior that is unconsciously being used to avoid experiencing a feeling that has been apprised as unwanted by others or dangerous based on past learning.

2. **Inquire or wonder out loud what the patient fears might happen if they did not use the defensive strategy.** Here we are asking the patient to imagine what they are actively avoiding.

---

### SKILL CRITERIA FOR EXERCISE 5

1. Point out the defensive strategy to the patient in an empathic and validating manner.
2. Inquire or wonder out loud what the patient fears might happen if they did not use the defensive strategy.

## Examples of Therapists Pointing Out Defenses

### Example 1

**PATIENT:** [*calmly*] I drive 2 hours to see my significant other every weekend; they never drive to see me. But I don't mind because I actually enjoy driving.

**THERAPIST:** It's a good thing you enjoy driving so much. (Criterion 1) I wonder what you imagine might happen if you didn't feel like driving. (Criterion 2)

### Example 2

**PATIENT:** [*cheerful*] I don't want to be a clingy partner. So whenever I am with my significant other, I put on a smiley face.

**THERAPIST:** It seems you need to put on a smiley face a lot when you are with him. (Criterion 1) Is there something you fear would happen if you came across as unhappy? (Criterion 2)

### Example 3

**PATIENT:** [*matter-of-fact*] At first I felt guilty about breaking up with my partner by text. Then I thought that it's really a kinder way to say goodbye.

**THERAPIST:** When you broke up by text you felt guilty; then you reasoned that it might actually be better for your partner. This made you feel less guilty. (Criterion 1) I wonder what you feared might happen if we explore your guilty feelings for breaking up by text? (Criterion 2)

| INSTRUCTIONS FOR EXERCISE 5 |
|---|

### Step 1: Role-Play and Feedback

- The patient says the first beginner patient statement. The therapist **improvises** a response based on the skill criteria.
- The trainer (or, if not available, the patient) provides **brief** feedback making sure that the therapist has met all the skill criteria.
- The patient then repeats the same statement, and the therapist again improvises a response. The trainer (or patient) again provides brief feedback based on the skill criteria.

### Step 2: Repeat

- Repeat Step 1 for all the statements **in the current difficulty level** (beginner, intermediate, or advanced).

### Step 3: Assess and Adjust Difficulty

- The therapist completes the Deliberate Practice Reaction Form (see Appendix A) and decides whether to make the exercise easier, to repeat the same difficulty level, or to go on to the harder difficulty level.

### Step 4: Repeat for Approximately 15 Minutes

- Repeat Steps 1 to 3 for at least 15 minutes.
- The trainees then switch therapist and patient roles and start over.

**Now it's your turn! Follow Steps 1 and 2 from the instructions.**

*Remember:* The goal of the role-play is for trainees to practice improvising responses to the patient statements in a manner that (a) uses the skill criteria and (b) feels authentic for the trainee. **Example therapist responses for each patient statement are provided at the end of this exercise. Trainees should attempt to improvise their own responses before reading the example responses.**

| BEGINNER-LEVEL PATIENT STATEMENTS FOR EXERCISE 5 |
| --- |
| *Beginner Patient Statement 1* |
| [**Casual**] My week has been alright—a little stressful. But what do you think of the current political stuff? |
| *Beginner Patient Statement 2* |
| [**Embarrassed**] Our landlord said we had to move. I drank too much that night. |
| *Beginner Patient Statement 3* |
| [**Irritated**] You know, all of my problems come from my partner. My partner is my problem! |
| *Beginner Patient Statement 4* |
| [**Cheerful**] I don't want to be a clingy partner. So, whenever I am with my significant other, I put on a smiley face. |
| *Beginner Patient Statement 5* |
| [**Adamant**] In session today, I'd like to focus on the future, not talk about my past. |

 **Assess and adjust the difficulty before moving to the next difficulty level (see Step 3 in the exercise instructions).**

| INTERMEDIATE-LEVEL PATIENT STATEMENTS FOR EXERCISE 5 |
| --- |
| *Intermediate Patient Statement 1* |
| [Surprised] When you asked me about school, I just kind of froze. It's like I have no feelings at all about it. |
| *Intermediate Patient Statement 2* |
| [Annoyed] I visited my parents and just bit my tongue the whole time. |
| *Intermediate Patient Statement 3* |
| [Boastful] When I applied to colleges, I considered applying to top schools like Harvard. But I decided I wouldn't apply to any Ivy League colleges because they rarely live up to their reputations. |
| *Intermediate Patient Statement 4* |
| [Self-doubting] At first I felt guilty about breaking up with my partner by text. Then I thought that it's really a kinder way to say goodbye. |
| *Intermediate Patient Statement 5* |
| [Matter-of-fact] I don't recall what we talked about last week. Can you remind me? |

🛑 **Assess and adjust the difficulty before moving to the next difficulty level (see Step 3 in the exercise instructions).**

| ADVANCED-LEVEL PATIENT STATEMENTS FOR EXERCISE 5 |
| --- |
| *Advanced Patient Statement 1* |
| [Critical] I've heard that people who become therapists are people who are pretty messed up. |
| *Advanced Patient Statement 2* |
| [Puzzled] Sorry I'm late. When I was driving here, I suddenly forgot where your building is. |
| *Advanced Patient Statement 3* |
| [Pleased and contemptuous] When I left the session last week where we talked about my boss, I immediately called them up and let them have it! My boss seemed surprised. Can you imagine that? |
| *Advanced Patient Statement 4* |
| [Angry and arrogant] I sent a manuscript to a journal in my field and they sent it back for revisions. When I received the journal's response, I was furious. I'm going to send a letter to the journal editor, complaining about the incompetence of his reviewers. |
| *Advanced Patient Statement 5* |
| [Dismissive] Thanks for letting me know what you think about my problem. That's a good observation. I'll have to think about that for a while. |

✋ **Assess and adjust the difficulty here (see Step 3 in the exercise instructions). If appropriate, follow the instructions to make the exercise even more challenging (see Appendix A).**

## Example Therapist Responses: Pointing Out Defenses

**Remember:** Trainees should attempt to improvise their own responses before reading the example responses. **Do not read the following responses verbatim unless you are having trouble coming up with your own responses!**

| EXAMPLE RESPONSES TO BEGINNER-LEVEL PATIENT STATEMENTS FOR EXERCISE 5 |
|---|
| *Example Response to Beginner Patient Statement 1* |
| Politics are important, but the more we discuss them, the less we focus on you. (Criterion 1) I wonder if you're concerned that something worrisome would happen if we focused on you? (Criterion 2) |
| *Example Response to Beginner Patient Statement 2* |
| So after the landlord said you needed to move, it sounds like you were looking for some relief by getting drunk. (Criterion 1) I wonder what you would have felt if you hadn't responded by drinking? (Criterion 2) |
| *Example Response to Beginner Patient Statement 3* |
| I can see why it's tempting to center your feelings on your partner. (Criterion 1) Is there something bad that you imagine occurring if we centered our work on you? (Criterion 2) |
| *Example Response to Beginner Patient Statement 4* |
| It seems you need to put on a smiley face a lot when you are with your significant other. (Criterion 1) Is there something you fear would happen if you came across as unhappy? (Criterion 2) |
| *Example Response to Beginner Patient Statement 5* |
| Of course, thinking about your future matters. (Criterion 1) But I'm wondering if there is part of you that imagines it not going so well if we also talked about your past? (Criterion 2) |

| EXAMPLE RESPONSES TO INTERMEDIATE-LEVEL PATIENT STATEMENTS FOR EXERCISE 5 |
| --- |
| ***Example Response to Intermediate Patient Statement 1*** |
| When I asked you about school, part of you "just froze," which stopped all your feelings. (Criterion 1) I wonder if there is something you fear would happen if you allowed yourself to have your feelings and didn't "freeze" them? (Criterion 2) |
| ***Example Response to Intermediate Patient Statement 2*** |
| By biting your tongue, you prevented yourself from speaking directly. (Criterion 1) It seems that you imagine bad things occurring if you were to tell your parents what you really feel. Is that right? (Criterion 2) |
| ***Example Response to Intermediate Patient Statement 3*** |
| It sounds like you gave a lot of thought to colleges you applied to. (Criterion 1) Was there some fear on your part as to what might happen if you applied to schools like Harvard? (Criterion 2) |
| ***Example Response to Intermediate Patient Statement 4*** |
| When you broke up by text, you felt guilty, then you reasoned that it might actually be *better* for your partner. This made you feel less guilty. (Criterion 1) I wonder what you fear might happen if we explore your guilty feelings for breaking up by text? (Criterion 2) |
| ***Example Response to Intermediate Patient Statement 5*** |
| Sure, I can remind you about last week's topic. Do you think forgetting might have saved you from having some disturbing thoughts or feelings during the week? (Criteria 1 and 2) |

| EXAMPLE RESPONSES TO ADVANCED-LEVEL |
| :---: |
| **PATIENT STATEMENTS FOR EXERCISE 5** |

**Example Response to Advanced Patient Statement 1**

There was something pleasing about hearing that therapists—including myself perhaps—are people who are really in need of help themselves. (Criterion 1) Is there something to fear if you believed the opposite—that I am capable of helping you? (Criterion 2)

**Example Response to Advanced Patient Statement 2**

On your way to see me for our therapy session, you forgot suddenly how to get here. In effect, that would prevent us from meeting. (Criterion 1) Maybe you are concerned that something bad might occur during this session? (Criterion 2)

**Example Response to Advanced Patient Statement 3**

It seems that our talking about your anger toward your boss provoked you to act—to immediately call your boss and "let them have it" as you put it. (Criterion 1) I wonder what you feared might occur if you didn't act immediately and instead examined how angry you were. (Criterion 2)

**Example Response to Advanced Patient Statement 4**

So you intensely focused on the incompetence of the reviewers when your paper got returned for revisions. (Criterion 1) If you didn't turn all your attention to their incompetence, where else might your attention have gone? (Criterion 2)

**Example Response to Advanced Patient Statement 5**

I'm glad you found my comments on target and want to think about them. (Criterion 1) However, I'm wondering if there's something about your immediate reaction that you are concerned about saying? (Criterion 2)

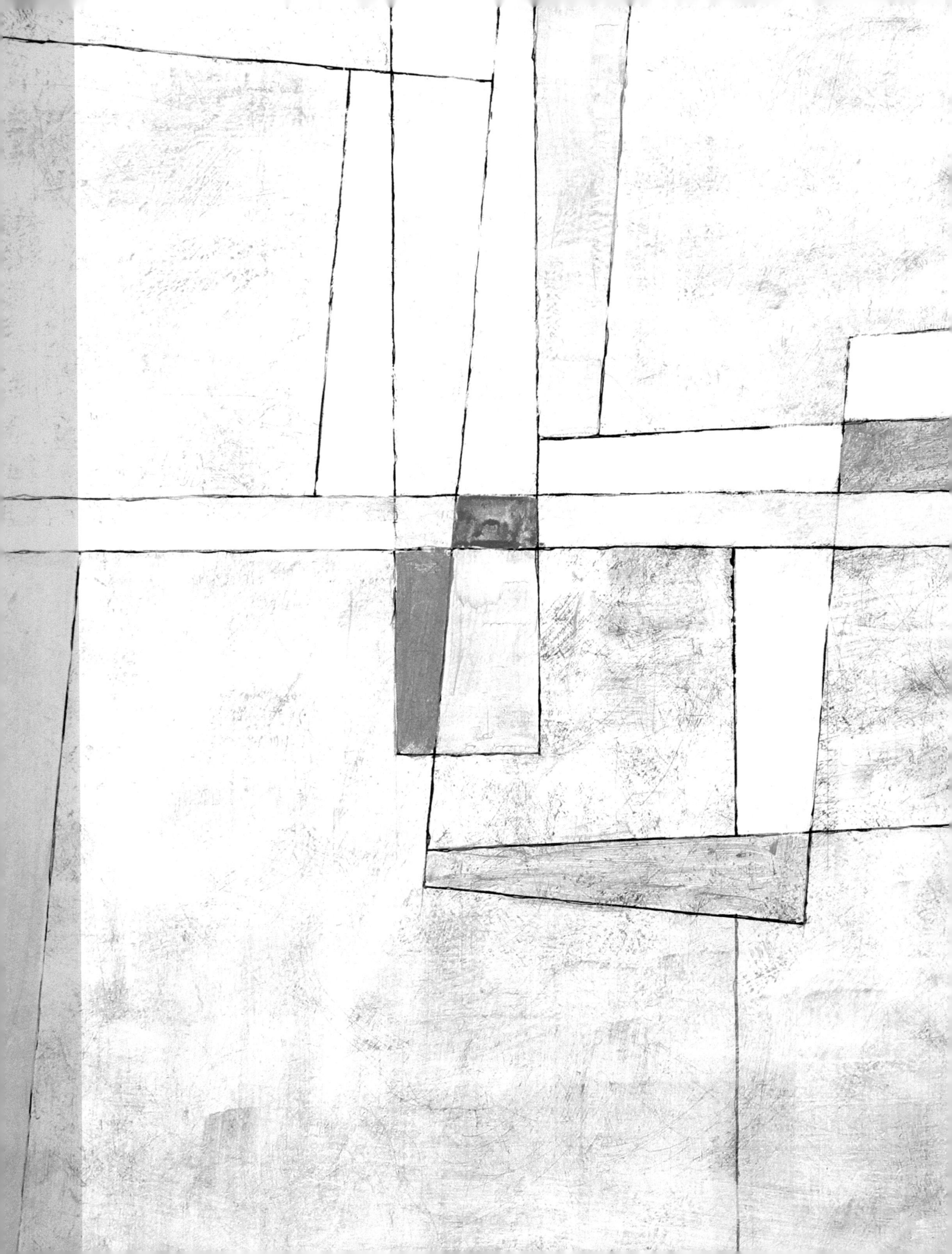

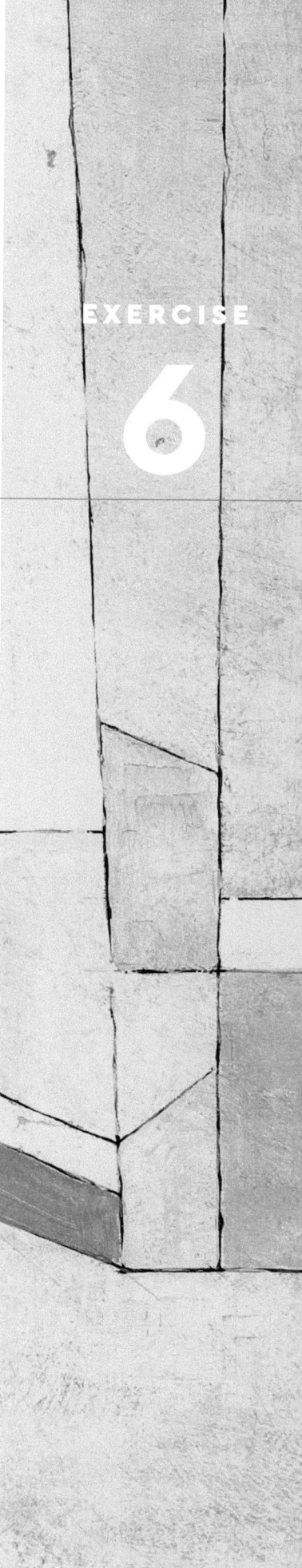

# Introducing the Rationale for Treatment

## Preparations for Exercise 6

1. Read the instructions in Chapter 2.

2. Download the Deliberate Practice Reaction Form and the Deliberate Practice Diary Form at https://www.apa.org/pubs/books/deliberate-practice-psychodynamic-psychotherapy (see the "Clinician and Practitioner Resources" tab; also available in Appendixes A and B, respectively).

## Skill Description

### Skill Difficulty Level: Intermediate

Often when people come into therapy, it's their first time. They may not know how therapy works. They certainly may not know how a relational psychodynamic therapist works. Typically, their idea of therapy is built from dramatic portrayals of therapy as shown on the big and small screen or in books. This exercise is designed to help trainees become more comfortable with explaining psychotherapy and psychodynamic concepts to patients who may have questions about what to expect. Therapists may need to concisely describe, in layperson's terms, how they conceptualize therapy, how they work in the hour, and/or how they view the goals of therapy. All these topics comprise what we are calling the *core elements*. Here is a list of such core elements of modern psychodynamic therapy organized into three groups:

- **Conceptualization:** This entails the role of conflicts and patterns of behavior and thinking (both between people and within oneself) and their attendant emotions, especially appreciating how relationship patterns in the past influence the perception of the behavior and intention of present significant others, including the therapist; the importance of past learning/development and trauma on present levels of functioning; unconscious processes; and the role of resistance.

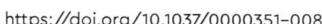

https://doi.org/10.1037/0000351-008

*Deliberate Practice in Psychodynamic Psychotherapy*, by H. Levenson, V. Gay, and J. L. Binder

- **Therapist interventions:** These include listening, supporting, empathizing, validating, collaborating, challenging, questioning, self-disclosing, and interpreting in the context of a safe-enough relationship. The therapist explores the patient's fantasies and daydreams and usually refrains from giving advice.

- **The goals of therapy:** These include gaining insight into and freedom from old patterns; reducing internal conflicts; promoting emotional awareness; bringing unconscious processes into conscious awareness; increasing the capacity for mentalization; and leading a more authentic, satisfying life.

The trainee should improvise a response to each patient description following these skill criteria:

1. **Validate or express appreciation for the patient's concern, question, or statement.** Often this opportunity will occur during the first few sessions, during a time when a therapeutic alliance will begin developing. Consequently, it is particularly important in this early stage of the therapeutic relationship to convey a respectful and collaborative attitude toward one's patient. An opportunity to convey this attitude may occur when responding to a patient's concern or question about how therapy works. Also, it is to be expected that this skill will not only be used at the beginning of therapy. It is also needed at various points in the work to address the patient's doubts that may emerge about certain interventions (e.g., interpreting the transference, which is covered in the next exercise), the goals of the therapy itself, or about the therapeutic bond with the therapist.

2. **Reflect the core element(s) behind the patient's concern.** Make sure you discern the patient's underlying concern. If there is any ambiguity in their communication, don't assume you know what the patient is asking. Instead, ask for more specificity or clarity (see Exercise 1, for example). Also, look for any implicit messages the patient might be conveying, with or without awareness, and address them. For example, imagine the patient says, "I've heard that in psychoanalytic therapy, everything is oedipal. Is that true?" First, you want to understand what the patient means by explicitly using the terms "everything" and "oedipal." Then, you want to be alert for an implicit message, such as a concern that you are going to ask the patient embarrassing questions about their sex life.

3. **Give a rationale for why that element is important.** Before seeing your first patient, have a clear and succinct theoretical framework (with little jargon) that describes how a psychodynamic therapist understands personality development, functioning and malfunctioning, and how this understanding is translated into therapy goals and is applied to the work of therapy. This framework provides you with a conceptual context for addressing many specific concerns or questions about psychodynamic therapy that may be expressed by the patient. While you will have some framework for discussing what is important in psychodynamic therapy and how it works, hold that information "lightly" so that you can address the specific concerns (implicit or explicit) of the patient. Having a "canned answer" is inconsistent with a psychodynamic approach that tailors every response with the specificity of the patient's dynamics, culture, and context (e.g., has there been a rupture in the alliance?).

4. **Ask how the patient feels about what you've said and/or if they find it relevant.** Any concerns or questions expressed by the patient about engaging in a psychodynamic therapy is as much a part of the ongoing therapeutic dialogue as anything else expressed by the patient. Therefore, as with any intervention, it is usually useful

to inquire about the patient's reaction to the intervention. Two immediate advantages of this inquiry are (a) the patient's answer provides clues about where the therapeutic alliance is heading, and (b) the chances are increased of spotting (and perhaps repairing) an imminent therapeutic rupture.

As noted in Chapter 1 of this volume, explaining the treatment rationale for psychodynamic therapy can be complicated, so we suggest practicing this exercise twice: once midway through the training process and a second time after completing all the other skill-based exercises.

---

### SKILL CRITERIA FOR EXERCISE 6

1. Validate or express appreciation for the patient's concern, question, or statement.
2. Reflect the core element(s) behind the patient's concern.
3. Give a rationale for why that element is important.
4. Ask how the patient feels about what you've said and/or if they find it relevant.

---

## Examples of Introducing the Rationale for Treatment

### Example 1

**PATIENT:** [*nervous*] Can't you just tell me what to do?

**THERAPIST:** That's a very understandable question! (Criterion 1) It seems to me you are a little bit lost and you need to see a map of your life situation with its possibilities so you can become more aware. (Criterion 2) I could help you see that map. When you see where you are, you will be able to envision some possibilities and figure out what you want to do. (Criterion 3) How does that sound to you? (Criterion 4)

### Example 2

**PATIENT:** [*irritated*] I don't want to be here, but my parents made me come; I had no voice in this thing!

**THERAPIST:** I appreciate your directness: You had no choice in seeing me. (Criterion 1) Seems you have strong feelings about your what parents did, about being here, and perhaps about me. (Criterion 2) If we work together, I would want to hear all your feelings and thoughts, including your anger. It would also be important to find a voice that can be heard by your parents. (Criterion 3) Does that seem like something you might want to work on with me? (Criterion 4)

### Example 3

**PATIENT:** [*cheerful*] I've really wanted to see how this whole therapy thing works. I have a pretty good life. I work for a bank part time, I'm in graduate school, and I have a long-distance relationship with my partner of 5 years.

**THERAPIST:** Thank you for so readily laying out your situation and motivation for therapy. (Criterion 1) So I am hearing that you are wondering how therapy works, and maybe what it's like. I'm wondering what you've heard about therapy and why you might be curious about therapy now. (Criteria 2 and 3) Does that sound like a good place to begin? (Criterion 4)

## INSTRUCTIONS FOR EXERCISE 6

### Step 1: Role-Play and Feedback

- The patient says the first beginner patient statement. The therapist **improvises** a response based on the skill criteria.
- The trainer (or, if not available, the patient) provides **brief** feedback based on the skill criteria.
- The patient then repeats the same statement, and the therapist again improvises a response. The trainer (or patient) again provides brief feedback.

### Step 2: Repeat

- Repeat Step 1 for all the statements **at the current difficulty level** (beginner, intermediate, or advanced).

### Step 3: Assess and Adjust Difficulty

- The therapist completes the Deliberate Practice Reaction Form (see Appendix A) and decides whether to make the exercise easier or harder or to repeat the same difficulty level.

### Step 4: Repeat for Approximately 15 Minutes

- Repeat Steps 1 to 3 for at least 15 minutes.
- The trainees then switch therapist and patient roles and start over.

**Now it's your turn! Follow Steps 1 and 2 from the instructions.**

*Remember:* The goal of the role-play is for trainees to practice improvising responses to the patient statements in a manner that (a) uses the skill criteria and (b) feels authentic for the trainee. **Example therapist responses for each patient statement are provided at the end of this exercise. Trainees should attempt to improvise their own responses before reading the example responses.**

| BEGINNER-LEVEL PATIENT STATEMENTS FOR EXERCISE 6 |
| --- |
| *Beginner Patient Statement 1* |
| [Curious] I've never been in therapy before. What do people usually talk about? |
| *Beginner Patient Statement 2* |
| [Sad] I'm having a hard time. I just started a new job, and it's been pretty stressful. I just need someone to talk to. Is that OK? |
| *Beginner Patient Statement 3* |
| [Matter-of-fact] I just need a few sessions; I need some tips on how to break up with this person I've been dating for a year. |
| *Beginner Patient Statement 4* |
| [Uncomfortable] Is this the kind of therapy where we talk about my mother and delve into my childhood? |
| *Beginner Patient Statement 5* |
| [Eager] I have lots of dreams. I never thought much of them, but I'm wondering if you would be interested in hearing about them? |

 **Assess and adjust the difficulty before moving to the next difficulty level (see Step 3 in the exercise instructions).**

| INTERMEDIATE-LEVEL PATIENT STATEMENTS FOR EXERCISE 6 |
| --- |
| **Intermediate Patient Statement 1** |
| [Anxious] I feel like I have no armor anymore. Everything just makes me feel so nervous. I never used to feel like this, so I don't know what's wrong with me. Can you help me? |
| **Intermediate Patient Statement 2** |
| [Irritated] I don't want to be here, but my parents made me; I had no voice in this thing! |
| **Intermediate Patient Statement 3** |
| [Ashamed] Our stupid dog ran away. And for some stupid reason I just can't stop crying about it. So I want to learn how to stop feeling so sad. It's so childish. And it's brought up a lot of other stuff I'd also like to forget. |
| **Intermediate Patient Statement 4** |
| [Apathetic] I'm only here because my spouse said they'd leave me if I didn't get better. I've been depressed my whole life. I don't really see how you can help me. What good is talking about it? |
| **Intermediate Patient Statement 5** |
| [Cheerful] I've really wanted to see how this whole therapy thing works. I have a pretty good life. I work for a bank part time, I'm in graduate school, and I have a long-distance relationship with my partner of 5 years. |

🖐 **Assess and adjust the difficulty before moving to the next difficulty level (see Step 3 in the exercise instructions).**

| ADVANCED-LEVEL PATIENT STATEMENTS FOR EXERCISE 6 |
| --- |
| *Advanced Patient Statement 1* |
| **[Hesitating]** I've heard that patients fall in love with their therapists. Does that really happen? |
| *Advanced Patient Statement 2* |
| **[Suspicious]** That's weird. You keep talking about "our relationship." We don't really have a relationship. This is like a business transaction. |
| *Advanced Patient Statement 3* |
| **[Critical]** Listen, I had a perfectly normal childhood. I don't need this Freudian crap. |
| *Advanced Patient Statement 4* |
| **[Irritable]** The doctors I go to keep treating me like an addict, so they won't refill my oxycodone. I keep telling them I'm not addicted, I just need it to feel more comfortable. I could really use some help with this, but I don't want you to think I'm an addict too. |
| *Advanced Patient Statement 5* |
| **[Guarded]** I've had some dark thoughts that I just can't get rid of. But I'm concerned that if I talk about them, you'll think I'm crazy. Can I trust you? |

 **Assess and adjust the difficulty here (see Step 3 in the exercise instructions). If appropriate, follow the instructions to make the exercise even more challenging (see Appendix A).**

## Example Therapist Responses: Introducing the Rationale for Treatment

*Remember:* Trainees should attempt to improvise their own responses before reading the example responses. **Do not read the following responses verbatim unless you are having trouble coming up with your own responses!**

| EXAMPLE RESPONSES TO BEGINNER-LEVEL PATIENT STATEMENTS FOR EXERCISE 6 |
|---|
| *Example Response to Beginner Patient Statement 1* |
| I appreciate your question. (Criterion 1) It's common for people just starting therapy to be curious about what it involves. (Criterion 2) People really talk about all kinds of things. Some start off by talking about parts of their lives that are troubling or difficult for them. Others focus on what brings them happiness and joy. Having the time set aside for the two of us to explore together the things that are on your mind is what really matters. (Criterion 3) How would you feel about our giving this a try? (Criterion 4) |
| *Example Response to Beginner Patient Statement 2* |
| I appreciate your being proactive in getting support for yourself. This is a perfect reason to seek out therapy. (Criterion 1) It sounds like something about this job has been more stressful than you thought it was going to be and you have a sense that talking to someone will be helpful. (Criterion 2) We can absolutely talk about your experiences in your new job. And I am here to listen, be curious, offer perspective, and ask questions that hopefully will help you have less stress. (Criterion 3) Sound like what you had in mind? (Criterion 4) |
| *Example Response to Beginner Patient Statement 3* |
| I appreciate your letting me know of your intended focus for the therapy and your time frame. (Criterion 1) Dynamic therapists find it useful to explore ways of looking at situations along with associated feelings and thoughts. For example, you already have a sense that you are going to solve this problem very soon and only need a few sessions. Although the focus on breaking up with this person you've been seeing for a while is definitely in alignment with what I do, I am hearing that you only want a few sessions. (Criterion 2) Sometimes issues can be dealt with in a short time frame, but I wouldn't want to mislead you into thinking I could guarantee that. (Criterion 3) Would you be interested in exploring why you want to end that relationship now and see where it takes us? (Criterion 4) |
| *Example Response to Beginner Patient Statement 4* |
| Thank you for that straightforward question (Criterion 1) about the importance of significant people in your life and the relevancy of one's childhood. (Criterion 2) You determine what we talk about in here. In psychodynamic therapy, we very much look at relationships you've had with significant people in your past and present. Often childhood comes up in therapy because we learn so much about what to expect from others and ourselves during these early years—sometimes before we even had language to think about it. (Criterion 3) So how does what I said sound? Does it make sense? (Criterion 4) |
| *Example Response to Beginner Patient Statement 5* |
| I really appreciate your question. (Criterion 1) What is important in here is that you decide on what we talk about and what we don't. If I seem particularly curious about something, it's because I think it might be helpful to discuss. (Criterion 2) Dynamic therapists are often interested in dreams because they might reflect your mind's trying to make sense of aspects of your life that you are interested in. (Criterion 3) Maybe talking about your dreams might allow you to see if they are relevant for your therapy goals. (Criterion 4) |

## EXAMPLE RESPONSES TO INTERMEDIATE-LEVEL PATIENT STATEMENTS FOR EXERCISE 6

### Example Response to Intermediate Patient Statement 1

Thank you for sharing with me about how vulnerable you have been feeling. (Criteria 1 and 2) Much of the work I do focuses on how people have learned to protect themselves from various threats—what you so descriptively call your armor. Maybe we can spend some of our time talking about what that armor used to feel like, and how and why you needed it. (Criterion 3) What do you think? (Criterion 4)

### Example Response to Intermediate Patient Statement 2

I appreciate your directness: You had no choice in seeing me. (Criterion 1) You have strong feelings about your parents, being here, and perhaps about me. (Criterion 2) If we work together, I would want to hear all your feelings and thoughts, including your anger. It would also be important to find a voice that can be heard by your parents. (Criterion 3) Does that seem like something you might want to work on with me? (Criterion 4)

### Example Response to Intermediate Patient Statement 3

It seems like your dog was really important to you. Your sadness over losing your dog makes so much sense. I don't see your sadness as childish, but I hear that you do. (Criterion 1) I use an approach to therapy that says every feeling and emotion matters, especially the ones we try to avoid. (Criterion 2) I see our emotions as providing valuable information about what is truly meaningful to us; like your tears tell me that you have lost something quite valuable to you. And your sadness also brought up what might be other important thoughts and feelings. (Criterion 3) I hear that this is not exactly what you were asking for, but what comes to your mind when you think about us taking that sort of approach in our work together? (Criterion 4)

### Example Response to Intermediate Patient Statement 4

Thanks for telling me your doubts about whether I can really help you. (Criteria 1 and 2) Whatever your feelings are in any moment, as well as your feelings about our interactions together, can be valuable for us to talk about. My clinical experience and research have indicated that talking about a problem and understanding the feelings that go with it can be really helpful for most people. (Criterion 3) I know it might sound vague in the abstract. Do you think you could give it a try and see what happens? (Criterion 4)

### Example Response to Intermediate Patient Statement 5

Thank you for so readily laying out your situation and motivation for therapy. (Criterion 1) So I am hearing that you are wondering how therapy works, and maybe what it's like. I'm wondering what you've heard about therapy and why you might be curious about therapy now. (Criteria 2 and 3) Does that sound like a good place to begin? (Criterion 4)

## EXAMPLE RESPONSES TO ADVANCED-LEVEL PATIENT STATEMENTS FOR EXERCISE 6

### Example Response to Advanced Patient Statement 1

I appreciate your asking directly. (Criterion 1) It is not unusual that during a therapy that delves into peoples' emotions, patients develop all kinds of strong feelings, sometimes even love, toward their therapists. (Criterion 2) This is not surprising given how important the person helping you might become over time. Examining your feelings about me and others can provide relevant clues as to how to have more meaningful relationships with people in your life. (Criterion 3) Could you imagine that working for you? (Criterion 4)

### Example Response to Advanced Patient Statement 2

That's an excellent question. (Criterion 1) I hear your concern about why I keep using the term *relationship*. (Criterion 2) And in some ways, this is a business relationship, where you are paying for my services. And yet, although we won't become friends, my guess is that we will develop a meaningful give-and-take relationship in our work together. By examining what goes on between the two of us in the here and now of the session and how you relate to other people as well, a lot can be learned. (Criterion 3) What would it be like for you to try this approach with me? (Criterion 4)

### Example Response to Advanced Patient Statement 3

I appreciate your directness (Criterion 1); you want to let me know upfront that your childhood was a normal one. (Criterion 2) We often focus on childhood in therapy because that is where we first learn a lot of important stuff about life and ourselves. But dynamic therapy has changed a lot since Freud. Maybe you could tell me more about the kind of "crap" you want to avoid, and I will be straight with you about how I work. Understanding what works for you and what doesn't is an important aspect of doing good therapy. (Criterion 3) Does that seem like a reasonable way to proceed? (Criterion 4)

### Example Response to Advanced Patient Statement 4

I appreciate you sharing your concern about what I think about you and the way you have been managing your pain. (Criteria 1 and 2) It also sounds like you have this concern with other providers as well. So that makes me think that we might be able to use our therapy to better understand how you think, feel, and act when people treat you like an addict. Exploring how this plays out between the two of us might help you figure out how to navigate the interactions with other providers more successfully—and perhaps even other relationships in your life too. (Criterion 3) How would it be for us to do that? (Criterion 4)

### Example Response to Advanced Patient Statement 5

I appreciate your telling me about your hesitancy to trust me. Your trust is something I will need to earn. (Criterion 1) Building trust between us is a necessary step to understand these "dark thoughts" you've been having. (Criterion 2) What I would invite from you is, when you are ready, you can talk with me frankly about your dark thoughts as well as any concerns you have about how I handle your dark thoughts. I will be transparent with you and let you know my honest reactions to whatever you tell me. (Criterion 3) How does that sound? (Criterion 4)

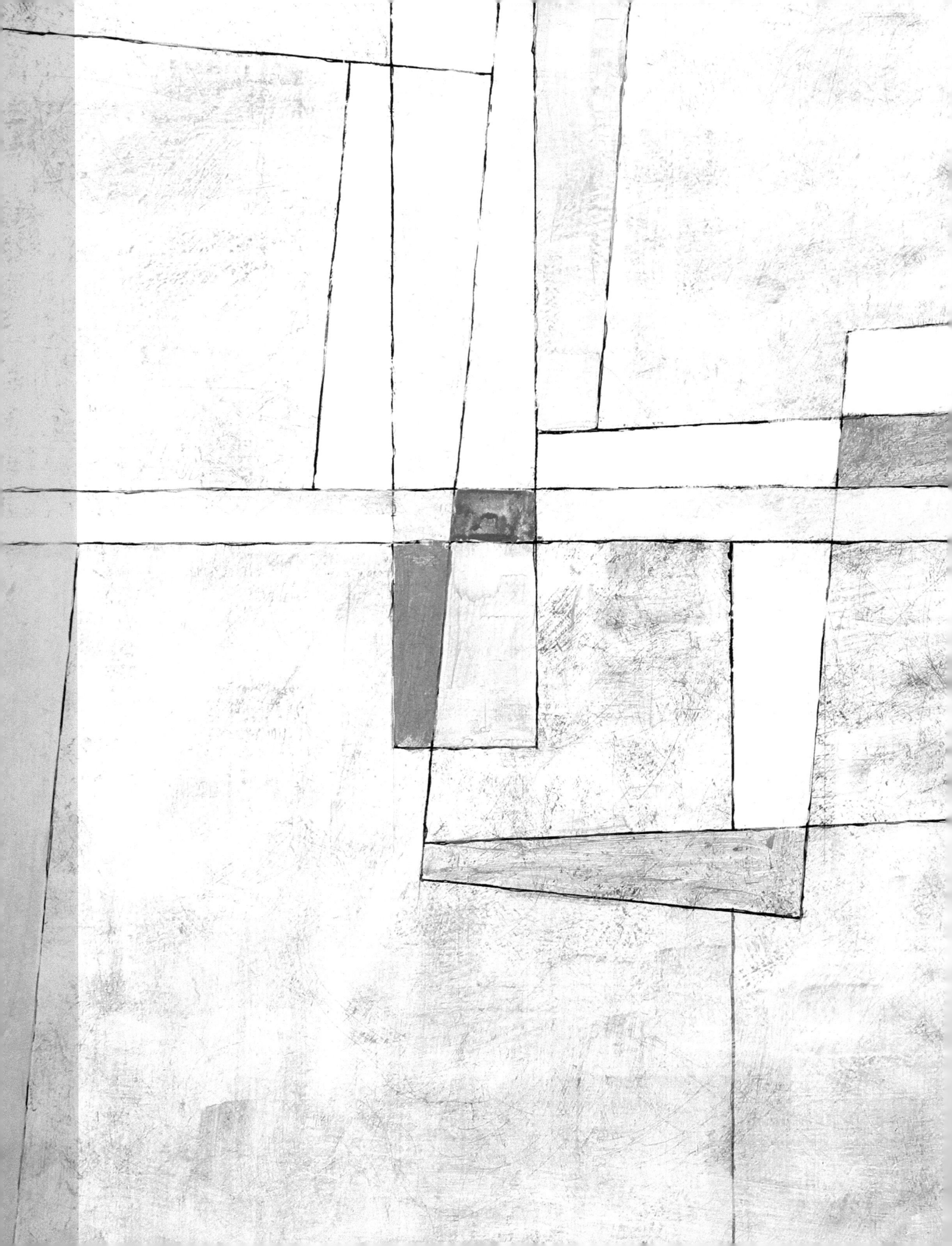

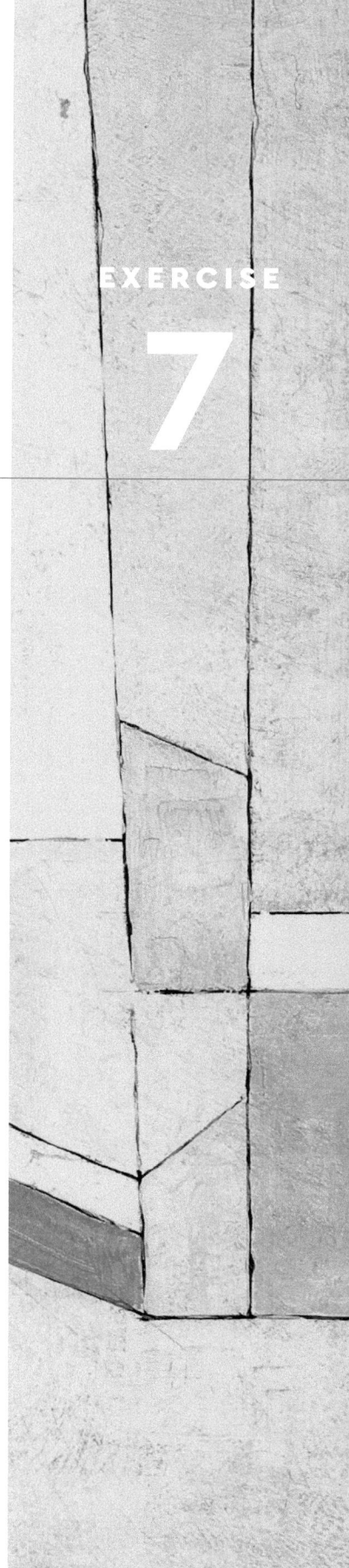

# Making Transference Interpretations

## Preparations for Exercise 7

1. Read the instructions in Chapter 2.

2. Download the Deliberate Practice Reaction Form and the Deliberate Practice Diary Form at https://www.apa.org/pubs/books/deliberate-practice-psychodynamic-psychotherapy (see the "Clinician and Practitioner Resources" tab; also available in Appendixes A and B, respectively).

## Skill Description

### Skill Difficulty Level: Advanced

Freud (1888) spoke of unconsciously transferring "displaceable energies" (strong feelings) about one person onto another (innocent) person. Just before he died, Freud (1937) wrote that such transferences were central to understanding how psychotherapy worked. He thought that the interpretation of the transference (whereby it is brought into the patient's consciousness) was a critical change agent.

Today psychodynamic therapists still use the concept of transference but within a contemporary definition: "a tendency in which representational aspects of important and formative relationships (such as with parents and siblings) can be both consciously experienced and/or unconsciously ascribed to other relationships" (Levy, 2009, p. 183). Some (e.g., Levy et al., 2019) make the differentiation between this *general transference* and *dynamic transference*, which is the same as general transference but involves conflicted or defensive components of the self. A modern definition of a transference

https://doi.org/10.1037/0000351-009

*Deliberate Practice in Psychodynamic Psychotherapy*, by H. Levenson, V. Gay, and J. L. Binder

interpretation is "a tactful comment[1] that clarifies and links the patient's experience of others outside of therapy with that of the therapist in therapy and to the patient's experience of past relationships with caregivers" (Levy, 2009, p. 183).

There is much excellent empirical evidence (from psychotherapy process/outcome research as well as social psychological studies) that transference in the real world is abundant—people see others in the present through a lens that is largely determined by their preexisting significant-other representations. As Sharpless et al. (2022) stated,

> Although the term appears to be quite abstract, and has undergone a number of definitional shifts over the years, . . . it nonetheless captures an intuitive reality. Namely, no one enters into a new relationship without the influence—conscious or otherwise—of prior relationships. (p. 81)

And there is also ample research indicating that a dynamic transference process (dealing with motivation, conflict, and defense) exists (Brumbaugh & Fraley, 2006).

Having established that transference exists in therapy, is it a good idea to inform the patient when it is occurring (i.e., make a transference interpretation) as Freud advocated? Here the answer at times has been controversial. Past research has suggested that transference interpretations lead to poor outcomes because patients often hear such interpretations as manifestations of the therapist's hostility and blaming attitude (Henry et al., 1990). Other research suggests that transference interpretations can have positive outcomes once the therapist has taken several factors into account (e.g., patient characteristics, timing, accuracy, therapeutic alliance).

More recent empirical studies indicate that low to moderate levels of transference interpretations are "highly effective" (Levy & Scala, 2012, p. 400). This seems to be particularly true for those with personality disorders (chronic, rigid cyclical maladaptive patterns; Clarkin et al., 2007; Fonagy & Bateman, 2006; Høglend et al., 2006; Levy & Scala, 2012). Our advice is to be aware of the transference dynamics in the session whether or not you chose to interpret them explicitly. This skill exercise was designed to help you do just that.

This exercise provides underlined context before each patient statement, which the trainee playing the patient should read aloud before reading the statement. The trainee playing the therapist should then improvise a response to each patient description and statement following these skill criteria:

1. **Start by internally (silently) considering if what the patient has said about, felt about, or done with others parallels what is going on in the here and now in your relationship with the patient.** When ready, perform the next three skill criteria by speaking out loud to the patient.

2. **Reflect back what you hear the patient has conveyed about their experience with others.** Focus on those things the patient has talked about that seem to parallel your experiences with the patient. For example, if the patient was demeaned by their father, have you noticed that they often feel demeaned by you?

3. **Offer a brief reflection that summarizes a possible parallel with you, the therapist.** Remembering the modern definition of a transference interpretation, make it a *tactful comment* that links the way the patient was treated by past or present significant others and how they feel treated by you or how they treat you.

4. **Ask an open-ended question about what the patient thinks or feels about what you have said.** Patients can hear these interpretations as blaming, hostile, or insensitive

---

1. Isaac Newton defined a "tactful comment" as making a point without making an enemy—or in psychotherapy terms, without rupturing the therapeutic alliance.

(e.g., "How dare you say I am mistaking you for my father?"), so it is always a good idea to check in with them to make sure they are not having a negative reaction to what you said. And if they did, to be prepared to make a repair (e.g., apologizing for phrasing your comments awkwardly or for being mistaken in your assumptions). Making a process comment (Exercise 4) can be helpful as a first step in repairing such ruptures.

---

**SKILL CRITERIA FOR EXERCISE 7**

1. Start by internally (silently) considering if what the patient has said about, felt about, or done with others parallels what is happening in your relationship with the patient.
2. Reflect back what the patient has conveyed about their experience with others.
3. Offer a brief, tactful reflection that summarizes a possible parallel with you, the therapist.
4. Ask an open-ended question about what the patient thinks or feels about what you have said.

---

## Example of Therapists Making Transference Interpretations

**Note:** Underlined text before each patient statement should be read aloud to provide context. Take your time in reading this slowly and repeating if necessary.

### Example 1

The patient sought therapy to deal with self-criticism and social anxiety. As a child, they were left under the care of an older sibling who viewed the patient as a "downer." The sibling often took the patient to unfamiliar places, where they sat alone, listening to the other kids laugh and have fun. Now, during this therapy session, the patient just noticed the therapist stifling a yawn.

**PATIENT:** [dejected] I know I can be boring. You even yawned a minute ago. Your other patients are probably much more interesting than I am.

**THERAPIST:** I could see why you would think that my yawn had something to do with you. If I remember correctly, one of your siblings viewed you as a drag, taking you to places where you were ignored while others had fun. (Criterion 2) So I can imagine that when I yawned, you could have readily assumed that I was bored with you. (Criterion 3) What do you think about what I've said? (Criterion 4)

### Example 2

In a previous session, the patient shared about how a teacher in high school helped them after school, for which they were very grateful.

**PATIENT:** [glad] I feel like you're helping me get through a lot. It's great to feel like you're on my side and I have some support.

**THERAPIST:** Thank you for your comments. They remind me of how you felt about the teacher who helped you through a tough time as a teenager. (Criterion 2) It seems like there are similarities between how grateful you were for the support you received from that teacher in high school and how you feel about the support you've received from me in therapy. (Criterion 3) Does that sound right? (Criterion 4)

## INSTRUCTIONS FOR EXERCISE 7

### Step 1: Role-Play and Feedback

- The patient reads the <u>underlined text</u> aloud, then the patient says the first beginner patient statement. The therapist **improvises** a response based on the skill criteria.
- The trainer (or, if not available, the patient) provides **brief** feedback based on the skill criteria.
- The patient then repeats the same statement, and the therapist again improvises a response. The trainer (or patient) again provides brief feedback.

### Step 2: Repeat

- Repeat Step 1 for all the statements **at the current difficulty level** (beginner, intermediate, or advanced).

### Step 3: Assess and Adjust Difficulty

- The therapist completes the Deliberate Practice Reaction Form (see Appendix A) and decides whether to make the exercise easier or harder or to repeat the same difficulty level.

### Step 4: Repeat for Approximately 15 Minutes

- Repeat Steps 1 to 3 for at least 15 minutes.
- The trainees then switch therapist and patient roles and start over.

**Now it's your turn! Follow Steps 1 and 2 from the instructions.**

*Remember:* The goal of the role-play is for trainees to practice improvising responses to the patient statements in a manner that (a) uses the skill criteria and (b) feels authentic for the trainee. **Example therapist responses for each patient statement are provided at the end of this exercise. Trainees should attempt to improvise their own responses before reading the example responses.**

 *Note:* <u>Underlined text</u> before each patient statement should be read aloud to provide context. Take your time in reading this slowly and repeating if necessary.

| BEGINNER-LEVEL PATIENT STATEMENTS FOR EXERCISE 7 |
| --- |
| ***Beginner Patient Statement 1*** |
| <u>The patient is in therapy to deal with anxiety and perfectionistic tendencies. They have previously shared about how their father had high standards, so they spent a great deal of time working hard to gain what little approval he gave.</u><br><br>PATIENT: [Anxious] The week was great! I spent 30 minutes each day reflecting on what you suggested last week. I think that's good progress, right? |
| ***Beginner Patient Statement 2*** |
| <u>Earlier in the therapy, the patient talked about how their parents used to tell them that they were immoral if they didn't always put others' needs first.</u><br><br>PATIENT: [Friendly] Wow, here we are at the end of the session, and I spent the whole time talking about myself; I didn't give you much of a chance to say anything. Next time, I'll be more considerate. |
| ***Beginner Patient Statement 3*** |
| <u>The patient previously described that as a child, they took care of their alcoholic mother, making sure she didn't choke on her own vomit. In relationships, the patient was used to "giving and giving."</u><br><br>PATIENT: [Anxiously] You're doing great. But I feel that my problems are so small. I think your time would be better off helping people who are more in need. |
| ***Beginner Patient Statement 4*** |
| <u>The patient has learned to be meek, apologetic, and passive because as a youngster, they feared their father, who could become physically abusive when disrespected.</u><br><br>PATIENT: [Ashamed] I know I got here a few minutes late. The traffic was terrible, and it was so hard to find a parking spot. I am so sorry. I won't let it happen again. |
| ***Beginner Patient Statement 5*** |
| <u>In a previous session, the patient shared about how a teacher in high school helped them after school for which they were very grateful.</u><br><br>PATIENT: [Glad] I feel like you're helping me get through a lot. It's great to feel like you're on my side and I have some support. |

 **Assess and adjust the difficulty before moving to the next difficulty level (see Step 3 in the exercise instructions).**

## INTERMEDIATE-LEVEL PATIENT STATEMENTS FOR EXERCISE 7

### Intermediate Patient Statement 1

The patient comes to therapy because of disdain toward their partner and is talking about possibly leaving them because they view the partner as incompetent and dumb. The patient has been seen by others as having "great intellectual gifts."

PATIENT: [Irritated] You know, I'm getting a bit frustrated with you. I've been coming for over a month, and you haven't told me anything about myself that I didn't already know.

### Intermediate Patient Statement 2

The patient has few friends yet boasts that their parents taught them to prioritize climbing the social ladder rather than making friends.

PATIENT: [Slightly condescending] You have been a fine therapist the past few sessions. However, I must admit that I had hoped to be seen by Dr. Cushman, the department chair. I think Dr. Cushman would be better equipped to help me.

### Intermediate Patient Statement 3

As a youth, the patient reported being nagged by their father to get everything done, so the patient rebelled by procrastinating. However, as an adult the patient struggles with feeling unproductive and holding a job.

PATIENT: [Withdrawn] I don't really know what there is to talk about . . .

### Intermediate Patient Statement 4

The patient sought therapy to deal with a chronic sense of inferiority. They felt that their parents gave most of their attention to their younger sibling, who is a talented volleyball player.

PATIENT: [Cheerful] I enjoyed reading that tennis magazine in your waiting room. You know, I am a pretty good tennis player.

### Intermediate Patient Statement 5

The patient's father would mock them for crying when they were a child, calling them a "crybaby." Now, during this session, the patient is upset and holding back tears.

PATIENT: [Sad] Damn it. I will not cry. I will not cry.

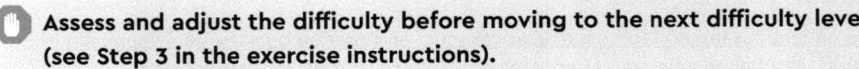 **Assess and adjust the difficulty before moving to the next difficulty level (see Step 3 in the exercise instructions).**

| ADVANCED-LEVEL PATIENT STATEMENTS FOR EXERCISE 7 |
| --- |

### Advanced Patient Statement 1

The patient sought therapy for help with anxiety and dissociation. They grew up in a religious commune in which their father was believed to possess mystical powers granted by God. They were recently ejected from the commune for looking at internet dating sites.

PATIENT: [Admiration] I was thinking so much this week about our last session, and I couldn't get over the fact that you knew exactly what I was feeling. You might not be able to tell me where you get your gift from, but you certainly have a gift.

### Advanced Patient Statement 2

In an earlier session, the patient shared about how a music teacher, once admired, taught them a lot, but then the music teacher made sexual advances during a lesson.

PATIENT: [Glad and anxious] I feel like you're helping me get through a lot. It's great to feel like you're on my side, but for some reason, it is also making me a little nervous.

### Advanced Patient Statement 3

Since childhood, the patient has held others at arm's length, preferring to isolate and be dependent on no one.

PATIENT: [Firmly] Is this work with me helping you to accomplish your goals?

### Advanced Patient Statement 4

The patient is coming to therapy because they want a relationship but feel "too ugly" to seek one. For years, their mother had repeatedly criticized their appearance, manners, and personality.

PATIENT: [Anxious] Every time I come to my appointment, I shudder to think what horrible things you think about me.

### Advanced Patient Statement 5

The patient has had several previous therapies with trainees at the counseling center.

PATIENT: [Challenging] So, you're the new therapist? Well, you should know that I've seen many therapists before you. And some helped. But then they always leave you, you know?

Assess and adjust the difficulty here (see Step 3 in the exercise instructions). If appropriate, follow the instructions to make the exercise even more challenging (see Appendix A).

## Example Therapist Responses: Making Transference Interpretations

*Remember:* Trainees should attempt to improvise their own responses before reading the example responses. **Do not read the following responses verbatim unless you are having trouble coming up with your own responses!**

| EXAMPLE RESPONSES TO BEGINNER-LEVEL PATIENT STATEMENTS FOR EXERCISE 7 |
|---|
| ***Example Response to Beginner Patient Statement 1*** |
| Sounds like you really want me to know how much effort you are making. (Criterion 2) This seems similar to how you learned you could get your father's approval. (Criterion 3) What do you think about my noticing some similarities? (Criterion 4) |
| ***Example Response to Beginner Patient Statement 2*** |
| I think I recall that your parents taught you to always put others first, right? (Criterion 2) By apologizing for talking about yourself for most of the session, I'm wondering if you are still trying to live up to their rules, even in your own therapy with me. (Criterion 3) What do you think about my mentioning that such a pattern might be playing out in the session right now? (Criterion 4) |
| ***Example Response to Beginner Patient Statement 3*** |
| You were so on the alert to make sure your mother was OK, your needs got lower and lower on the list. (Criterion 2) I'm wondering if the same dynamic is happening here with me in the session, where you are trying to make sure that my time is spent wisely even at a cost to you. (Criterion 3) What do you think about my observing that dynamic operating here? (Criterion 4) |
| ***Example Response to Beginner Patient Statement 4*** |
| With all of your apologies, I have the feeling that you think I am angry with you for arriving late, much like your father, who would get irate and become abusive. (Criterion 3) I am wondering if you are seeing me right now as your father who might emotionally or physically hurt you if I think you are being disrespectful. (Criterion 2) Does that make sense? (Criterion 4) |
| ***Example Response to Beginner Patient Statement 5*** |
| Thank you for your comments. They remind me of how you felt about the teacher who helped you through a tough time as a teenager. (Criterion 2) It seems like there are similarities between how grateful you were for the support you received from that teacher in high school and how you feel about the support you've received from me in therapy. (Criterion 3) Does that sound right? (Criterion 4) |

| **EXAMPLE RESPONSES TO INTERMEDIATE-LEVEL PATIENT STATEMENTS FOR EXERCISE 7** |
|---|
| *Example Response to Intermediate Patient Statement 1* |
| I know you take pride in your intelligence and are put off by your partner's incompetence. (Criterion 2) It's interesting that I am letting you down intellectually like your partner does. (Criterion 3) What do you feel about what I have said concerning a possible way we both disappoint you? (Criterion 4) |
| *Example Response to Intermediate Patient Statement 2* |
| You've mentioned that your parents taught you to associate with people who were of high social status. (Criterion 2) Certainly Dr. Cushman's credentials are impeccable. If I don't have those credentials, it sounds like working with me would be disappointing—maybe even insulting. (Criterion 3) What do you make of my wondering that what your parents taught you is getting played out between us? (Criterion 4) |
| *Example Response to Intermediate Patient Statement 3* |
| Might you be shutting down in here? I know your father pushed you to be productive above everything else. (Criterion 2) Perhaps you felt that I was pushing you toward your goals, which started to feel too much like your father's pressure, so you've shut down in response. (Criterion 3) What do think about my conjecture? (Criterion 4) |
| *Example Response to Intermediate Patient Statement 4* |
| Oh, I didn't know that. I do remember that you told me your sibling is a gifted volleyball player who gets a lot of parental attention because of their athleticism. (Criterion 2) Do you think it's possible that you wanted me to know that you're a pretty good tennis player so I might be more interested in you like your parents are in your sibling? (Criterion 3) Does my bringing up this possibility seem likely to you? (Criterion 4) |
| *Example Response to Intermediate Patient Statement 5* |
| I see you holding back your tears. And yet you are feeling very sad right now. I am wondering if you are hearing your father's mocking voice in your ear: "Crybaby!" (Criterion 2) Perhaps you are wondering if you let yourself fully cry, I also will brand you as a crybaby. (Criterion 3) Does my conjecture have meaning for you? (Criterion 4) |

## EXAMPLE RESPONSES TO ADVANCED-LEVEL PATIENT STATEMENTS FOR EXERCISE 7

### Example Response to Advanced Patient Statement 1

I'm really glad you felt that I understood you. (Criterion 3) I promise you it's not a mystical power. Yet I understand why you might believe that about me, given how you viewed your father. (Criterion 2) Does it make sense, that you might see similarities between your father and me? (Criterion 4)

### Example Response to Advanced Patient Statement 2

I remember your telling me about the music teacher who helped you learn a lot but then tried to take advantage of you sexually. (Criterion 2) I am wondering if as you feel the support from me, you get worried that I might try to violate you like your teacher did. (Criterion 3) What do you think about my putting forward this idea? (Criterion 4)

### Example Response to Advanced Patient Statement 3

I do recall that you like being self-sufficient and not depending on anyone. (Criterion 2) Does focusing on my goals rather than on you and your goals make it easier not to feel dependent on me in therapy? (Criterion 3) What do you think? (Criterion 4)

### Example Response to Advanced Patient Statement 4

It's almost like you assume that I am thinking terrible things about you, (Criterion 3) much like your mother who was hyper-focused on finding fault with everything about you. (Criterion 2) Does this make sense to you? Do you think there could be an overlap between what you got from your mother and now expect from me? (Criterion 4)

### Example Response to Advanced Patient Statement 5

I hear you've had many therapists in the past here at the clinic, but they all leave. (Criterion 2) I'm wondering if you are already preparing for my leaving before we have even begun. (Criterion 3) What do you think about what I've said? (Criterion 4)

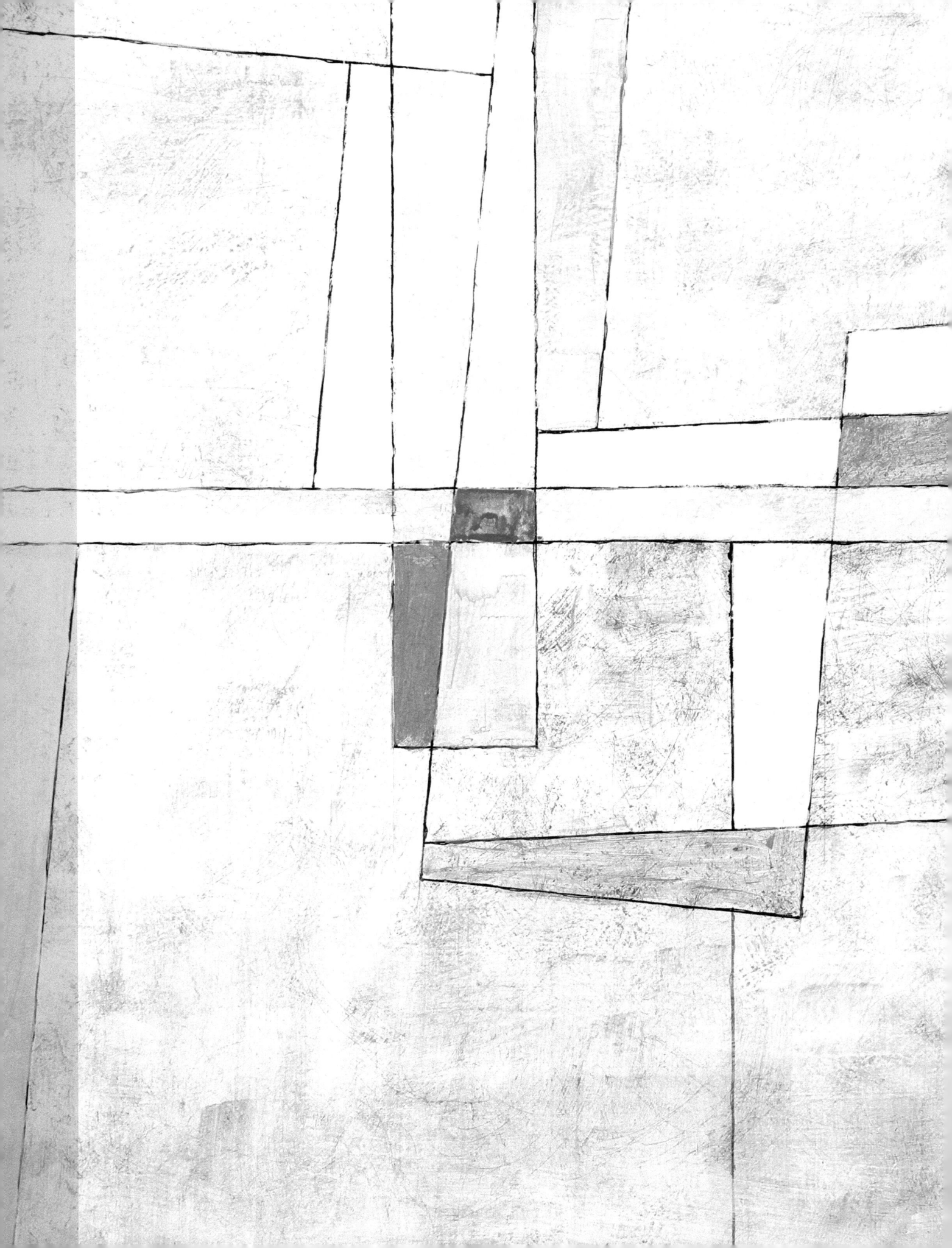

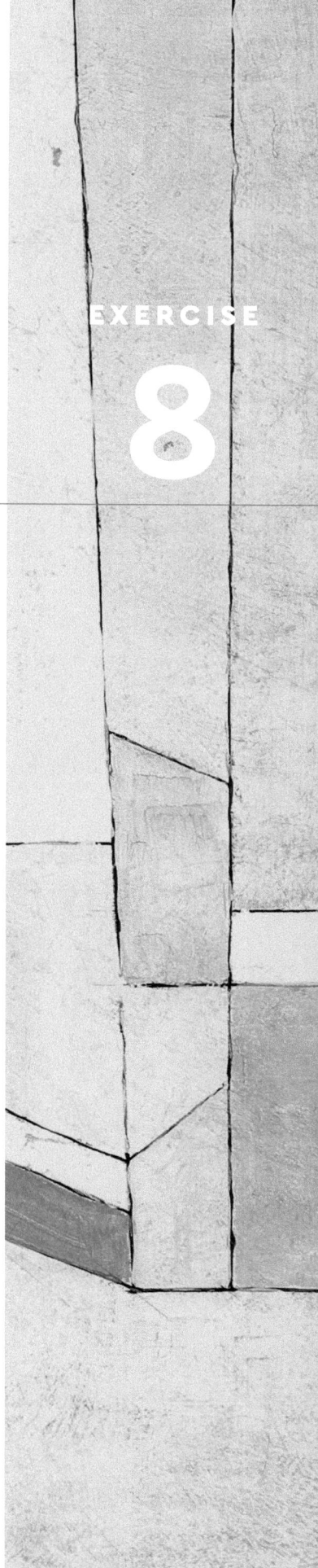

# Using Metaphors

## Preparations for Exercise 8

1. Read the instructions in Chapter 2.

2. Download the Deliberate Practice Reaction Form and the Deliberate Practice Diary Form at https://www.apa.org/pubs/books/deliberate-practice-psychodynamic-psychotherapy (see the "Clinician and Practitioner Resources" tab; also available in Appendixes A and B, respectively).

## Skill Description

### Skill Difficulty Level: Advanced

Metaphors are deceptively simple. We use metaphors every day; often they become such common phrases that we don't realize we are using them—like, "When I contradicted Deborah, she attacked me" or "Sam broke down and cried." In the first example, Deborah is not actually attacking the speaker, but perhaps that's what it felt like to the speaker. In the second example, Sam cried, but was not "breaking down," yet this is how it might have felt to Sam—that he was no longer functional. Because emotion so often infiltrates metaphors and because of their power to convey how the speaker feels, exploring metaphors in a psychodynamic therapy is invaluable. Furthermore, metaphors are another road to understanding unconscious processes by expressing something that the speaker isn't even aware of yet. Furthermore, metaphors can paint a picture when words alone are inadequate to convey one's experience, and they allow the speaker to say things more tactfully.

In therapy, metaphors used by both the patient and the therapist help the dyad understand, explore, and communicate at conscious and unconscious levels. Perhaps you can see the use of metaphor and transference (see Exercise 7) as one and the

https://doi.org/10.1037/0000351-010
*Deliberate Practice in Psychodynamic Psychotherapy*, by H. Levenson, V. Gay, and J. L. Binder

same—both serving as a stand-in for "something else" in the clinical session. In a paper titled "Metaphor and the Psychoanalytic Situation," Arlow (1979) stated the following:

> The word metaphor comes from the two Greek words meaning "to carry over," and refers to a set of linguistic processes whereby aspects of one object are carried over or transferred to another object so that the second object is spoken of *as if it were* the first. (p. 367)

Therapists can listen to patients' metaphors and gain insights into what patients might be saying on a deeper level. (The astute reader might have recognized that even our using the word *deeper* is a metaphor.) Therapists can also explore metaphors with patients to help patients understand something on the edge of awareness. And therapists can generate metaphors in therapy to communicate with patients more implicitly than explicitly. This exercise will give trainees the opportunity to practice these three ways of using metaphors: (a) staying within the patient's metaphor to elicit deeper meaning, (b) exploring the patient's metaphor to recognize something on the edge of awareness, and (c) creating metaphors to conjecture and even interpret in a tactful manner.[1]

Over time, metaphors become part of the shared language between therapist and patient—shorthand ways of saying a lot with very little. They become ways to foster alliances and a sense of we-ness as well as furthering therapeutic progress itself. In short, metaphors are like winning lottery tickets waiting to be redeemed, or maybe they are diamonds in the rough, waiting for the experienced eye to notice, eventually to be mined, cut, and polished so they can be appreciated for the treasures they are. You get the idea.

The trainee should improvise a response to each patient description following these skill criteria:

1. **For the beginner patient statements:** Explore the patient's metaphor while staying within the metaphor.

2. **For the intermediate patient statements:** State an implicit message behind the metaphor and explore the unstated feelings and thoughts that might have generated the metaphor.

3. **For the advanced patient statements:** Create and suggest metaphors that try to capture the patient's unstated experience.

---

**SKILL CRITERIA FOR EXERCISE 8**

1. **For the beginner patient statements:** Ask a question using aspects of the patient's metaphor that would likely prompt them to expand their feelings or understanding in some way.
2. **For the intermediate patient statements:** Tentatively say the implicit message behind the metaphor back to the patient. Finish by asking if that sounds right.
3. **For the advanced patient statements:** Tentatively use a metaphor that captures the meaning of something the patient is saying, doing, or feeling that would be likely to click into focus their feelings or understandings in some way. Finish by asking about the usefulness of the metaphor.

---

1. Remember Isaac Newton's definition of saying things in a tactful manner from Exercise 7.

## Examples of Clinicians Using Metaphors in Therapy

### Example 1: Staying Within the Metaphor

**PATIENT:** [*frightened*] They looked at me with piercing eyes.

**THERAPIST:** When their eyes pierce you, what do they see?

### Example 2: Stating an Implicit Message Behind the Metaphor

**PATIENT:** [*frightened*] They looked at me with piercing eyes.

**THERAPIST:** That makes it sound like you are so vulnerable to them. Is that the way it feels to you?

### Example 3: Creating Metaphors

**PATIENT:** [*frustrated*] I have a hard time making up my mind and taking any action.

**THERAPIST:** I imagine you standing in front of a bakery counter and going hungry because you cannot choose a pastry. Does that image fit?

## INSTRUCTIONS FOR EXERCISE 8

### Step 1: Role-Play and Feedback

- The patient says the first beginner patient statement. The therapist **improvises** a response based on the skill criteria.
- The trainer (or, if not available, the patient) provides **brief** feedback based on the skill criteria.
- The patient then repeats the same statement, and the therapist again improvises a response. The trainer (or patient) again provides brief feedback.

### Step 2: Repeat

- Repeat Step 1 for all the statements **at the current difficulty level** (beginner, intermediate, or advanced).

### Step 3: Assess and Adjust Difficulty

- The therapist completes the Deliberate Practice Reaction Form (see Appendix A) and decides whether to make the exercise easier or harder or to repeat the same difficulty level.

### Step 4: Repeat for Approximately 15 Minutes

- Repeat Steps 1 to 3 for at least 15 minutes.
- The trainees then switch therapist and patient roles and start over.

**Now it's your turn! Follow Steps 1 and 2 from the instructions.**

*Remember:* The goal of the role-play is for trainees to practice improvising responses to the patient statements in a manner that (a) uses the skill criteria and (b) feels authentic for the trainee. **Example therapist responses for each patient statement are provided at the end of this exercise. Trainees should attempt to improvise their own responses before reading the example responses.**

| BEGINNER-LEVEL PATIENT STATEMENTS FOR EXERCISE 8: STAYING WITHIN THE METAPHOR |
| --- |
| *Beginner Patient Statement 1* |
| [Anxious] My partner is a porcupine. |
| *Beginner Patient Statement 2* |
| [Frightened] They looked at me with piercing eyes. |
| *Beginner Patient Statement 3* |
| [Indignant] My spouse is my rock. |
| *Beginner Patient Statement 4* |
| [Embarrassed] I cart around so much baggage from my previous life! |
| *Beginner Patient Statement 5* |
| [Sad, failing to make eye contact] I feel like I am in the last act of my life. |

 **Assess and adjust the difficulty before moving to the next difficulty level (see Step 3 in the exercise instructions).**

| INTERMEDIATE-LEVEL PATIENT STATEMENTS FOR EXERCISE 8: STATING AN IMPLICIT MESSAGE BEHIND THE METAPHOR |
| --- |
| *Intermediate Patient Statement 1* |
| [Frustrated] My partner is a porcupine. |
| *Intermediate Patient Statement 2* |
| [Frightened] They looked at me with piercing eyes. |
| *Intermediate Patient Statement 3* |
| [Proudly] My spouse is my rock. |
| *Intermediate Patient Statement 4* |
| [Ashamed] I cart around so much baggage from my previous life. |
| *Intermediate Patient Statement 5* |
| [Downhearted] I feel like I am in the last act of my life. |

✋ **Assess and adjust the difficulty before moving to the next difficulty level (see Step 3 in the exercise instructions).**

| ADVANCED-LEVEL PATIENT STATEMENTS FOR EXERCISE 8: CREATING METAPHORS |
|---|
| *Advanced Patient Statement 1* |
| **[Frightened]** When I hear my father's car in the driveway, I tense up. |
| *Advanced Patient Statement 2* |
| **[Frustrated]** I have a hard time making up my mind and taking any action. |
| *Advanced Patient Statement 3* |
| **[Matter-of-fact]** I am a very resilient person. |
| *Advanced Patient Statement 4* |
| **[Pleased]** I always try to look on the bright side of things. |
| *Advanced Patient Statement 5* |
| **[Proudly]** I'm the only one in my family that stands up to our parents. |

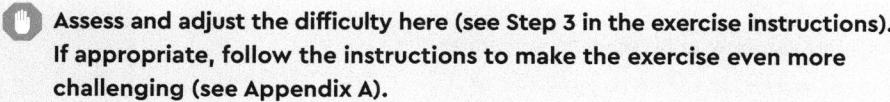 **Assess and adjust the difficulty here (see Step 3 in the exercise instructions). If appropriate, follow the instructions to make the exercise even more challenging (see Appendix A).**

## Example Therapist Responses: Using Metaphors

*Remember:* Trainees should attempt to improvise their own responses before reading the example responses. **Do not read the following responses verbatim unless you are having trouble coming up with your own responses!**

| EXAMPLE RESPONSES TO BEGINNER-LEVEL PATIENT STATEMENTS FOR EXERCISE 8: STAYING WITHIN THE METAPHOR |
| --- |
| *Example Response to Beginner Patient Statement 1* |
| If you wanted to stroke a porcupine, how would you do it? |
| *Example Response to Beginner Patient Statement 2* |
| When their eyes pierce you, what do they see? |
| *Example Response to Beginner Patient Statement 3* |
| Can you snuggle with a rock? |
| *Example Response to Beginner Patient Statement 4* |
| Do you have to carry them by yourself? |
| *Example Response to Beginner Patient Statement 5* |
| What is the title of the play that is your life? |

## EXAMPLE RESPONSES TO INTERMEDIATE-LEVEL PATIENT STATEMENTS FOR EXERCISE 8: STATING AN IMPLICIT MESSAGE BEHIND THE METAPHOR

**Example Response to Intermediate Patient Statement 1**

It sounds like approaching your partner feels scary. You'd have to be so careful. Is that your experience?

**Example Response to Intermediate Patient Statement 2**

That makes it sound like you are so vulnerable to them. Is that the way it feels to you?

**Example Response to Intermediate Patient Statement 3**

Sounds like your spouse is strong, but kind of impenetrable. Does that feel true?

**Example Response to Intermediate Patient Statement 4**

That sounds like you are exhausted. Are you?

**Example Response to Intermediate Patient Statement 5**

It sounds like you feel most of your life is over. Do I have that right?

**EXAMPLE RESPONSES TO ADVANCED-LEVEL PATIENT STATEMENTS
FOR EXERCISE 8: CREATING METAPHORS**

*Example Response to Advanced Patient Statement 1*

You are a deer in the headlights. Does that capture something of your feeling?

*Example Response to Advanced Patient Statement 2*

I see you standing in front of a bakery counter and going hungry because you cannot choose a pastry. Does that image fit?

*Example Response to Advanced Patient Statement 3*

I see you as one of those bobo dolls that you punch, and it keeps bouncing back. Does that fit for you?

*Example Response to Advanced Patient Statement 4*

I hear that, but sometimes I picture you painting on a smiley face even when you feel sad. Does my image make any sense to you?

*Example Response to Advanced Patient Statement 5*

You are the lone sheriff of your town protecting the residents from the bad guy. Is that what it feels like sometimes?

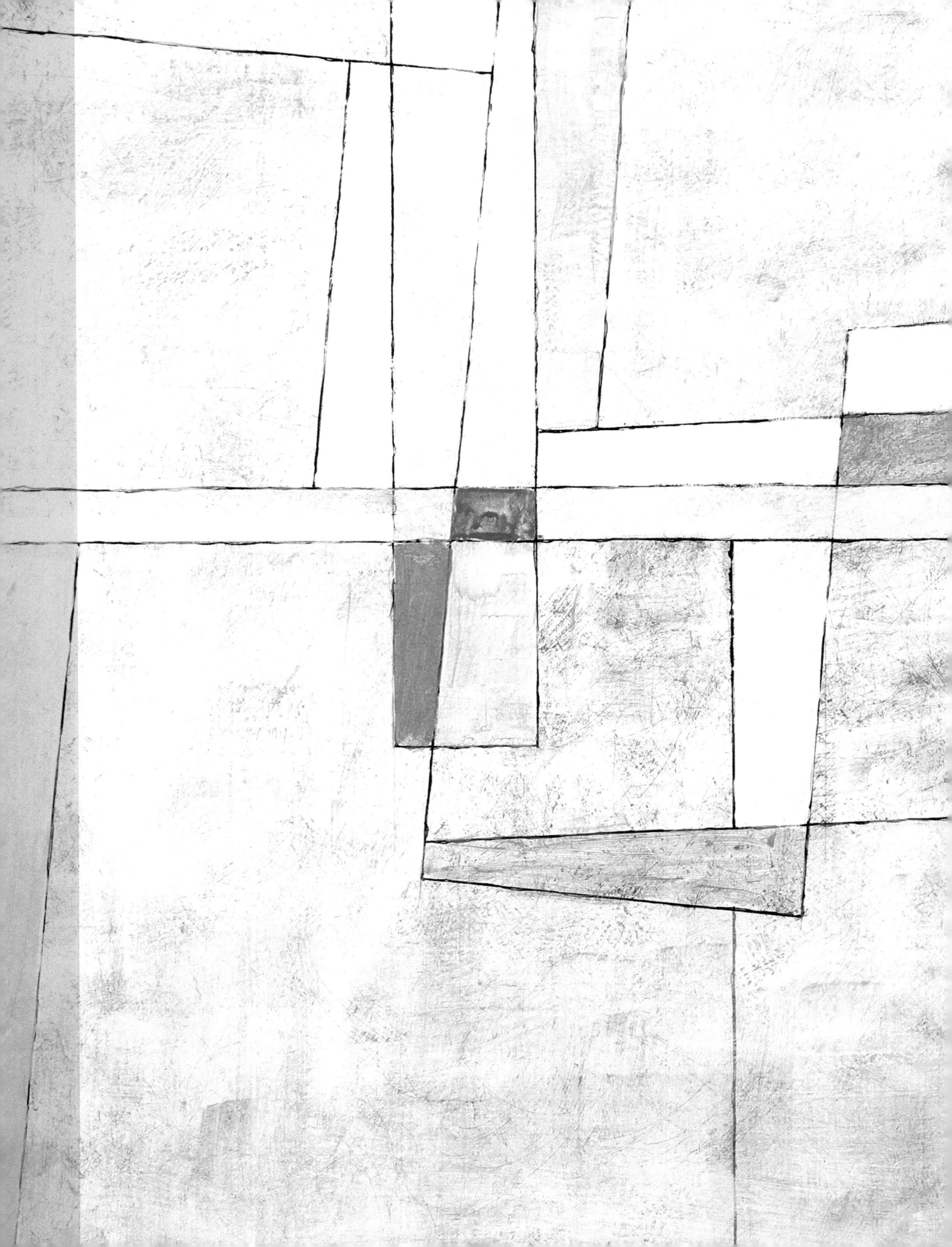

# Exploring Fantasy

## Preparations for Exercise 9

1. Read the instructions in Chapter 2.

2. Download the Deliberate Practice Reaction Form and the Deliberate Practice Diary Form at https://www.apa.org/pubs/books/deliberate-practice-psychodynamic-psychotherapy (see the "Clinician and Practitioner Resources" tab; also available in Appendixes A and B, respectively).

## Skill Description

### Skill Difficulty Level: Advanced

Dynamic clinicians explore patients' fantasies (daydreams, favorite TV shows, movies, and such) because fantasies can reveal so much about one's needs, wishes, and desires. A teenage patient who feels powerless may have daydreams about becoming a super-hero. A depressed older male patient may be captivated by movies about regained youth. A young female patient harmed by a cruel man may find herself watching revenge movies over and over. In each case, a favorite fantasy illuminates an essential conflict in the patient's life.

The easiest fantasies to understand are ones in which the patient is self-aware and says, "I have this fantasy" or "I wish" or "I have this dream." The more difficult fantasies to understand are ones in which the patient is less direct, less self-aware, and uses less mature defenses such as denial. The most difficult fantasies to understand are ones in which the patient is indirect, not self-aware, and embeds the fantasy in lengthy, some-times confusing stories.

Exploring fantasies in the therapy hour is not only a powerful way to understand the dynamics of patients, but it also helps patients appreciate the relevance and meaning of their own internal experience. Looking at daydreams in particular can be "a relatively

https://doi.org/10.1037/0000351-011

*Deliberate Practice in Psychodynamic Psychotherapy*, by H. Levenson, V. Gay, and J. L. Binder

non-threatening path to self-understanding [especially] for individuals who come into therapy without [a strong] capacity for introspection, tolerance of affect, and sense of agency" (Barth, 1997, p. 265).

This exercise provides underlined context before each patient statement, which the trainee playing the patient should read aloud before reading the statement. Some patients—Mr. Hiram Johnson, Ms. Ann Lee, and Dr. Nevell Ingram—were originally presented in Exercise 4 and will appear again in Exercises 10 and 12 to give you a sense of how cases develop in psychodynamic therapy.

The trainee playing the therapist should then improvise a response to each patient description and statement following these skill criteria:

1. **Identify and name the conflict between the patient's present circumstances and what they ideally want.** How do the patient's difficulties conflict with what they wish for?

2. **Name the implicit or explicit fantasy.** Explicitly state the patient's dream, daydream, hopes, or imaginings.

3. **Ask if the fantasy resolves the conflict.** Ask if the fantasy's ending seems to satisfy the patient's hopes or wishes.

---

### SKILL CRITERIA FOR EXERCISE 9

1. Identify and name the conflict between the patient's present circumstances and what they ideally want.
2. Name the implicit or explicit fantasy.
3. Ask if the fantasy resolves the conflict.

---

## Example of Therapist Exploring Fantasy

**Note:** Underlined text before each patient statement should be read aloud to provide context. Take your time in reading this slowly and repeating if necessary.

### Example 1

The patient is a high school student.

PATIENT: [*nervous*] I struggle with my schoolwork in class. Next thing I know is I am on a lake in a canoe. It is so peaceful. Then the bell rings, and class is over.

THERAPIST: You are struggling in school and wish it was easier. (Criterion 1) And then you start daydreaming about being in a canoe where it is so peaceful instead of so effortful. (Criterion 2) Did the peaceful canoe ride give you some relief from those classroom struggles? (Criterion 3)

### Example 2

The patient is a veterinary assistant who is afraid of speaking up to her boss.

PATIENT: [*meek, quiet voice*] I love my job. I even have some ideas about how to make the office function better. But it's scary to think of bringing them up with the doctor. When I was finishing up my day today, I imagined the doctor asking me, "Do you have any ideas how we could improve what we do here?"

**THERAPIST:** You would love to share your good ideas with your boss, but you are afraid to put yourself out there. (Criterion 1) In your imagination, the doctor solicits your advice. (Criterion 2) Did this relieve you of your anxiety and let you assert yourself? (Criterion 3)

**Example 3**

The patient is newly divorced with primary care of two children.

**PATIENT:** [*worried*] The divorce was OK enough. We've got enough support, me and the kids, to make it. But I see myself alone for a long, long time. [*Cheerful*] Except, this new person moved next door and seems really nice—and good-looking too! I can picture us going out.

**THERAPIST:** You see yourself alone for a long time, which sounds lonely to you. (Criterion 1) Suddenly, a new, attractive person appears. In your mind's eye, you and the new person get together. (Criterion 2) Does it seem this person could be the answer to your worries? (Criterion 3)

## INSTRUCTIONS FOR EXERCISE 9

### Step 1: Role-Play and Feedback

- The patient reads the <u>underlined text</u> aloud before each patient prompt.
- The patient says the first beginner patient statement. The therapist **improvises** a response based on the skill criteria.
- The trainer (or, if not available, the patient) provides **brief** feedback based on the skill criteria.
- The patient then repeats the same statement, and the therapist again improvises a response. The trainer (or patient) again provides brief feedback.

### Step 2: Repeat

- Repeat Step 1 for all the statements **in the current difficulty level** (beginner, intermediate, or advanced).

### Step 3: Assess and Adjust Difficulty

- The therapist completes the Deliberate Practice Reaction Form (see Appendix A) and decides whether to make the exercise easier or harder or to repeat the same difficulty level.

### Step 4: Repeat for Approximately 15 Minutes

- Repeat Steps 1 to 3 for at least 15 minutes.
- The trainees then switch therapist and patient roles and start over.

**Now it's your turn! Follow Steps 1 and 2 from the instructions.**

*Remember:* The goal of the role-play is for trainees to practice improvising responses to the patient statements in a manner that (a) uses the skill criteria and (b) feels authentic for the trainee. **Example clinician responses for each patient statement are provided at the end of this exercise. Trainees should attempt to improvise their own responses before reading the example responses.**

   *Note:* Underlined text before each patient statement should be read aloud to provide context. Take your time in reading this slowly and repeating if necessary.

| BEGINNER-LEVEL PATIENT STATEMENTS FOR EXERCISE 9 |
| --- |
| *Beginner Patient Statement 1* |
| The patient is a 15-year-old high school student who has moved to a new school.<br><br>**[Distressed]** Our family moved in August, and now I have to attend a new school where I don't know anyone. Every day I keep imagining that my parents will say, "Hey, guess what? We're moving back to our old house!" |
| *Beginner Patient Statement 2* |
| The patient is a 12-year-old girl referred by her school for "constant daydreaming" in class.<br><br>**[Aloof, looking around the room]** Class is so boring and confusing. I just kind of "space out" and go over scenes from my favorite movie. |
| *Beginner Patient Statement 3* |
| The patient is a 65-year-old man, now jobless and "angry all the time."<br><br>**[Agitated, fidgety]** I don't recognize my city anymore. There are all these young people moving in—taking our jobs, destroying our neighborhoods! I can visualize myself at 35, you know, showing them how it should be done! |
| *Beginner Patient Statement 4* |
| The patient is a 29-year-old assistant in a veterinary office who is afraid of speaking up to their boss.<br><br>**[Meek, quiet voice]** I love my job. I even have some ideas about how to make the office function better. But it's scary to think of bringing them up with the doctor. When I was finishing up my day today, I imagined the doctor asking me, "Do you have any ideas how we could improve what we do here?" |
| *Beginner Patient Statement 5* |
| The patient is a 49-year old father of three children who works as a grocery clerk.<br><br>**[Excited]** I'd like to have enough money to send my kids to college, but I just don't make enough at my job. So I've started buying 25 lottery tickets every week and am feeling pretty lucky. I can just picture me with them in their caps and gowns and how happy they would be. |

 **Assess and adjust the difficulty before moving to the next difficulty level (see Step 3 in the exercise instructions).**

| INTERMEDIATE-LEVEL PATIENT STATEMENTS FOR EXERCISE 9 |
| --- |
| ***Intermediate Patient Statement 1*** |
| The patient is a 16-year-old high school student whose younger sister was recently diagnosed with a fatal illness. |
| **[Forlorn]** Last spring my sister got real sick. She is constantly in pain. I am so frightened and sad. Now the doctors say it's a matter of months until she dies. After I heard that, I started thinking about cutting on myself and imagining what it would be like for me to feel real pain. |
| ***Intermediate Patient Statement 2*** |
| The patient is a 28-year-old resident of a group home for intellectually challenged adults. |
| **[Sad]** Ah, there's a new girl in our dormitory, her name is Debbie. She makes friends with everyone, except me. I keep hoping that she will suddenly talk to me. |
| ***Intermediate Patient Statement 3*** |
| The patient is a depressed and anxious 38-year-old who sells cars for a living. |
| **[Annoyed, sullen]** Business is bad, at least for me. The other people in the showroom are doing great! So I took a weekend program at a hotel called "Super Selling!" They promised all kinds of great things. But it was a real rip-off. |
| ***Intermediate Patient Statement 4*** |
| The patient is a 35-year-old and is recently divorced with custody of two children. |
| **[Worried]** The divorce was OK; we've got enough support, me and the kids, to make it. But I see myself alone for a long, long time. **[Cheerful]** Except, this new person moved next door and seems really nice—and good-looking too! I can picture us going out to some romantic spot. |
| ***Intermediate Patient Statement 5*** |
| Mr. Johnson is a 72-year-old, depressed widower with four grown children. |
| **[Meek]** Ah, my doctor said that you'd know how to solve my many problems. I've seen lots of brilliant doctors on TV, you know. I had a premonition that you would be like one of them. |

 **Assess and adjust the difficulty before moving to the next difficulty level (see Step 3 in the exercise instructions).**

## ADVANCED-LEVEL PATIENT STATEMENTS FOR EXERCISE 9

### Advanced Patient Statement 1

Ann Lee is a 22-year-old who complains about "giving and giving and not getting anything in return." She is outwardly cheerful but inwardly feeling depressed and worthless.

[Smiling] I felt a lot better after our first session. I was thinking that if I could learn how to handle my boyfriend better, we could have a really great relationship.

### Advanced Patient Statement 2

Dr. Ingram is a 35-year-old sociology professor at a nearby university who does not feel appreciated by the students or fellow teachers. His department chair recommended he go to therapy because of his off-putting behavior.

[Haughty, sitting very erect] I was wondering if you've presented my "case" to your supervisors yet. No doubt you are a good student, but, you know, senior clinicians might be helpful to you.

### Advanced Patient Statement 3

The patient is a 19-year-old high school graduate.

[Conflicted] Part of me thinks I should go to work and earn some money for my family. But I want to become a great math teacher like the lead in my favorite movie. That teacher came from a community like mine. And they went to college and were greatly admired.

### Advanced Patient Statement 4

The patient is a 20-year-old African American, female college student.

[Appears anxious and eager to speak] My parents gave me two goals: get a great education and marry a Black man. I am doing the first thing. But the guy I like, Arthur, is not Black. I told my parents about Arthur, and they wanted to meet him. They don't know that he's a White Jewish guy from Chicago. Last night I had this marvelous dream: Arthur and I traveled to meet his parents in Chicago. While there, I see an old photo of his great grandmother, who was born in Egypt, in a beautiful silver frame. She is clearly mixed race. I imagine telling my parents.

### Advanced Patient Statement 5

The patient is a 33-year-old attorney, struggling to expand their solo professional practice.

[Animated] I did well in college and law school; I got used to writing and performing for my professors. Now, I'm in my home office all day, alone. Maybe I should chuck it all and go get a PhD or start a premed program?

 **Assess and adjust the difficulty here (see Step 3 in the exercise instructions). If appropriate, follow the instructions to make the exercise even more challenging (see Appendix A).**

## Example Therapist Responses: Exploring Fantasy

*Remember:* Trainees should attempt to improvise their own responses before reading the example responses. **Do not read the following responses verbatim unless you are having trouble coming up with your own responses!**

| EXAMPLE RESPONSES TO BEGINNER-LEVEL PATIENT STATEMENTS FOR EXERCISE 9 |
|---|
| *Example Response to Beginner Patient Statement 1* |
| You miss your old school and are at a new school where you don't know anyone. (Criterion 1) You imagine that your parents grant a wish: You get to move back to your old school. (Criterion 2) Could it be that with that move, all your friends and everything you miss is restored? (Criterion 3) |
| *Example Response to Beginner Patient Statement 2* |
| Class feels confusing and boring and you would so like it to be different. (Criterion 1) In your daydream, you watch scenes from a favorite movie. (Criterion 2) Does this allow you to escape from your bad feelings about class and feel happier? (Criterion 3) |
| *Example Response to Beginner Patient Statement 3* |
| So many young people are "moving in." This used to be your neighborhood. (Criterion 1) You'd like to be much younger and show them. You take charge! Sounds like an exciting image. (Criterion 2) Does this make you feel any better? (Criterion 3) |
| *Example Response to Beginner Patient Statement 4* |
| You would love to share your good ideas with your boss, but you are afraid to put yourself out there. (Criterion 1) In your imagination, the doctor solicits your advice. (Criterion 2) As you imagine this, does it relieve you of your anxiety and let you assert yourself? (Criterion 3) |
| *Example Response to Beginner Patient Statement 5* |
| You want so much to see your kids get a good education but don't see how you will finance it. (Criterion 1) So you are imagining winning the lottery and watching your kids graduate. (Criterion 2) Would that feel to you like a great accomplishment in your life—seeing them in their caps and gowns? (Criterion 3) |

| EXAMPLE RESPONSES TO INTERMEDIATE-LEVEL PATIENT STATEMENTS FOR EXERCISE 9 |
| --- |

### Example Response to Intermediate Patient Statement 1

You don't want anything bad to happen to your sister, but now she has been diagnosed with a fatal illness. (Criterion 1) You started imagining cutting on yourself and what it would be like to feel real pain. (Criterion 2) Could there be some way your being in pain would help you deal with what is happening with your sister? (Criterion 3)

### Example Response to Intermediate Patient Statement 2

You like Debbie, but you don't know if she likes you. (Criterion 1) You hope Debbie reaches out to you. (Criterion 2) If she did that, would you know she likes you? (Criterion 3)

### Example Response to Intermediate Patient Statement 3

Selling cars at this moment is frustrating, and you're concerned about your capacity to do so. (Criterion 1) You had hoped the program "Super Selling!" would change all of that. (Criterion 2) Could it be that the "Super Selling!" program promised a way to solve your problems and quickly? (Criterion 3)

### Example Response to Intermediate Patient Statement 4

You see yourself alone for a long time which sounds lonely to you. (Criterion 1) Suddenly, a new, attractive person appears. In your mind's eye, you and the new person get together. (Criterion 2) Does it seem this person could be the answer to your worries? (Criterion 3)

### Example Response to Intermediate Patient Statement 5

You are burdened by your "many problems" and have not been able to solve them on your own. (Criterion 1) You had a sense I would be like one of those brilliant TV doctors. (Criterion 2) So you are hoping that I will be able to solve your problems? (Criterion 3)

**EXAMPLE RESPONSES TO ADVANCED-LEVEL PATIENT STATEMENTS FOR EXERCISE 9**

### Example Response to Advanced Patient Statement 1

You are having difficulties in your relationship with your boyfriend and feel stuck. (Criterion 1) You felt a lot better after our first session and were thinking things would get better with your boyfriend as a result. (Criterion 2) Do you imagine that if we worked together in therapy, you would end up having a really great relationship? (Criterion 3)

### Example Response to Advanced Patient Statement 2

You wish to be appreciated but do not feel understood by students and peers at your university. (Criterion 1) You are suggesting that I call in senior clinicians to help me help you. (Criterion 2) If I did that, would these senior clinicians recognize how special and complex you are? (Criterion 3)

### Example Response to Advanced Patient Statement 3

Part of you wants to become a math teacher, but another part feels you should earn money right now for your family instead. (Criterion 1) You greatly enjoy a movie about a math teacher from a community like yours. (Criterion 2) Does the movie's outcome resolve your dilemma and encourage you follow in that person's footsteps? (Criterion 3)

### Example Response to Advanced Patient Statement 4

You seem caught between your feelings for Arthur and pleasing your parents. (Criterion 1) In your dream, you discover that Arthur's family also has African roots and is proud of them. (Criterion 2) Does this dream give you some relief from your distress about introducing Arthur to your parents? (Criterion 3)

### Example Response to Advanced Patient Statement 5

Your job sounds burdensome and lonely, not like what it felt like when you were in school. (Criterion 1) The idea of going back to school for another degree is appealing. (Criterion 2) If you did go back to school, do you think you would do well like you did the first time? (Criterion 3)

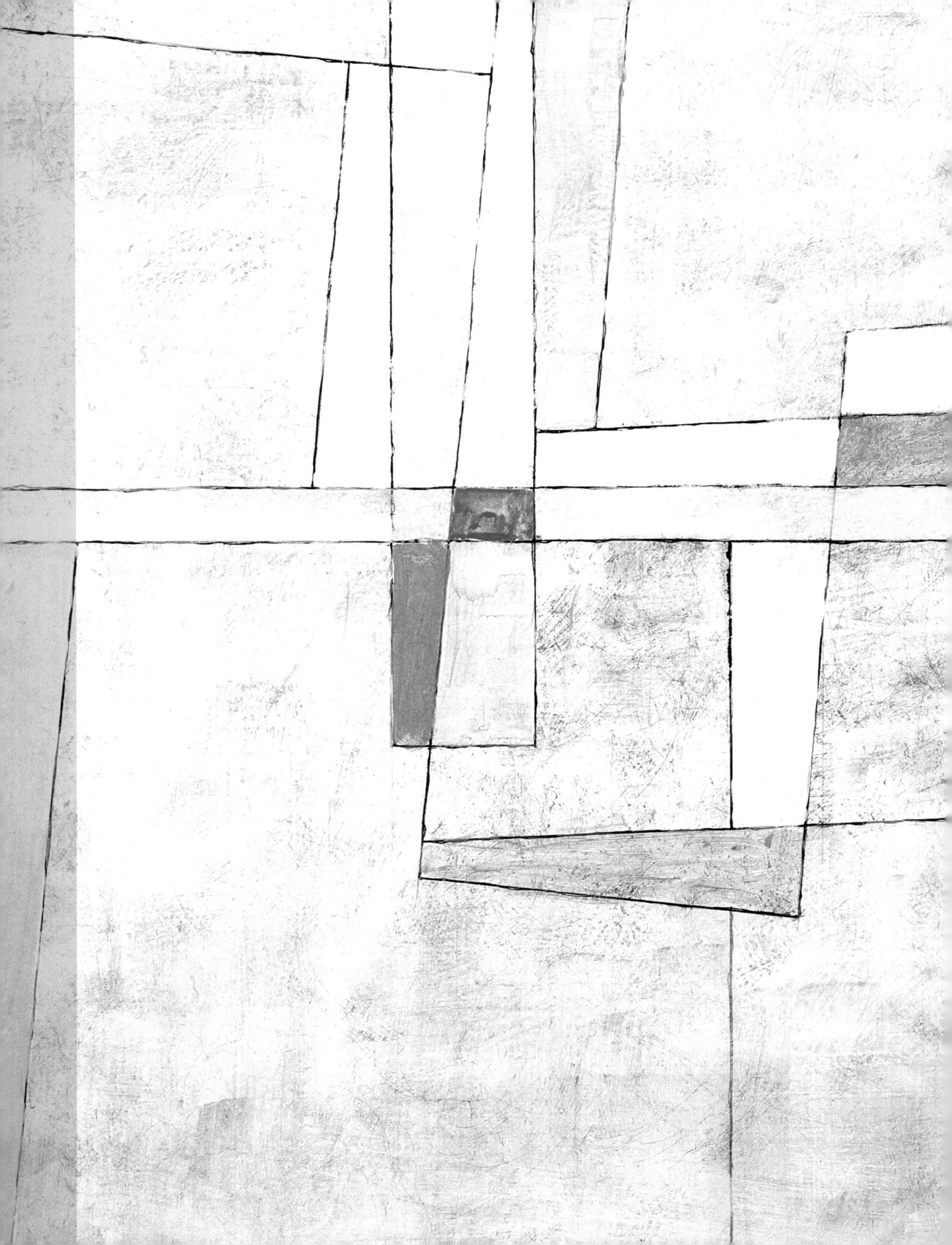

# Case Formulation: Gathering Data for the Cyclical Maladaptive Pattern

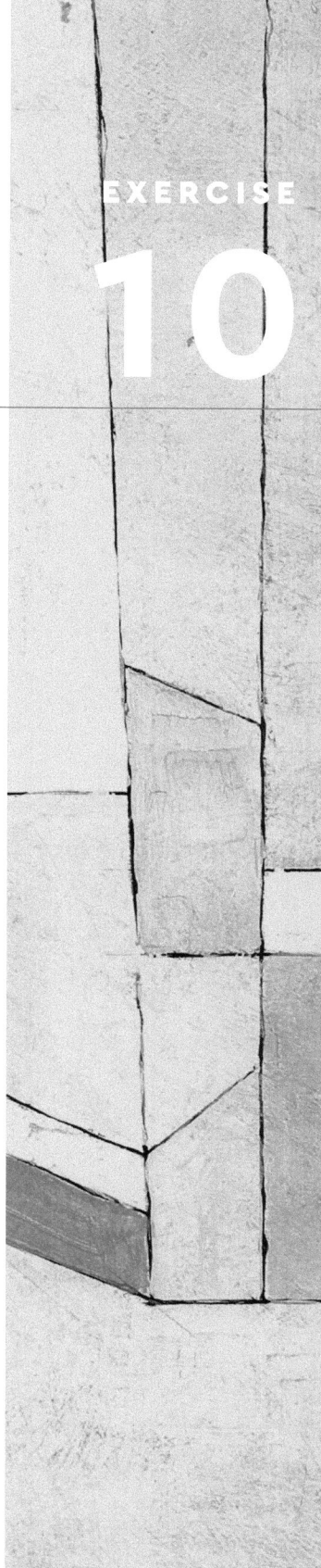

## Preparations for Exercise 10

1. Read the instructions in Chapter 2.

2. Download the Deliberate Practice Reaction Form and the Deliberate Practice Diary Form at https://www.apa.org/pubs/books/deliberate-practice-psychodynamic-psychotherapy (see the "Clinician and Practitioner Resources" tab; also available in Appendixes A and B, respectively).

## Skill Description

### Skill Difficulty Level: Advanced

Case formulations are clinicians' efforts to provide a cause-and-effect account of their patients' suffering. Why is this person depressed, anxious, or lonely, for example? In interpersonal–psychodynamic therapies (and with time-limited dynamic psychotherapy [TLDP] in particular), we assume that patients are suffering because they have become stuck in maladaptive patterns of interpersonal and intrapsychic cycles that feed on each other (Levenson, 2003, 2017; Levenson & Strupp, 2007). As the patient tells their spontaneous narrative, the therapist is listening and probing for such patterns. In TLDP, this reorganization of the patient's narrative into a pattern is called the cyclical maladaptive pattern (CMP; Levenson, 1995; Strupp & Binder, 1984); thus, the CMP describes a repetitive, dysfunctional configuration of feelings, thoughts, and behaviors that usually occur across time, person, and place.

In this exercise, trainees practice distinct ways to discover the four components of the patient's CMP by asking a series of questions about (a) the patient's thoughts, feelings, wishes, or behaviors (acts of the self); (b) what the patient expects from others (expectations of others' responses); (c) how the patient views their treatment by others (perceived acts of others); and (d) how the patient views and treats one's

https://doi.org/10.1037/0000351-012
*Deliberate Practice in Psychodynamic Psychotherapy*, by H. Levenson, V. Gay, and J. L. Binder

FIGURE E10.1. **The Cyclical Maladaptive Pattern**

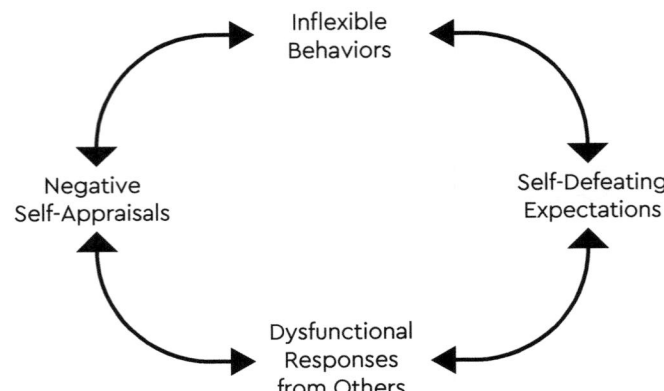

*Note.* From "Enlivening Psychodynamic Brief Therapy With Emotion-Focused Interventions: An Integrative Therapist's Approach," by H. Levenson, 2020, *Clinical Social Work Journal, 48*(3), p. 271 (https://doi.org/ 10.1007/s10615–020–00762-z). Copyright 2020 by Springer Nature. Reprinted with permission

self (introject). By getting the answers to these four sets of questions, the therapist can weave a causal narrative ("story") about the patient's pattern of interpersonal inter- actions and intrapsychic representations of self and other. That story describes how the patient's inflexible actions are generated in response to self-defeating expecta- tions of what others will do; these actions in turn lead to dysfunctional behaviors from others, which then serve to amplify the patient's negative introject (self-appraisal). That introject causes further inflexible actions, and the cycle repeats (see Figure E10.1), creating a self-fulfilling prophecy. Such maladaptive cyclical patterns often begin in childhood (where the acts of others usually pertain to parental figures) driven by the child's attachment needs and longings. Although patients are stuck in these repeated patterns, they are largely unaware of them; that is, they are unconscious. To elicit the information necessary for developing a formulation, therapists must become adept at asking good questions about these four aspects of the CMP. Asking such good ques- tions is the focus of this exercise.

Rather than following the standard statement–response format used in previous exer- cises, this one involves back-and-forth dialogues between the patient and the therapist. Some of the patients in this exercise—Mr. Hiram Johnson, Ms. Ann Lee, and Dr. Nevell Ingram[1]—were originally presented in Exercises 4 and 9 will appear again in Exercise 12 to give you a sense of how cases develop in psychodynamic therapy.

The therapist should improvise a response to each patient statement following these skill criteria:

1. **Ask about one act of the self (thought, feeling, wish, or behavior).** When the oppor- tunity arises, the therapist will intervene to obtain relevant information about the patient's thoughts, feelings, wishes, and/or behaviors usually around some relational content. Note that the therapist should only ask about **one** act of self. However, the exercise can be made more difficult by having the therapist give more than one act.

---

1. The identities of all patients in the exercise have been disguised to protect their confidentiality. Ann is based on a real patient whose CMP has previously been discussed and published (Levenson, 2017). In addition, there is a video of all six sessions done with Ann that is commercially available (Levenson & Carlson, 2010), as well as a two-session version containing an interview with Hanna Levenson discussing the case from a deliberate practice point of view (Levenson & Friedlander, in production). A transcript of the two sessions can be found in Exercise 13. There have also been four published studies using the Ann video that can be found in the references.

2. **Ask about the patient's expectations of others' responses.** Here the therapist will ask about how the patient imagines others will act toward them.

3. **Ask how the patient perceives the acts of others toward the patient.** This perception typically involves assuming the *intentions* behind others' behavior.

4. **Ask how the patient views and treats themselves (introject).** This component is based on two fundamental principles of interpersonal theory: (a) how one views oneself is a product of the "reflected appraisals" of significant others, and (b) how one treats oneself is determined by one's perception of how significant others have treated oneself.

| SKILL CRITERIA FOR EXERCISE 10 |
| --- |
| 1. Ask about one act of the self (thought, feeling, wish, or behavior).<br>2. Ask about the patient's expectations of others' responses.<br>3. Ask how the patient perceives the acts of others toward the patient.<br>4. Ask how the patient views or treats themselves (introject). |

## Example of Gathering Data for the Cyclical Maladaptive Pattern

| EXAMPLE: A PATIENT REFERRED FOR ANXIETY ABOUT POTENTIALLY LOSING THEIR SIGNIFICANT OTHER |
| --- |
| **PATIENT:** [*anxious*] My significant other seems like they're going to leave me; they're so distant. |
| Criterion 1: Ask about an act of the self (thought, feeling, wish, or behavior).<br>**THERAPIST:**<br>• When you see them acting distant, what do you notice yourself thinking about? (Thought)<br>• How do you feel about the prospect of losing this intimate relationship? (Feeling)<br>• What do you wish would happen to make things better? (Wish)<br>• Is there anything you could do differently to make the situation better? (Behavior) |
| **PATIENT:** [*frustrated*] They want me to do everything around our apartment, and then they complain when things aren't done. |
| Criterion 2: Ask about the patient's expectations of others' responses.<br>**THERAPIST:** Did you expect your significant other to be more appreciative of your efforts? |
| **PATIENT:** [*nervous*] I am afraid to say anything to my significant other. |
| Criterion 3: Ask how the patient perceives the acts of others toward the patient.<br>**THERAPIST:** When you say something to them, how do they respond? |
| **PATIENT:** [*dejected*] I try to talk to my significant other, but they don't care. |
| Criterion 4: Ask about how the patient views or treats themself (introject).<br>**THERAPIST:** What do you feel about yourself in trying to navigate all of this? |

## COMMON MISTAKES

1. Make sure that when you ask about actions of the self (Criterion 1) you do **not** accept how the patient acts toward themselves, which should be classified under the introject (Criterion 4).

2. You only need to ask about **one** of the four components for act of the self. However, as previously stated, the exercise can be made more difficult by having the therapist give more than one component.

3. When asking about how the patient **expects** to be treated (Criterion 2), do not accept how the patient **wishes** to be treated, which should be classified under acts of the self (Criterion 1).

| INSTRUCTIONS FOR EXERCISE 10 |
|---|

**Step 1: Role-Play With Therapist Improvisation**

- The patient initiates the dialogue by reading the first statement in the initial beginner dialogue.
- The therapist improvises a response following the first skill criterion.
- The patient reads the next statement in the same dialogue, and the therapist responds using the second criterion. This continues until the dialogue has been completed.

**Step 2: Assess and Adjust Difficulty**

- The therapist completes the Deliberate Practice Reaction Form (see Appendix A) and decides whether to make the exercise easier or harder or to repeat the same dialogue.

**Step 3: Repeat for Approximately 15 Minutes**

- Repeat Steps 1 and 2 for at least 15 minutes.
- The trainees then switch therapist and patient roles and start over.

> **Now it's your turn! Follow Steps 1 and 2 from the instructions.**

*Remember:* The goal of the role-play is for trainees to practice improvising responses to the patient statements in a manner that (a) uses the skill criteria and (b) feels authentic for the trainee. **Example clinician responses for each patient statement are provided at the end of this exercise. Trainees should attempt to improvise their own responses before reading the example responses.**

| BEGINNER-LEVEL DIALOGUE 1:<br>HIRAM JOHNSON, 72, RETIRED |
|---|
| **PATIENT: [Frustrated]** We got a notice that the landlord was going to move into our apartment and we would have to move out. So I started looking for a place to live. I would look every day through the real estate listings. I just couldn't find anything. |
| **THERAPIST PROMPT (CRITERION 1):** Ask about one act of the self (thought, feeling, wish, or behavior). |
| **PATIENT: [Ashamed]** My daughter had me admitted to the psychiatric hospital. I was there for a couple of weeks and then they sent me here to the outpatient clinic. |
| **THERAPIST PROMPT (CRITERION 2):** Ask about the patient's expectations of others' responses. |
| **PATIENT: [Sad]** My father was a drinker, and he'd get really angry toward my mother and the kids when he was drunk. |
| **THERAPIST PROMPT (CRITERION 3):** Ask how the patient perceives the acts of others toward the patient. |
| **PATIENT: [Ashamed]** I should have done a better job finding a house that would have kept us all together. |
| **THERAPIST PROMPT (CRITERION 4):** Ask how the patient views or treats themself (introject). |

| **BEGINNER-LEVEL DIALOGUE 2:**<br>**ANN LEE, 22, SINGLE, IN A RELATIONSHIP** |
|---|
| **PATIENT:** **[Cheery]** When I visit my boyfriend, he spends more time with his friends than with me. But I pretend like I'm okay with it. |
| **THERAPIST PROMPT (CRITERION 1):** Ask about one act of the self (thought, feeling, wish, or behavior). |
| **PATIENT:** **[Nervous]** I would like to ask my boyfriend to spend more time with me when I visit him, but I am afraid to. |
| **THERAPIST PROMPT (CRITERION 2):** Ask about the patient's expectations of others' responses. |
| **PATIENT:** **[Ashamed]** My boyfriend has said he doesn't like "clingy people." So I act like I don't mind being alone. |
| **THERAPIST PROMPT (CRITERION 3):** Ask how the patient perceives the behavior of others toward the patient. |
| **PATIENT:** **[Sad]** My boyfriend and my friends don't often ask me to do things with them. I don't know why. |
| **THERAPIST PROMPT (CRITERION 4):** Ask how the patient views and treats themselves (introject). |

**BEGINNER-LEVEL DIALOGUE 3:**
**NEVELL INGRAM, PhD, 32, ASSISTANT PROFESSOR AT A UNIVERSITY**

| |
|---|
| **PATIENT: [Frustrated]** My department chair was abrupt with me. I asked them to support my grant application, due tomorrow. They were rude. |
| **THERAPIST PROMPT (CRITERION 1):** Ask about one act of the self (thought, feeling, wish, or behavior). |
| **PATIENT: [Proud, then annoyed]** I've been an exemplary employee, and I was in a hurry; I had this deadline. The department chair should have known this. |
| **THERAPIST PROMPT (CRITERION 2):** Ask about the patient's expectations of others' responses. |
| **PATIENT: [Indignant]** Well, I think my request would be reasonable to anyone with half a mind. |
| **THERAPIST PROMPT (CRITERION 3):** Ask how the patient perceives the acts of others toward the patient. |
| **PATIENT: [Angry]** I can tell you that I always jump when someone in authority says "jump!" |
| **THERAPIST PROMPT (CRITERION 4):** Ask how the patient views or treats themselves (introject). |

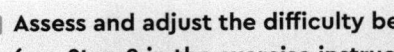 **Assess and adjust the difficulty before moving to the next difficulty level (see Step 2 in the exercise instructions).**

| INTERMEDIATE-LEVEL DIALOGUE 1: |
| :---: |
| LYDIA LUDLOW, 45, MARRIED BUT SEPARATED FROM HER HUSBAND[2] |

**PATIENT: [Frustrated]** When I've needed help the most, I've had to wait and wait to get to see you. I don't hate therapists. I just have never found them very helpful.

**THERAPIST PROMPT (CRITERION 1):** Ask about one act of the self (thought, feeling, wish, or behavior).

**PATIENT: [Exasperated]** I've been compulsively overeating ever since I was a child. I keep hoping someone will come along who can help me lose weight.

**THERAPIST PROMPT (CRITERION 2):** Ask about the patient's expectations of others' responses.

**PATIENT: [Proud]** You've probably never seen anyone as complex as me before, so I think we are going to have to meet two or three times a week if you are going to figure me out.

**THERAPIST PROMPT (CRITERION 3):** Ask how the patient perceives the acts of others toward the patient.

**PATIENT: [Irritated]** My parents focused on my physical defects. They just wanted to fix me.

**THERAPIST PROMPT (CRITERION 4):** Ask how the patient views or treats themself (introject).

2. This patient's CMP has previously been discussed and published (Levenson, 1995).

| INTERMEDIATE-LEVEL DIALOGUE 2: TIM WONG, 52, DIVORCED, SALESPERSON |
|---|
| **PATIENT:** **[Friendly]** I've been in therapy before, [address the therapist by their first name]. |
| **THERAPIST PROMPT (CRITERION 1):** Ask about one act of the self (thought, feeling, wish, or behavior). |
| **PATIENT:** **[Upbeat]** I like to keep things informal and friendly. |
| **THERAPIST PROMPT (CRITERION 2):** Ask about the patient's expectations of others' responses. |
| **PATIENT:** **[Defensive]** My philosophy is that formality can sour a relationship very quickly. |
| **THERAPIST PROMPT (CRITERION 3):** Ask how the patient perceives the acts of others toward the patient. |
| **PATIENT:** **[Uncomfortable]** Well, one of the reasons I came to see you is that sometimes my friendliness works out fine, but too often my friendliness gets misunderstood. |
| **THERAPIST PROMPT (CRITERION 4):** Ask how the patient views or treats themself (introject). |

| INTERMEDIATE-LEVEL DIALOGUE 3: CHRIS ROBERTO, 48, PARTNER HAS THREATENED TO LEAVE |
| --- |
| **PATIENT:** **[Demanding]** Make my partner stay with me! |
| **THERAPIST PROMPT (CRITERION 1):** Ask about one act of the self (thought, feeling, wish, or behavior). |
| **PATIENT:** **[Ashamed]** Sometimes, my partner gets depressed or something. Then I feel really helpless. |
| **THERAPIST PROMPT (CRITERION 2):** Ask about the patient's expectations of others' responses. |
| **PATIENT:** **[Hopeless]** Well, I don't know. It's overwhelming for me, I guess. |
| **THERAPIST PROMPT (CRITERION 3):** Ask how the patient perceives the acts of others toward the patient. |
| **PATIENT:** **[Nervous]** Lots of people are untrustworthy. They can turn on you suddenly. |
| **THERAPIST PROMPT (CRITERION 4):** Ask how the patient views or treats themself (introject). |

 **Assess and adjust the difficulty before moving to the next difficulty level (see Step 2 in the exercise instructions).**

| **ADVANCED-LEVEL DIALOGUE 1:** <br> **BEVERLY VICTOR, 47, MARRIED, WITH TWO YOUNG ADULT CHILDREN[3]** |
| --- |
| **PATIENT:** [Matter-of-fact] My internist sent me here because he thinks I am depressed. |
| **THERAPIST PROMPT (CRITERION 1):** Ask about one act of the self (thought, feeling, wish, or behavior). |
| **PATIENT:** [Flat affect] I have a very nice life, a good family, married for 26 years, two great sons, and we have a nice home. I don't think I'm depressed. |
| **THERAPIST PROMPT (CRITERION 2):** Ask about the patient's expectations of others' responses. |
| **PATIENT:** [Curious] I do have some stomach problems. They got worse around the time my younger son left for college. |
| **THERAPIST PROMPT (CRITERION 3):** Ask how the patient perceives the acts of others toward the patient. |
| **PATIENT:** [Earnest] Once when I was a child, I was whining about not having something. My mother told me, "Don't complain and be glad for what you have." My brother was blind, so that advice set me straight. |
| **THERAPIST PROMPT (CRITERION 4):** Ask how the patient views or treats themselves (introject). |

---

3. This patient's CMP has previously been discussed and published as a chapter (Levenson, 2018). In addition, there is a video enactment of session vignettes from this therapy that is available and linked to the published chapter.

| ADVANCED-LEVEL DIALOGUE 2: |
| :--- |
| **MRS. VERONIQUE FOLLETTE, 59, DIVORCED, WITH TWO GROWN DAUGHTERS[4]** |
| **PATIENT: [Irritated]** My aunt and my sisters are aloof and uncaring. I don't like it when other people get too close to me. |
| **THERAPIST PROMPT (CRITERION 1):** Ask about one act of the self (thought, feeling, wish, or behavior). |
| **PATIENT: [Changing the subject]** Is seeing me in therapy helping you to accomplish your goals? |
| **THERAPIST PROMPT (CRITERION 2):** Ask about the patient's expectations of others' responses. |
| **PATIENT: [Matter-of-fact]** Like I mentioned in our last session, it was hard to say that my stepfather was sexually inappropriate with me. But what I hadn't told you was that I've tried to tell my aunts about this. |
| **THERAPIST PROMPT (CRITERION 3):** Ask how the patient perceives the acts of others toward the patient. |
| **PATIENT: [Matter-of-fact]** My daughters have each other; they don't need me. |
| **THERAPIST PROMPT (CRITERION 4):** Ask how the patient views or treats themself (introject). |

4. This patient is modeled on a real patient whose identity has been disguised and whose CMP has previously been discussed and published (Levenson, 1995).

| ADVANCED-LEVEL DIALOGUE 3:<br>HENRY BELOTTI, 38, MAN WHOSE MOTHER CONSTANTLY CRITICIZED HIM |
| --- |
| **PATIENT:** [Panicky] My partner broke up with me! |
| **THERAPIST PROMPT (CRITERION 1):** Ask about one act of the self (thought, feeling, wish, or behavior). |
| **PATIENT:** [Worried] My ex-partner just never got me. |
| **THERAPIST PROMPT (CRITERION 2):** Ask about the patient's expectations of others' responses. |
| **PATIENT:** [Dejected] It's like my ex-partner felt that I was never good enough for them. |
| **THERAPIST PROMPT (CRITERION 3):** Ask how the patient perceives the acts of others toward the patient. |
| **PATIENT:** [Sad] When my ex said they were leaving, I just couldn't speak. I just stood there. |
| **THERAPIST PROMPT (CRITERION 4):** Ask how the patient views or treats themself (introject). |

✋ **Assess and adjust the difficulty here (see Step 2 in the exercise instructions). If appropriate, follow the instructions to make the exercise even more challenging (see Appendix A).**

## Example Therapist Responses: Gathering Data for the Cyclical Maladaptive Pattern

*Remember:* Trainees should attempt to improvise their own responses before reading the example responses. **Do not read the following responses verbatim unless you are having trouble coming up with your own responses!**

| EXAMPLE RESPONSES TO BEGINNER-LEVEL DIALOGUE 1: MR. JOHNSON |
| --- |
| **PATIENT: [Frustrated]** We got a notice that the landlord was going to move into our apartment and we would have to move out. So I started looking for a place to live. I would look every day through the real estate listings. I just couldn't find anything. |
| **THERAPIST:**<br>• While you were going out every day looking for a place to live, what was going through your mind? (Thought)<br>• What were you feeling during your searching and searching for a place to live? (Feeling)<br>• Did you have any hopes during your searching? (Wish)<br>• What was your behavior like before the notice of eviction? (Behavior) |
| **PATIENT: [Ashamed]** My daughter had me admitted to the psychiatric hospital. I was there for a couple of weeks, and then she sent me here to the outpatient clinic. |
| **THERAPIST:** Did you expect your daughter would have you admitted to the hospital? |
| **PATIENT: [Sad]** My father was a drinker, and he'd get really angry toward my mother and the kids when he was drunk. |
| **THERAPIST:** What did he do to you? |
| **PATIENT: [Ashamed]** I should have done a better job finding a house that would have kept us all together. |
| **THERAPIST:** As you say that, how are you feeling about yourself? |

| EXAMPLE RESPONSES TO BEGINNER-LEVEL DIALOGUE 2: ANN LEE |
| --- |
| **PATIENT:** [Cheery] When I visit my boyfriend, he spends more time with his friends than with me. But I pretend like I'm OK with it. |
| **THERAPIST:** <br> • What are your thoughts about his behavior? (Thought) <br> • I hear you act like you are OK with it, but how does it really make you feel? (Feeling) <br> • What do you hope will happen when you visit him? (Wish) <br> • When you act like you are okay with it, what exactly do you do? (Behavior) |
| **PATIENT:** [Nervous] I would like to ask my boyfriend to spend more time with me when I visit him, but I am afraid to. |
| **THERAPIST:** What do you imagine his reaction would be if you told him how you feel? |
| **PATIENT:** [Ashamed] My boyfriend has said they don't like "clingy people." So I act like I don't mind being alone. |
| **THERAPIST:** When you appear to be very self-sufficient, how do people usually treat you? |
| **PATIENT:** [Sad] My boyfriend and my friends don't often ask me to do things with them. I don't know why. |
| **THERAPIST:** How does their behavior leave you feeling about yourself? |

| EXAMPLE RESPONSES TO BEGINNER-LEVEL DIALOGUE 3: NEVELL INGRAM, PhD |
| --- |
| **PATIENT: [Frustrated]** My department chair was abrupt with me. I asked them to support my grant application, due tomorrow. They were rude. |
| **THERAPIST:**<br>• What did you think when your chair was rude? (Thought)<br>• What did you feel when your chair was rude? (Feeling)<br>• What do you wish your chair would do now? (Wish)<br>• What will you do now? (Behavior) |
| **PATIENT: [Proud, then annoyed]** I've been an exemplary employee, and I was in a hurry; I had this deadline. My chair should have known this. |
| **THERAPIST:** Based on their past behavior, did you expect your chair to act swiftly? |
| **PATIENT: [Indignant]** Well, I think my request would be reasonable to anyone with half a mind. |
| **THERAPIST:** How do other people usually respond to your requests? |
| **PATIENT: [Angry]** I can tell you, that I always jump when someone in authority says "jump!" |
| **THERAPIST:** If you didn't jump, what would that mean about you? |

| EXAMPLE RESPONSES TO INTERMEDIATE-LEVEL DIALOGUE 1: LYDIA LUDLOW |
| --- |
| **PATIENT:** [**Frustrated**] When I've needed help the most, I've had to wait and wait to get to see you. I don't hate therapists. I just have never found them very helpful. |
| **THERAPIST:**<br>• When you say you've never found therapists helpful, what do you mean? (Thought)<br>• You say you don't hate therapists; what *is* your feeling toward them? (Feeling)<br>• Sounds like you were hoping to be seen right away. Is that right? (Wish)<br>• What do you do while you are waiting and waiting? (Behavior) |
| **PATIENT:** [**Exasperated**] I've been compulsively overeating ever since I was a child. I keep hoping someone will come along who can help me lose weight. |
| **THERAPIST:** I hear that you are hoping someone will come along, but are you expecting that they will? |
| **PATIENT:** [**Proud**] You've probably never seen anyone as complex as me before, so I think we are going to have to meet two or three times a week if you are going to figure me out. |
| **THERAPIST:** Did the other therapists you saw see you so frequently? |
| **PATIENT:** [**Irritated**] My parents focused on my physical defects. They just wanted to fix me. |
| **THERAPIST:** Do you treat yourself like you need of fixing? |

| EXAMPLE RESPONSES TO INTERMEDIATE-LEVEL DIALOGUE 2: TIM WONG |
|---|
| **PATIENT:** **[Friendly]** I've been in therapy before, [address the therapist by their first name]. |
| **THERAPIST:**<br>• Oh, do you think I prefer to be called by my first name? (Thought)<br>• What would it feel like if I told you I prefer that you use my last name? (Feeling)<br>• I wonder if there is a wish behind using my first name. (Wish)<br>• Did you call your previous therapist by their first name as well? (Behavior) |
| **PATIENT:** **[Upbeat]** I like to keep things informal and friendly. |
| **THERAPIST:** What do you imagine would happen if we keep our relationship a bit more formal? |
| **PATIENT:** **[Defensive]** My philosophy is that formality can sour a relationship very quickly. |
| **THERAPIST:** How do people usually react to your informality? |
| **PATIENT:** **[Uncomfortable]** Well, one of the reasons I came to see you is that sometimes my friendliness works out fine, but too often my friendliness gets misunderstood. |
| **THERAPIST:** What do you say to yourself when you get misunderstood? |

| EXAMPLE RESPONSES TO INTERMEDIATE-LEVEL DIALOGUE 3: CHRIS ROBERTO |
|---|
| **PATIENT:** **[Demanding]** Make my partner stay with me! |
| **THERAPIST:**<br>• What makes you think your partner intends to leave you? (Thought)<br>• What feelings come up when you think they could leave? (Feeling)<br>• What do you wish would happen to make things better? (Wish)<br>• Is there anything you could do differently at home to improve the situation? (Behavior) |
| **PATIENT:** **[Ashamed]** Sometimes my partner gets depressed or something. Then I feel really helpless. |
| **THERAPIST:** Do you expect your partner will leave regardless of anything you do? |
| **PATIENT:** **[Hopeless]** Well, I don't know. It's overwhelming for me, I guess. |
| **THERAPIST:** Have other people walked away from a relationship with you? |
| **PATIENT:** **[Nervous]** Lots of people are untrustworthy. They can turn on you suddenly. |
| **THERAPIST:** How do you think about yourself in those moments? |

| EXAMPLE RESPONSES TO ADVANCED-LEVEL DIALOGUE 1: BEVERLY VICTOR |
|---|
| **PATIENT:** **[Matter-of-fact]** My internist sent me here because they think I am depressed. |
| **THERAPIST:**<br>• What do you think? (Thought)<br>• How did it feel when your doctor told you they thought you were depressed? (Feeling)<br>• Did you wish your doctor would have said something different? (Wish)<br>• Looks like you readily followed your doctor's instructions in coming here. Is this typical for you? (Behavior) |
| **PATIENT:** **[Flat affect]** I have a very nice life, a good family, married for 26 years, two great sons, and we have a nice home. I don't think I'm depressed. |
| **THERAPIST:** It sounds like it was quite unexpected for your doctor to say you were depressed. |
| **PATIENT:** **[Curious]** I do have some stomach problems. They got worse around the time my younger son left for college. |
| **THERAPIST:** When did your son leave for college? |
| **PATIENT:** **[Earnest]** Once when I was a child, I was whining about not having something. My mother told me, "Don't complain and be glad for what you have." My brother was blind, so that advice set me straight. |
| **THERAPIST:** Do you find that you criticize yourself frequently given your mother's advice? |

| **EXAMPLE RESPONSES TO ADVANCED-LEVEL DIALOGUE 2:** |
| **MRS. VERONIQUE FOLLETTE** |
| PATIENT: **[Irritated]** My aunt and my sisters are aloof and uncaring. I don't like it when other people get too close to me. |
| THERAPIST:<br>• Why do you think your relatives are aloof and uncaring? (Thought)<br>• How do you feel when your aunt and sisters are aloof and uncaring? (Feeling)<br>• How do you wish they would react to you? (Wish)<br>• How do you behave when your aunt is aloof toward you? (Behavior) |
| PATIENT: **[Changing the subject]** Is seeing me in therapy helping you to accomplish your goals? |
| THERAPIST: What do you expect are my goals? |
| PATIENT: **[Matter-of-fact]** Like I mentioned in our last session, it was hard to say that my stepfather was sexually inappropriate with me. But what I hadn't told you was that I've tried to tell my aunts about this. |
| THERAPIST: How did they respond? |
| PATIENT: **[Matter-of-fact]** My daughters have each other; they don't need me. |
| THERAPIST: As you hear yourself say that, how do you feel about yourself? |

| EXAMPLE RESPONSES TO ADVANCED-LEVEL DIALOGUE 3: HENRY BELOTTI |
| --- |
| **PATIENT: [Panicky]** My partner broke up with me! |
| **THERAPIST:**<br>• How do you understand your ex-partner's actions? (Thought)<br>• What feelings did that arouse in you? (Feeling)<br>• What do you wish would happen to make things better for you? (Wish)<br>• Is there anything you could do differently to improve the situation? (Behavior) |
| **PATIENT: [Worried]** My ex-partner just never got me. |
| **THERAPIST:** Did you ever think they would? |
| **PATIENT: [Dejected]** It's like my ex felt that I was never good enough for them. |
| **THERAPIST:** Do other people treat you like you are not good enough? |
| **PATIENT: [Sad]** When my ex said they were leaving, I just couldn't speak. I just stood there. |
| **THERAPIST:** Did you say anything to yourself about yourself at that moment? |

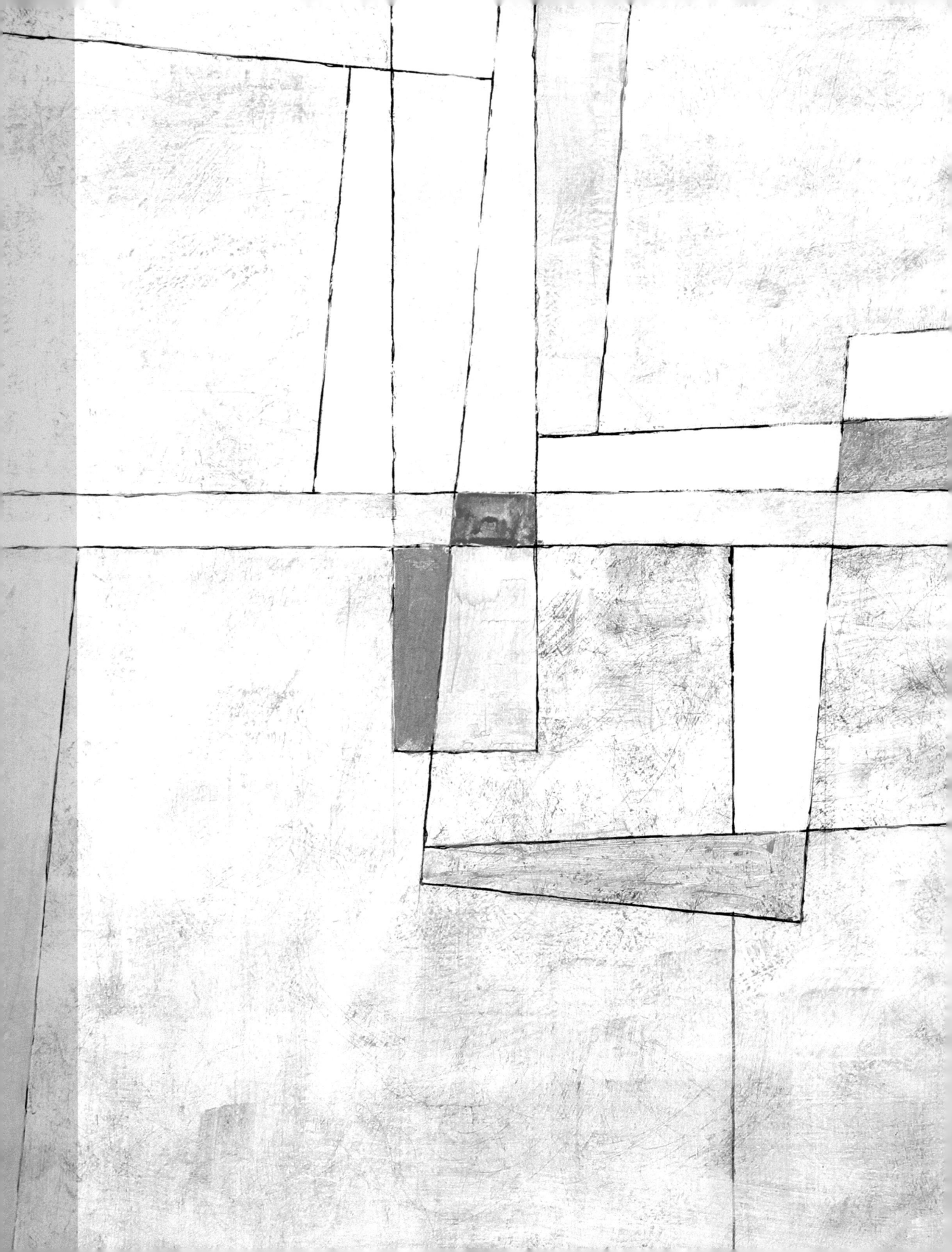

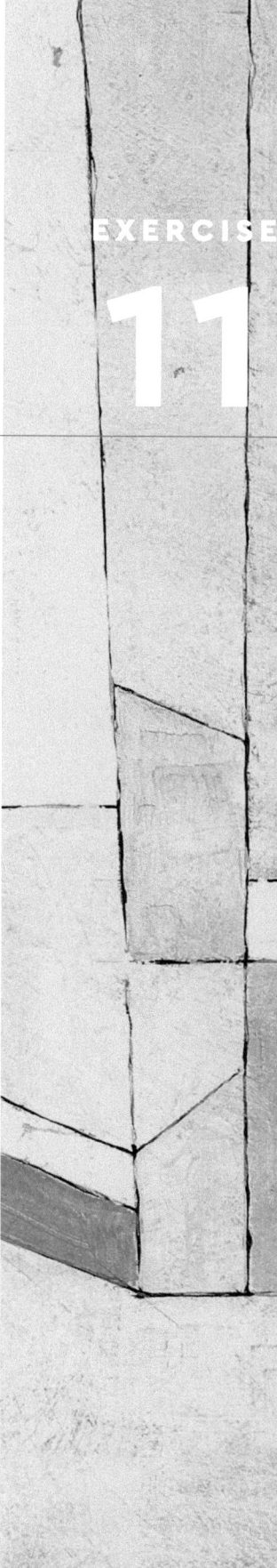

# Using Supervision to Recognize Reenactments

## Preparations for Exercise 11

1. Read the instructions in Chapter 2.

2. Download the Deliberate Practice Reaction Form and the Deliberate Practice Diary Form at https://www.apa.org/pubs/books/deliberate-practice-psychodynamic-psychotherapy (see the "Clinician and Practitioner Resources" tab; also available in Appendixes A and B, respectively).

## Skill Description

### Skill Difficulty Level: Advanced

Exercise 2 focused on helping trainees practice becoming aware of their counter-transference (CT). This exercise builds on that one. In this exercise, we focus on thera-pists' sharing with their supervisors their complementary CTs engendered by specific patients, and the "pull" the therapists feel to interact with patients in ways that inadver-tently (iatrogenically) end up recreating the very problem the patients are struggling with—their cyclical maladaptive patterns. For example, a therapist's complementary CT to dealing with a hostile and demeaning patient with a history of neglect may be anger and anxiety. Their CT may then result in the therapist's unconsciously reenacting the patient's experience of others (i.e., neglect) by "accidentally" forgetting a session. Talking about one's CT in supervision is an excellent way to deal with such potential or actual reenactments by bringing the dynamic into awareness.

Unfortunately, many trainees do not bring their difficult feelings to supervision. Researchers (Cook et al., 2020; Ladany et al., 1996) found that more than 95% of super-visees at some point intentionally avoid such discussions with their supervisors. Trainees withhold information for several reasons—for example, not knowing what is appropriate to discuss, embarrassment over in-session mistakes, impression management, imposter

https://doi.org/10.1037/0000351-013

*Deliberate Practice in Psychodynamic Psychotherapy*, by H. Levenson, V. Gay, and J. L. Binder

syndrome, or fears of being evaluated negatively. Trainees suppress the information generated by their CT because they have not been trained sufficiently to (a) recognize their reactions in nuanced and complex situations that require supervisory help, (b) normalize their occurrence, and (c) know how to discuss their CT reactions with their supervisors.

A consequence of such withholding is that supervisees miss out on much-needed help. It also means that they cannot acquire the more advanced skills of using one's CT to derive case formulations, choose interventions, or assess progress. Discussing one's CT in supervision can be scary. Therapists brave enough to do so require compassionate supervision, and the supervisor must be diligent about maintaining appropriate boundaries within supervision.

In this exercise, we focus on recognizing one's countertransferential feelings, naming what triggers them, and communicating that to one's supervisor. We hope that practicing these skills will encourage trainees to bring their CT to actual supervision sessions. In real supervision sessions, supervisors can then help trainees process and metabolize their CT feelings and the behavioral urges that accompany them.

Instead of role-playing a patient as in previous exercises, in this exercise one trainee acts as a supervisor and the other trainee, role-playing a therapist-in-training, shares their CT experiences of a patient (as described in the clinical context provided). Note that this exercise does not involve training supervisors on how to respond to therapists. The supervisor only needs to read aloud the underlined clinical context. The trainee playing the therapist then improvises a response to each clinical context following these skill criteria:

1. **Share with your clinical supervisor your complementary countertransferential response(s) to something that the patient has said or done.** Describe in some detail the feelings, thoughts, and somatic responses you experienced being with the patient. Remember that the goal here is to process your difficult reactions, not just the "nice" ones.

2. **Specify what the patient said or did to evoke that reaction.** As best you can figure out, let your supervisor know what the patient did that triggered your responses.

3. **State the urge you had to say or do something in the moment in response to the patient.** If you haven't mentioned it already, include in your presentation to your supervisor what *you felt like doing* in response to the patient's behavior. Remember that these are not actions that you actually carried out with the patient. Rather, they are your experiential reactions that you want the supervisor's help in understanding and containing.

---

**SKILL CRITERIA FOR EXERCISE 11**

1. Share with your clinical supervisor your complementary countertransferential response(s) to something that the patient has said or done.
2. Specify what the patient said or did to evoke that reaction.
3. State the urge you had to say or do something in the moment in response to the patient.

## Examples of Therapists Using Supervision to Recognize Reenactments

***Note:*** <u>Underlined text</u> before each patient statement should be read aloud to provide context. Take your time in reading this slowly and repeating if necessary.

### Example 1

<u>In the therapy session, the patient brought up a conflict with a colleague, and you mentioned a similar "conflict" the patient had with their secretary that the patient described in a previous session. At this point, the patient said sternly and forcefully to you, "I did not say it was a 'conflict'; I said that my secretary had a problem, not that I had a conflict."</u>

**THERAPIST TO SUPERVISOR:** When the patient confronted me, (Criterion 2) I felt admonished and demeaned. (Criterion 1) I felt really defensive and like I wanted to convince them that they really did have a conflict. I wanted to show them how wrong they were! (Criterion 3)

### Example 2

<u>After five sessions of therapy, a patient unexpectedly started off the session saying to you, "This is our last session."</u>

**THERAPIST TO SUPERVISOR:** I was devastated to hear that and disappointed too. (Criterion 1) I was so sure that our work was going well, but the patient wanted to end. (Criterion 2) I thought of saying, "OK, let's end it right now!" (Criterion 3)

### Example 3

<u>A patient queried you about your knowledge of research: "Perhaps you can tell me about the empirical evidence for why you do what you do in therapy."</u>

**THERAPIST TO SUPERVISOR:** I felt like the patient was examining me rather than letting me get to know them as a person. I really felt on the spot. (Criterion 1) When they said "empirical evidence," I felt pushed to defend every aspect of my training. (Criterion 2) My impulse was to say, "Look, I'm here to help you, not debate theories of therapy!" (Criterion 3)

**INSTRUCTIONS FOR EXERCISE 11**

### Step 1: Role-Play and Feedback

- The trainee role-playing the supervisor reads the first clinical context. The therapist **improvises** a response based on the skill criteria imagining they are talking to their supervisor.
- The trainee role-playing the supervisor provides **brief** feedback based on the skill criteria.
- The supervisor repeats the same clinical context, and the therapist again improvises a response. The supervisor again provides brief feedback.

### Step 2: Repeat

- Repeat Step 1 for the next clinical context and proceed through all the contexts **in the current difficulty level** (beginner, intermediate, or advanced).

### Step 3: Assess and Adjust Difficulty

- When indicated, the therapist completes the Deliberate Practice Reaction Form (see Appendix A) and decides whether to go on to the harder segment or to make the exercise easier or to repeat the same difficulty level.

### Step 4: Repeat for Approximately 20 Minutes

- Repeat Steps 1 to 3 for at least 20 minutes.
- The trainees then switch therapist and supervisor roles and start over.

**Now it's your turn! Follow Steps 1 through 4 from the exercise instructions.**

**Remember:** The goal of the role-play is for trainees to practice improvising responses in supervision given the therapy context in a manner that (a) uses the skill criteria and (b) feels authentic for the trainee. **Example therapist responses for each clinical context are provided at the end of this exercise. Trainees should attempt to improvise their own responses before reading the example responses.**

    **Note:** Underlined text before each patient statement should be read aloud to provide context. Take your time in reading this slowly and repeating if necessary.

| BEGINNER-LEVEL CLINICAL CONTEXTS FOR EXERCISE 11 |
| --- |
| *Beginner Clinical Context 1* |
| After requesting an early morning appointment, the patient came 20 minutes late for the third time in a row. |
| *Beginner Clinical Context 2* |
| In the first session, the patient asked detailed questions about your training and wondered out loud, "Do you think you have sufficient training to be of help to me?" |
| *Beginner Clinical Context 3* |
| An anxious and dependent college student brought their mother to the initial session. In the waiting room, the mother did most of the talking. The patient sat still with downcast eyes. |
| *Beginner Clinical Context 4* |
| A patient asked if you have ever been in therapy. |
| *Beginner Clinical Context 5* |
| After five sessions of therapy, a patient started off the sixth session saying, "This is our last session." |

 **Assess and adjust the difficulty before moving to the next difficulty level (see Step 3 in the exercise instructions).**

## INTERMEDIATE-LEVEL CLINICAL CONTEXTS FOR EXERCISE 11

### *Intermediate Clinical Context 1*

In a session a day before Valentine's Day, a patient brought you a surprise present—an expensive bottle of champagne, saying seductively, "I know we can't be more than patient and therapist, but I thought maybe you could have this champagne tomorrow and think of me. I know I'll be thinking of you."

### *Intermediate Clinical Context 2*

You show your supervisor a video of a session. In it, you speak in a stern tone to your patient: "If you aren't going to do the homework, this therapy isn't going to work for you."

### *Intermediate Clinical Context 3*

A patient came to therapy begging you to tell them what to do about their child's serious drug use: "You are my only hope!"

### *Intermediate Clinical Context 4*

The patient said, "In a dream I had last night, you and I were kind of dating, and you invited me to your place. So today I got curious as to where you lived and googled you."

### *Intermediate Clinical Context 5*

The patient learned you are only 26 years old. In response, they said, "Well that's pretty young to be a therapist. By the way, I skipped two grades in elementary school."

✋ **Assess and adjust the difficulty before moving to the next difficulty level (see Step 3 in the exercise instructions).**

| ADVANCED-LEVEL CLINICAL CONTEXTS FOR EXERCISE 11 |
|---|
| ***Advanced Clinical Context 1*** |
| After 10 sessions, a patient, who is coming for treatment mandated by their employer because the patient treats customers disrespectfully, demanded of you, "I want to speak to your supervisor!" |
| ***Advanced Clinical Context 2*** |
| After seeing you for two sessions, a patient who appears to be of a different race than you, wondered if the two of you were "a good fit." |
| ***Advanced Clinical Context 3*** |
| A new patient whose partner recently died cried throughout the first three sessions, and you had difficulty ending the sessions on time. |
| ***Advanced Clinical Context 4*** |
| A patient came to an early morning session without eating breakfast. They said meekly, "I can't concentrate because I am hungry. Do you happen to have anything I could eat?" |
| ***Advanced Clinical Context 5*** |
| Out of respect for privacy, you greet a new patient in the clinic waiting room using their first name. The patient, who has a PhD, responded in a stern, reprimanding tone, "People call me Dr." |

**Assess and adjust the difficulty here (see Step 3 in the exercise instructions). If appropriate, follow the instructions to make the exercise even more challenging (see Appendix A).**

## Example Therapist Statements: Using Supervision to Recognize Reenactments

**Remember:** Trainees should attempt to improvise their own responses before reading the example responses. **Do not read the following responses verbatim unless you are having trouble coming up with your own responses!**

| EXAMPLE STATEMENTS IN SUPERVISION: BEGINNER-LEVEL CLINICAL CONTEXTS FOR EXERCISE 11 |
| --- |
| *Example Therapist Statement to Supervisor—Beginner Clinical Context 1* |
| I really felt irritated (Criterion 1) when the patient was 20 minutes late for the third time in a row. (Criterion 2) I felt like warning them that I would not wait again. (Criterion 3) |
| *Example Therapist Statement to Supervisor—Beginner Clinical Context 2* |
| I felt criticized by the patient (Criterion 1) when the patient examined my worthiness. (Criterion 2) I felt like saying, "I wonder if *you* are adequate." (Criterion 3) |
| *Example Therapist Statement to Supervisor—Beginner Clinical Context 3* |
| I felt really upset with the patient (Criterion 1) who did nothing to stop their intrusive parent. (Criterion 2) I felt like shaking them and saying, "When are you going to stand up for yourself!" (Criterion 3) |
| *Example Therapist Statement to Supervisor—Beginner Clinical Context 4* |
| I felt very invited in (Criterion 1) when the patient asked if I've ever been in therapy. (Criterion 2) I was really tempted to tell them about my experiences and how the therapy really helped me get over my depression. (Criterion 3) |
| *Example Therapist Statement to Supervisor—Beginner Clinical Context 5* |
| I was devastated to hear that and disappointed too. (Criterion 1) I was so sure that our work was going well, but the patient wanted to end. (Criterion 2) I thought of pleading for them to come back for one more session. (Criterion 3) |

| EXAMPLE STATEMENTS IN SUPERVISION: INTERMEDIATE-LEVEL CLINICAL CONTEXTS FOR EXERCISE 11 |
| --- |
| ***Example Therapist Statement to Supervisor—Intermediate Clinical Context 1*** |
| I felt confused and kind of unsettled (Criterion 1) by the gift and the part about thinking about them. (Criterion 2). I turned down the champagne, but I did end up thinking about them on Valentine's Day. (Criterion 3) |
| ***Example Therapist Statement to Supervisor—Intermediate Clinical Context 2*** |
| I was angry at the patient's lack of follow-through. (Criterion 1) Not doing the homework after I've said repeatedly how important it is seems irresponsible. (Criterion 2) But my tone with them was stronger than I intended. I guess I'm worried that you [the supervisor] will see how poorly I'm doing. (Criterion 3) |
| ***Example Therapist Statement to Supervisor—Intermediate Clinical Context 3*** |
| I feel overwhelmed by the patient. (Criterion 1) They were so insistent—like it was up to me if their child lived or died! (Criterion 2) I'm wondering if maybe I should tell them we are not a good match. I'm not an expert in drug counseling. (Criterion 3) |
| ***Example Therapist Statement to Supervisor—Intermediate Clinical Context 4*** |
| That distressed me a lot. (Criterion 1) The "dating" part of the dream felt creepy. And then their googling me really bothered me. (Criterion 2) I had the urge to present the ethics and rules of therapy. (Criterion 3) |
| ***Example Therapist Statement to Supervisor—Intermediate Clinical Context 5*** |
| When the patient told me about skipping grades in elementary school, (Criterion 2) I felt like they were behaving like a child trying to compete with me. (Criterion 1) I had an urge to laugh at how ridiculous they were being. I also felt a little sad. (Criterion 3) |

| EXAMPLE STATEMENTS IN SUPERVISION: ADVANCED-LEVEL CLINICAL CONTEXTS FOR EXERCISE 11 |
|---|
| ***Example Therapist Statement to Supervisor—Advanced Clinical Context 1*** |
| That came from nowhere! I was shocked. (Criterion 1) The patient seemed so calm, but I felt like it was a command. (Criterion 2) I've been worried about what the patient might want to tell you and had the urge not to come to supervision today. (Criterion 3) |
| ***Example Therapist Statement to Supervisor—Advanced Clinical Context 2*** |
| When the patient brought up whether we were a "good fit," (Criterion 2) I really felt on the spot. (Criterion 1) I asked a lot of questions about what they meant, but truthfully, I didn't want to discuss it at all. (Criterion 3) |
| ***Example Therapist Statement to Supervisor—Advanced Clinical Context 3*** |
| When the patient starts crying, (Criterion 2) I find myself tearing up a little. (Criterion 1) I just feel I'm being mean and withholding if I kept a strict time limit. (Criterion 1) I'd like to just let them stay as long as they want. (Criterion 3) |
| ***Example Therapist Statement to Supervisor—Advanced Clinical Context 4*** |
| When the patient told me they hadn't eaten breakfast, (Criterion 2) I felt irritated. (Criterion 1) I felt like saying we needed to have the session, especially since I thought they were avoiding something, but instead I kind of froze. (Criterion 3) |
| ***Example Therapist Statement to Supervisor—Advanced Clinical Context 5*** |
| When the patient chastised me, (Criterion 2) I felt both embarrassed and defensive. (Criterion 1) I really wanted both to apologize profusely and to defend myself by saying it was an honest mistake. (Criterion 3) |

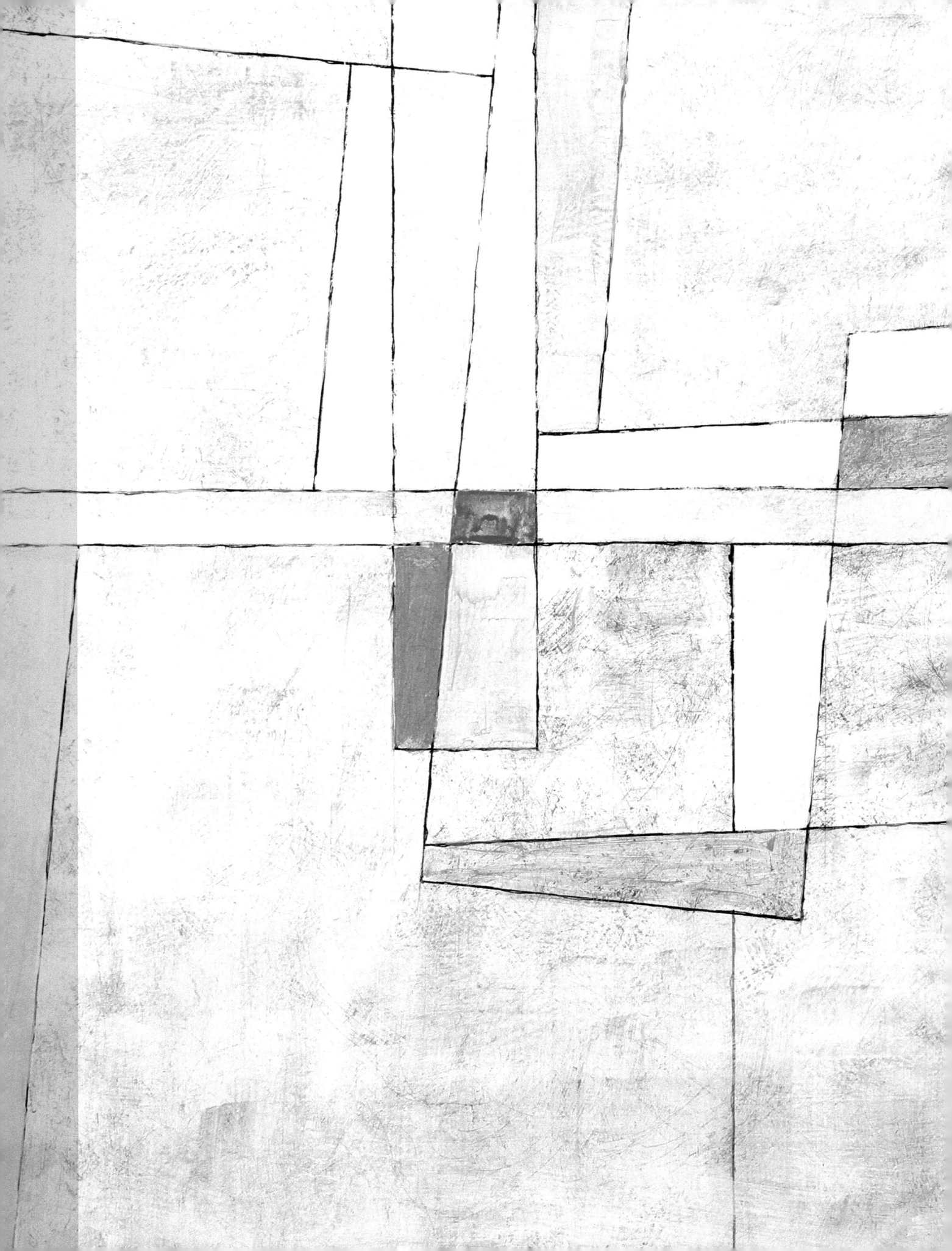

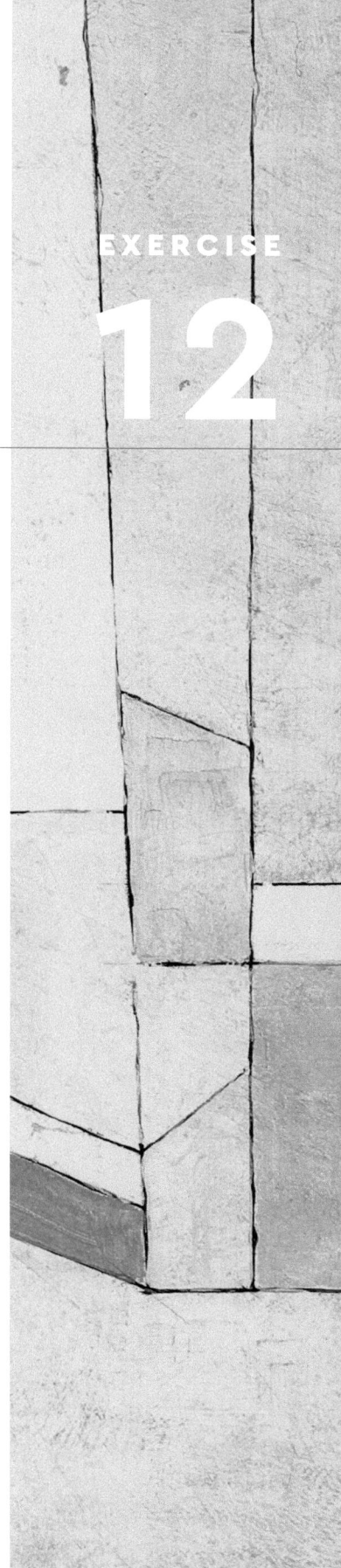

# Providing a Corrective Emotional Experience

## Preparations for Exercise 12

1. Read the instructions in Chapter 2.

2. Download the Deliberate Practice Reaction Form and the Deliberate Practice Diary Form at https://www.apa.org/pubs/books/deliberate-practice-psychodynamic-psychotherapy (see the "Clinician and Practitioner Resources" tab; also available in Appendixes A and B, respectively).

## Skill Description

### Skill Difficulty Level: Advanced

Analysts Alexander and French (1946) are credited with developing the concept of the *corrective emotional experience*. While psychoanalytic thought at the time held that interpretations leading to insight were the main curative intervention, Alexander and French opined that only the "actual experiencing of a new outcome" that is "the exact opposite" of the patient's expectation could "give the patient the conviction that a new solution is possible and [induce] him to give up the old . . . patterns" (p. 115). They reasoned that an opportune setting for gaining this type of life-changing experience was within the therapeutic relationship.

Let's see how this might work in a session. Take, for example, Sandra B., a hypothetical patient, who learned to relinquish her healthy assertiveness as a child because behaviors such as saying "no" were not tolerated by her strict and stern parents. She therefore grew up to be a submissive, anxiety-ridden adult. What if, as Sandra feels safer in therapy, she goes counter to her well-worn pattern of timidity and lets her therapist know she does not want to do something the therapist suggests? Sandra might be expecting the therapist to become quite angry with her noncompliance, like her parents did. Suppose instead that her therapist said, "I feel so much more connected with you now when you tell me what you really do not want in your therapy." Such a remark would come as a big surprise to Sandra, who was expecting she might be rejected or punished. Her therapist's attuned response potentially becomes part of a corrective emotional experience that encourages further positive shifts in her behavior, thoughts, and feelings, sense of self, and expectations of others.

In this exercise, you will have the chance to practice detecting and responding to glimmers of when a patient is breaking with an old pattern and use the opportunity to say something significant about the effect this is having on you, the therapeutic relationship, or the patient's progress. Such feedback is especially important because often patients tend to minimize or not even recognize the forays they make into healthier behavior. Additionally, sometimes therapists get so used to pointing out what the patient is doing wrong that they miss chances to affirm the patient's previously relinquished parts when they show up in subtle behaviors or fleeting moments within a session. However, attuning to and highlighting such shifts can permit the patient to reintegrate a previously disowned part of themselves. Bowlby (1985) said it best:

> Our [the therapist's] role is in sanctioning the patient to think thoughts that his parents have discouraged or forbidden him to think, to experience feelings his parents have discouraged or forbidden him to experience, and to consider actions that his parents have forbidden him to contemplate. (p. 198)

Each set of patient statements follows a different clinical context based on the three recurring patients from Exercises 4, 9, and 10. The beginner statements follow Ann, the intermediate statements follow Dr. Ingram, and the advanced statements follow Mr. Johnson.

The trainee should improvise a response to each patient statement following these skill criteria:

1. **Mention the way the patient had to adapt to caregivers growing up (i.e., acts of self-protection) by forfeiting a healthy and normal part of the self to remain connected.** This comment sets the stage for the patient to see how they usually act and why they had to act that way. It is a compassionate, informative, and understanding statement from the therapist.

2. **Describe how glimmers of this healthy part just appeared in the patient's statements, feelings, or actions.** This describes how that healthy part of them was just manifested in their lives or in the session and is so opposite of how they usually act (i.e., they have broken from their own mold).

3. **Affirm why this healthy part is a good (helpful) thing.** Often patients do not know why that part of them that significant others would not tolerate is really a good thing. Affirming this for them in the session will contribute to their new learning as they own parts they previously warded off and become more their authentic self.

4. **Inquire how the patient felt about showing this previously forfeited part of the self.** Because patients are often quite scared to show these previously suppressed parts, checking in with them to acknowledge their risk-taking can be a supportive and encouraging intervention.

| SKILL CRITERIA FOR EXERCISE 12 |
| --- |

1. Mention the way the patient had to adapt to caregivers growing up (i.e., acts of self-protection) by forfeiting a healthy and normal part of the self to remain connected.
2. Describe how glimmers of this healthy part show up in the patient's present statements, feelings, or actions.
3. Affirm why this healthy part is a good (helpful) thing.
4. Inquire how the patient felt about showing this previously forfeited part of the self.

## Examples of Therapists Providing a Corrective Emotional Experience

**Note:** Underlined text before the first patient statement should be read aloud to provide context. This context applies to all statements that follow. Take your time in reading this slowly and repeating if necessary.

### Example 1: The Case of Ann

As a child, Ann would watch over her mother to make sure she wouldn't choke on her own vomit if she had too much to drink. Ann, therefore, became a hypervigilant child trying to keep those around her safe and happy. She felt most like herself when she was self-sacrificing, unaware of having given up her own wants and needs in the process. In therapy, she talked a lot about fears her boyfriend might leave her.

**PATIENT:** [*hesitant*] To be a good person, I need to keep other people in mind. But in today's session, I really wasn't thinking much about you; in fact, I really didn't think about you at all. I'm sorry about that.

**THERAPIST:** You grew up putting others' needs before your own, (Criterion 1) so talking about yourself without thinking about me and my needs is quite a shift for you. (Criterion 2) I really enjoyed hearing you talk today in a more free-flowing manner. (Criterion 3) What was it like concentrating on you for a change? (Criterion 4)

### Example 2: The Case of Ann, Continued

**PATIENT:** [*anxious*] I'm afraid my boyfriend will leave me. He told me he doesn't want a clingy girlfriend. [*irritated*] But as I'm talking about him in here with you, I'm feeling really angry and fed up with his drunken behavior.

**THERAPIST:** Growing up you felt so concerned about your mother but could never say anything about her drinking. (Criterion 1) I can imagine you are tired of pretending to be happy when you are really angry inside. (Criterion 2) Knowing you are fed up with your boyfriend's behavior sounds like a really important first step in achieving a more authentic relationship with him. (Criterion 3) How was it for you to realize how angry you are? (Criterion 4)

### Example 3: The Case of Ann, Continued

**PATIENT:** [*with trepidation*] When I began therapy, it was important to me to have you like me; now I don't think about that so much. Does that mean I'm becoming a less of a kind person?

**THERAPIST:** Quite the contrary! You have really taken chances in this therapy and been able to be more your authentic self without worrying about my reaction. This has been a new experience for you. (Criterion 2) Given how you learned to please everyone in your family rather than be your independent self, (Criterion 1) I know it must come as quite a surprise that you find yourself able to react without worrying about my reactions. (Criterion 3) Is that true? (Criterion 4)

## INSTRUCTIONS FOR EXERCISE 12

### Step 1: Role-Play and Feedback

- The patient reads the <u>underlined text</u> aloud then says the first beginner patient statement. The therapist **improvises** a response based on the skill criteria.
- The trainer (or, if not available, the patient) provides **brief** feedback based on the skill criteria.
- The patient then repeats the same statement, and the therapist again improvises a response. The trainer (or patient) again provides brief feedback.

### Step 2: Repeat

- Repeat Step 1 for all the statements **in the current difficulty level** (beginner, intermediate, or advanced).

### Step 3: Assess and Adjust Difficulty

- The therapist completes the Deliberate Practice Reaction Form (see Appendix A) and decides whether to make the exercise easier or harder or to repeat the same difficulty level.

### Step 4: Repeat for Approximately 15 Minutes

- Repeat Steps 1 to 3 for at least 15 minutes.
- The trainees then switch therapist and patient roles and start over.

> **Now it's your turn! Follow Steps 1 through 4 from the exercise instructions.**

*Remember:* The goal of the role-play is for trainees to practice improvising responses to the patient statements in a manner that (a) uses the skill criteria and (b) feels authentic for the trainee. **Example therapist responses for each patient statement are provided at the end of this exercise. Trainees should attempt to improvise their own responses before reading the example responses.**

*Note:* Underlined text before each patient statement should be read aloud to provide context. This context before the first statement applies to all following statements in the same difficulty level, and some statements provide additional context. Take your time in reading this slowly and repeating if necessary.

| BEGINNER-LEVEL PATIENT STATEMENTS FOR EXERCISE 12: THE CASE OF ANN |
|---|
| ***Beginner Patient Statement 1*** |
| As a child, Ann would watch over her mother to make sure she wouldn't choke on her own vomit if she had too much to drink. Ann, therefore, became a hypervigilant child trying to keep those around her safe and happy. She felt most like herself when she was self-sacrificing, unaware of her having given up her own wants and needs in the process. In therapy, she talked a lot about fears her boyfriend might leave her. <br><br> **[Cheerful]** To be a good friend, I need to listen to my friends' complaints. But yesterday I started telling them about me without listening first. **[Hesitant]** Maybe I shouldn't have done that. |
| ***Beginner Patient Statement 2*** |
| **[Sad but with energy in her voice]** I just give and give . . . and sometimes I want something back! |
| ***Beginner Patient Statement 3*** |
| **[Anxious]** I'm afraid my boyfriend will leave me. He told me he doesn't want a clingy girlfriend. **[Irritated]** But I am tired of pretending to be happy while he's out drinking; I'm really angry and fed up with his drunken behavior. |
| ***Beginner Patient Statement 4*** |
| **[Matter-of-fact]** It is important for me to be strong and independent in all respects, and I pretty much am—**[anxious]** although leaning on you for support in here has been a lifesaver. |
| ***Beginner Patient Statement 5*** |
| **[With trepidation]** When I began therapy, it was important to me to have you like me; now I don't think about that so much. Does that mean I'm becoming less of a nice person? |

 **Assess and adjust the difficulty before moving to the next difficulty level (see Step 3 in the exercise instructions).**

### INTERMEDIATE-LEVEL PATIENT STATEMENTS FOR EXERCISE 12: THE CASE OF DR. INGRAM

**Intermediate Patient Statement 1**

Dr. Ingram is 32, married, and a professor at a major university. He prides himself on his accomplishments and evaluates others based on theirs. Many people find him arrogant and self-centered. His father, who was a dental assistant, worked long hours to provide for his wife and their only son. His mother, who was more formal than her husband, took her young son to museums and libraries dressed as a miniature adult. She instructed him on the importance of dignity and being in charge—not like his father, "who has to be an assistant to others." In therapy, as in life, it is hard for him to show his softer, more vulnerable side.

**[Nostalgic]** My dad gave me a "junior" lab coat when I was a kid; I wore it every night to sleep until the fabric wore out. But **[sterner]** I see that it was silly now. It didn't mean anything in the long-term view of things.

**Intermediate Patient Statement 2**

Before the session, the therapist saw Dr. Ingram in the waiting room a few minutes early, approached him, and said warmly, "Good morning. I'm glad to see you." Dr. Ingram smiled back warmly then stiffened.

**[Soft]** I was surprised that you said you were glad to see me in the waiting room. **[Gruffer]** Is that appropriate for a therapist? Weren't you trained to look and act like a professional at all times? I think that's important.

**Intermediate Patient Statement 3**

**[Irritated]** My colleague got his photo on the cover of our alumni magazine. For a moment I was jealous, and then I reminded myself that I have more publications than he does and will make tenure at an earlier age.

**Intermediate Patient Statement 4**

**[Compassionate]** I was sorry to hear you felt ill and needed to cancel our session last week. I hope you're feeling better. I almost brought you some local honey. It has medicinal properties. **[Abrupt formality]** Let's see, what do we have on the agenda for today?

**Intermediate Patient Statement 5**

**[Warmly]** I parked next to an old Honda in your parking lot. I remembered dad always drove those. For a moment I thought it must be yours. He was a good man. **[Sudden haughtiness]** However, it looks out of place next to my Mercedes.

 **Assess and adjust the difficulty before moving to the next difficulty level (see Step 3 in the exercise instructions).**

---

### ADVANCED-LEVEL PATIENT STATEMENTS FOR EXERCISE 12:
### THE CASE OF MR. JOHNSON[1]

*Advanced Patient Statement 1*

As a child, Mr. Johnson feared his father, who could become physically abusive when drunk. Mr. Johnson therefore became a meek, placating, and quiet child, growing up to be a depressed and passive man in his relationships. He felt safer in his passiveness even though he was unaware of the price he paid in giving up his assertiveness. Early in therapy, Mr. Johnson complied with everything the therapist said. He uttered no complaints about any aspect of the therapy.

[Tentative] I didn't quite like that suggestion you made last week about writing down the place and time when I feel like a drink.

*Advanced Patient Statement 2*

Mr. Johnson was a few minutes late for his session.

[Apologetic] Sorry I am late for our session, but the street parking near your office is really difficult.

*Advanced Patient Statement 3*

The therapist asked Mr. Johnson to check in with his body to see how he felt about lending money to his daughter so she could take a vacation without him.

[Irritated] Right now I feel constipated! Why didn't you tell me the medication I'm taking causes constipation?

*Advanced Patient Statement 4*

The therapist has asked Mr. Johnson repeatedly how he is feeling in the moment without getting a clear answer.

[Uncomfortable and stammering] I wa-wa-want to keep my feelings hidden!

*Advanced Patient Statement 5*

Mr. Johnson came at his regular time and discovered that his therapist was occupied with another patient for some 15 minutes. Once his session began, he said:

[Visibly frustrated] I wonder if, uh, I should come less often. I realize that you've got other patients to see.

 **Assess and adjust the difficulty here (see Step 3 in the exercise instructions). If appropriate, follow the instructions to make the exercise even more challenging (see Appendix A).**

---

1. In addition to publications about Mr. Johnson (Levenson, 1995, 2017), there is a video enactment of session vignettes from this therapy that is commercially available (https://www.psychotherapy.net/).

## Example Therapist Responses: Providing a Corrective Emotional Experience

*Remember:* Trainees should attempt to improvise their own responses before reading the example responses. **Do not read the following responses verbatim unless you are having trouble coming up with your own responses!**

---

| EXAMPLE RESPONSES TO BEGINNER-LEVEL PATIENT STATEMENTS FOR EXERCISE 12: THE CASE OF ANN |
| --- |
| *Example Response to Beginner Patient Statement 1* |
| You grew up putting others' needs before your own, (Criterion 1) so talking about yourself first is quite a shift for you. (Criterion 2) I can understand it might have felt uneasy to do that, (Criterion 4) but I wonder if now they appreciate knowing a bit more about who you are. (Criterion 3) What was it like to put yourself first for a change? (Criterion 4) |
| *Example Response to Beginner Patient Statement 2* |
| Given how you grew up needing to be so watchful and concerned about others, (Criterion 1) saying your own true needs out loud is newer for you. (Criterion 2) Hearing that you want something back, I now have a better idea of what we should work on in therapy. (Criterion 3) How did it feel for you to tell me what you need? (Criterion 4) |
| *Example Response to Beginner Patient Statement 3* |
| Growing up you felt so concerned about your mother but could never say anything about her drinking. (Criterion 1) I can imagine you are tired of pretending to be happy when you are really angry inside. (Criterion 2) Knowing you are fed up with your boyfriend's behavior sounds like a really important first step in achieving a more authentic relationship with him. (Criterion 3) How was it for you to realize how angry and fed up you are? (Criterion 4) |
| *Example Response to Beginner Patient Statement 4* |
| Wow! Hearing that means a lot to me. (Criterion 3) You have allowed yourself to receive my support in here and have grown from the experience. This has been a new experience for you. (Criterion 2) Given how you grew up watching over your mother when it should have been the other way around, (Criterion 1) I could imagine it might not have been easy to say how much my support means to you. Yeah? (Criterion 4) |
| *Example Response to Beginner Patient Statement 5* |
| Quite the contrary! You have really taken chances in this therapy and been able to be more your authentic self without worrying about my reaction. This has been a new experience for you. (Criterion 2) Given how you learned to please everyone in your family rather than be your independent self, (Criterion 1) I know it must come as quite a surprise that you find yourself able to react without obsessing about my reactions. (Criterion 3) Is that true? (Criterion 4) |

## EXAMPLE RESPONSES TO INTERMEDIATE-LEVEL PATIENT STATEMENTS FOR EXERCISE 12: THE CASE OF DR. INGRAM

### Example Response to Intermediate Patient Statement 1

Given the pressure your mother put on you to be more successful than your father and how little you got to see him, (Criterion 1) I can imagine that gift meant a lot to you as a boy. Your tenderness talking about the junior lab coat is new for you to express. (Criterion 2) I can see another side to you today that helps me understand more fully who you are. (Criterion 3) What was it like letting down your guard just a bit in here just now? (Criterion 4)

### Example Response to Intermediate Patient Statement 2

With your mother, you felt a lot of pressure to appear dignified at all times. (Criterion 1) I can imagine that my casualness in the waiting room might have taken you by surprise. Your warm smile back felt really good to me (Criterion 3) even if it felt unusual for you. (Criterion 2) Did it feel like a risk to let me see your warmer side? (Criterion 4)

### Example Response to Intermediate Patient Statement 3

Your mother made you constantly compare your level of success to your father's. (Criterion 1) So I can imagine that feeling any sense of not measuring up can feel unacceptable to you. (Criterion 2) But your letting me know of your jealousy, showing me how you really feel— even for a moment—was a real gift of trust and openness. (Criterion 3) What was it like letting us both see your authentic feelings in here just now? (Criterion 4)

### Example Response to Intermediate Patient Statement 4

I really appreciate your compassion and thoughtfulness toward me. It makes me feel much closer to you. (Criterion 3) I recognize that growing up your mother taught you to keep your real feelings toward others behind a wall of professionalism, (Criterion 1) but showing more of this softer side of you might help you feel more connected with others and vice versa. (Criterion 2) I know you want to move on to our agenda, but I'm wondering if we could pause for a moment—what was it like to let me see your compassionate side? (Criterion 4)

### Example Response to Intermediate Patient Statement 5

You seemed happy when you connected me to your dad. (Criterion 2) Then you seemed to disown that feeling of connection. I wonder if at times you had to disown your emotional ties to your father. (Criterion 1) Yet feeling connected to me—to our shared values—helps our work. (Criterion 3) Can you say how what I am saying strikes you? (Criterion 4)

## EXAMPLE RESPONSES TO ADVANCED-LEVEL PATIENT STATEMENTS FOR EXERCISE 12: THE CASE OF MR. JOHNSON

### Example Response to Advanced Patient Statement 1

Since you had to be so cautious around your father when you were growing up, (Criterion 1) I appreciate your being more direct with me. By telling me of your displeasure with my suggestion, (Criterion 2) we can take a look at it and see why it didn't sit right with you. (Criterion 3) How did you feel telling me you didn't like my suggestion? (Criterion 4)

### Example Response to Advanced Patient Statement 2

I realize that it might not be easy to tell me about difficulties parking in my neighborhood (Criterion 2) given that you grew up needing to be so quiet and meek around your father. (Criterion 1) But it really helps me understand what led to you being late for today's session. (Criterion 3) How was it for you to let me know about the parking difficulties near my office? (Criterion 4)

### Example Response to Advanced Patient Statement 3

As a kid, you couldn't point out your father's behavior without serious repercussions, (Criterion 1) so it's a shift for you to hold me accountable for not warning you about the medication side effects. (Criterion 2) Your direct question to me lets me know how I need to do a better job to meet your needs. (Criterion 3) What was it like for you to hold me accountable just then? (Criterion 4)

### Example Response to Advanced Patient Statement 4

Oh, I thought you were having difficulty telling me how you were feeling, not that you wanted to keep your feelings private. (Criterion 2) Now I understand, and we can move to a different topic if you like. Thank you for that. (Criterion 3) I want to honor your need to hold a boundary on your terms, which was something your father didn't let you do when you were young. (Criterion 1) I can imagine it wasn't easy to tell me straight out what you wanted. Is that right? (Criterion 4)

### Example Response to Advanced Patient Statement 5

I feel that you are frustrated with me. However, that seems dangerous to say since I might get angry at you, the way your father could. (Criterion 1) Yet you did comment, indirectly, on my seeming to favor "other patients." (Criterion 2) It was like you were dipping your toe in the water, letting me know you didn't appreciate my lateness. I am sorry I was late and appreciate your commenting. When I can hear all your feelings—especially your angry feelings—it helps me understand you better. (Criterion 3) How was it for you to show a bit of your frustration to me today? (Criterion 4)

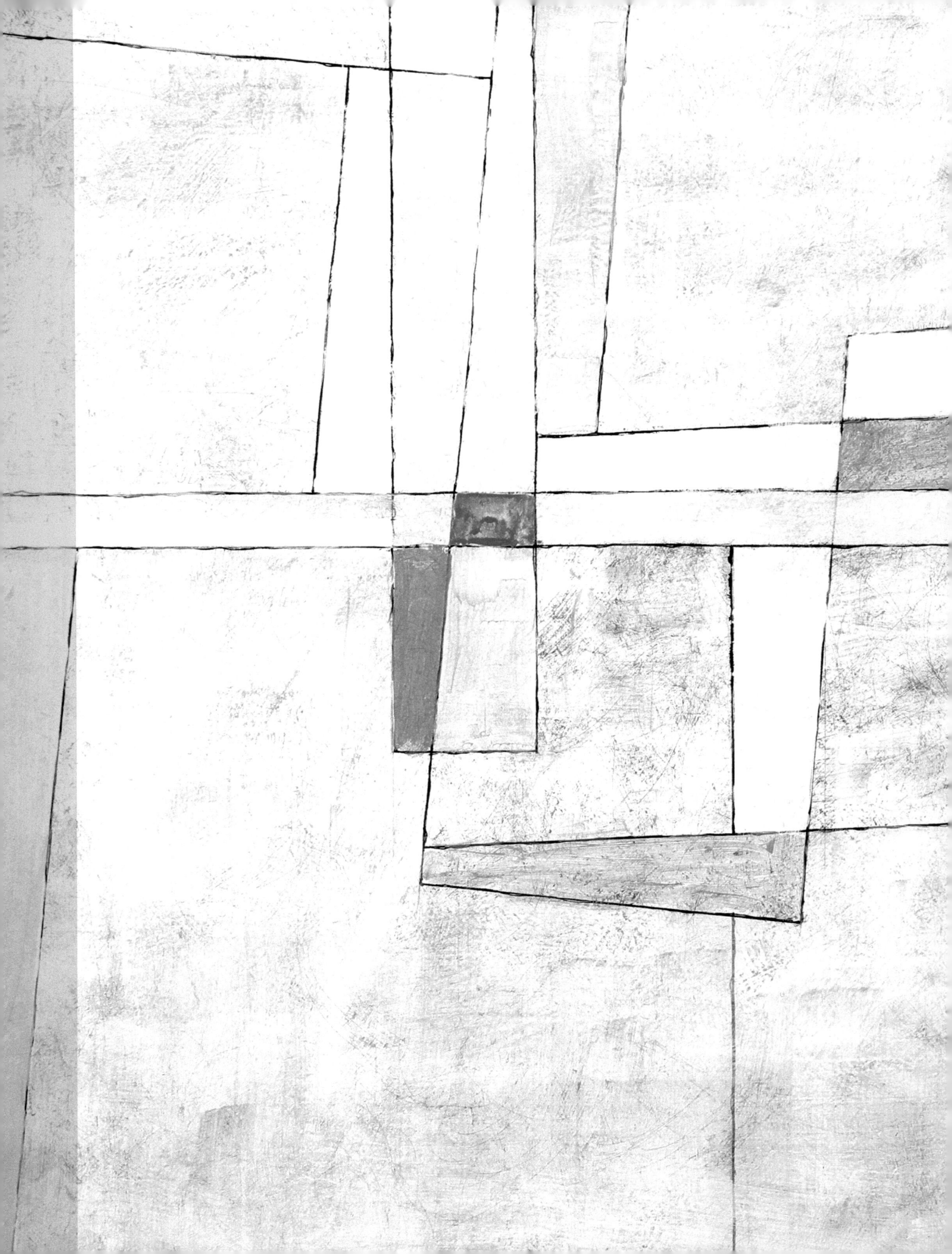

# Annotated Interpersonal–Psychodynamic Therapy Session Transcripts

## Practice Session Transcripts

It is now time to see how all the skills you have learned come together in the flow of actual sessions. This exercise presents transcripts from two therapy sessions conducted with the same patient—Ann Lee,[1] who was featured in Exercises 4, 9, 10, and 12. By using these transcripts, trainees can offer psychodynamic interventions in ways that simulate the complexity of actual therapy sessions.

In some respects, the conditions under which the sessions took place were unusual. The American Psychological Association (APA) invited the first author (H. L.) to record six sessions with someone seeking psychological help as part of APA's Psychotherapy in Six Sessions Video Series. All sessions (completed in 3 months in the summer of 2010) were done on a soundstage with bright lights and three camera operators. Each session was recorded in its entirety. Although the context of the sessions was unusual, the sessions were typical of the work conducted in Levenson's private office. In a companion book to the video series (Levenson, 2017), Levenson explained that the six-session limit imposed by APA "[was] not set up to be a complete brief dynamic therapy. . . . Nonetheless, I think the work effectively illustrates many of the concepts and interventions of a modern brief dynamic therapy" (p. 94).

These two sessions illustrate all 12 deliberate practice psychodynamic skills. However, they are valuable for several other reasons: (a) Videos of all six sessions and the first two sessions are commercially available; (b) immediately following each video session, the series editor interviews Dr. Levenson about her perspectives on the developing case; (c) there is a voiceover for all six sessions explicating the therapist's experience

---

1. Details about the patient have been changed to protect her confidentiality. Ann is based on the case of a real patient whose case has previously been discussed and published (Levenson, 2017). In addition, there is a video of all six sessions done with this patient that is commercially available (Levenson & Carlson, 2010), as well as a two-session version containing an interview with the first author (H. L.) discussing the case from a skills-based point of view (Levenson & Friedlander, in production). There have also been four published studies using the transcripts from the 2010 video that can be found in the references (Friedlander et al., 2018, 2020; Levenson, 2020; Levenson et al., 2020).

https://doi.org/10.1037/0000351-015

*Deliberate Practice in Psychodynamic Psychotherapy*, by H. Levenson, V. Gay, and J. L. Binder

with the patient minute by minute; (d) in the two-session video, there is a discussion of using deliberate practice in skill development; and (e) the sessions have been the focus of several published studies. In those studies, researchers analyzed the therapy in clinically rich ways (e.g., moment-to-moment coding to identify indicators of a corrective experience, noting verbal and emotion markers of shifts in the patient's "same old story," and observations of the patient's and therapist's behavioral contributions to the working alliance).

The two sessions provided in this exercise contain examples of common therapeutic factors (e.g., validation of the patient's perceptions), the specific skills of dynamic therapy (e.g., pointing out the patient's defenses), and the therapist's idiosyncratic style (e.g., repeating the patient's key words for emphasis). The first transcript reflects a typical first session in interpersonal–psychodynamic psychotherapy; the second transcript reflects a typical midphase session. Where possible, each therapist statement is annotated to indicate which psychodynamic skill from Exercises 1 through 12 is used. Trainees may use parts or all this exercise for practice. Appendix B includes a Deliberate Practice Diary Form that can be used to monitor trainees' experiences after performing this exercise (also available at the "Clinician and Practitioner Resources" tab online at https://www.apa.org/pubs/books/deliberate-practice-psychodynamic-psychotherapy).

## Instructions

As in most of the previous exercises, one trainee plays the patient while the other plays the therapist. As much as possible, the trainee who plays the patient should try to adopt an emotional tone like an actual patient. Before starting, both therapist and patient should read the entire transcript through on their own. The second time through, both partners can read aloud verbatim from the transcript with one trainee reading for the therapist and the other for the patient.

After two complete readings, partners can try it again—this time, the patient reads from the script while the therapist improvises the interventions. Trainees may also profit from reading some of the research or watching a video of the session to see how these 12 skills are woven into the fabric of psychodynamic therapy. They also may wish to get input from their professor or supervisor and go through the transcripts again.

### Note to Therapists

First, be aware of your countertransference, both complementary (e.g., how the patient's words and behavior pull or push you emotionally) and classical (e.g., is there something from your background that is triggered in the clinical exchange?). Second, be aware of your vocal quality, tone, and nonverbal behaviors when responding to a patient. Much of psychodynamic therapy has to do with how something is said (or not said). Throughout the transcripts, we have suggested a tone for some therapist responses alongside the skill itself. However, we encourage trainees to use whichever tone they think is best and most appropriate. Please note that there are several points in the transcript where the patient cries. At these points, the trainee playing the patient can express sad anguish but should not feel pressured to have to produce actual tears.

You will notice differences in the skills employed as the therapy progresses. Although some skills appear throughout treatment (e.g., Skill 1: Engaging in a Therapeutic Inquiry), advanced skills are more frequent in the later session. As you learn more about the patient, you can tailor your responses to the patient's personality and attachment style. And as the dynamics in the therapeutic relationship unfold, you can draw on other skills to attune to the patient better and repair any ruptures in the working alliance. In fact, over time, with more and more deliberate practice, your interventions should become more responsive to a variety of factors in the treatment.

## Annotated Psychodynamic Therapy Transcript 1: Session 1

**THERAPIST 1:** Well, hi, Ann, I'm Hanna Levenson. (Hi, Hanna.) And I really appreciate you being here today. I know this is a kind of strange way to (Right.) start off an intimate discussion with lights and cameras and so forth, but they will fade. My experience is they'll fade into the background as you and I kind of get into the reason you're here today. (OK.) We'll have 45 minutes to meet today and if it looks like I can be of help to you then we'll be able to meet another five times. (Oh, great!) I really don't know anything about you, or what brings you here. So maybe you can fill me in. (Skill 6: Introducing the Rationale for Treatment)

**PATIENT 1:** [*said in a run-on, cheerful manner with a big smile*] Well, I am currently a student at W. University. I'm going for my master's in public health. (Oh.) So when I got the call about this, I was really excited. Wanted to see how this all worked so. And so I'm going full time for that and that requires two summer classes and I'm kind of a little bit stressed about that right now. So basically full time for the next 2 years. (Wow!) It's getting intense, but it's good to—I want to get it done so I can go on to my PhD like you have. So, I'm really excited. (Well, terrific.) And then I currently work at a real estate office, you know, just as part time to have some income coming in and that's been kind of stressful too. Just a lot of different things happening at work. We've had a few people leave and you know, I'm part time but I'm really working a full-time schedule and doing school. (Wow.) So it's just a lot of work. So I'm kind of dealing with that right now. And then in the meantime I have a boyfriend. He lives about an hour from here. So about an hour from my house. And that's a little stressful just getting there and back and just trying to fit everything into my schedule so. That's the big three main issues I think that are affecting . . . are big issues in my life right now.

**THERAPIST 2:** [*soft, solid tone*] Right. So you're going to school full-time. You've almost got a full-time job and you've got a full-time relationship. (Skill 10: Case Formulation—Actions of the Self; Skill 2: Being Aware of Countertransference Reactions; <u>her bubbly presentation makes me wonder about the absence of her pain</u>.)

**PATIENT 2:** Right. Yes, it's a lot of full-time stuff. (Sounds like it.) There's not enough hours in the day. So, just dealing with that.

**THERAPIST 3:** And is there something in particular in trying to juggle all of that that concerns you? (Skill 1: Engaging in a Therapeutic Inquiry—Clarification of Details; Skill 2: Being Aware of Countertransference Reactions—<u>I am bothered by her eager, accommodating, smiling mode that does not match her words</u>.)

**PATIENT 3:** Just the stress level. I have a really, I don't think I get stressed out too easily, but I feel like my stress level is just getting higher and higher, especially since the summer semester is almost over. So all the projects are coming due and you know the papers and then work keeps getting crazy. So it's just my stress level is going up and getting pretty a lot of anxiety you know over it. Because I'm in a class where we have to present in front of the class so. So I mean I like doing that but you know, there's always anxiety with that when you're in front of a bunch of people and so that's, I think it's my anxiety level.

**THERAPIST 4:** Right. And when you get really anxious Ann, what goes on for you? What, how does that manifest itself? How do you feel at, what happens? (Skill 1: Engaging in a Therapeutic Inquiry—Clarification of Details and Implications; Skill 2: Being Aware of Countertransference Reactions—I am aware of my own personal countertransference of performance anxiety caused by being in front of cameras and lights and wanting to do my best for the commercial video recording.)

**PATIENT 4:** Well, I definitely feel my heart racing. I'll get, especially if, I tend to think a lot in my head. Like I drive a lot with the hour drive everywhere it seems like and I'll think about what to do next week or what I have to, I have going on in an hour or when I need to do this, when I need to do that. So it just gets me all tense and you know hard, it's not hard to breathe but you know, breathing heavier and I just notice that I'm getting all tense and not like tearing up or anything, but just a little overwhelmed. So that way and then my thoughts start racing about am I going to get this done? I have no choice. I have no time you know. And then you know, just it's just anxiety I guess. A little.

**THERAPIST 5:** So you feel it in your body. Your heart starts pumping and then you also feel it in your mind. You start thinking about all these thoughts and then they make you feel more anxious and you have more thoughts and more heart pumping and. (Skill 10: Case Formulation—Introject)

**PATIENT 5:** Right and it just doesn't, it's a vicious circle. (Yeah, yeah.) Especially I notice when I try to lay down and sleep. I have a hard time actually falling asleep because I'm thinking about what's coming, what I have due even the next day.

**THERAPIST 6:** Yeah, so your sleep is being affected by this as well? (Skill 1: Engaging in a Therapeutic Inquiry—Clarification of Details)

**PATIENT 6:** Yeah. Yeah, it's, it's, I have a hard time falling asleep and then I tend to wake up in the night. Oh, I wake up at least three times with just, I freak out because I think I missed my alarm. But I'll wake up at like 3 o'clock in the morning and be like oh my god, did I miss my alarm? Because at the real estate office, you have to be there exactly when it opens; then if I'm not there then I'm really letting someone down and I can't do it. That's just how I am. So I wake up about three times during the night and it's sometimes more depending on where I'm at. If I'm staying at my boyfriend's, probably more, just because he, his alarm is not dependable so I have to put my alarm on my phone and you know, it's just, I just got to make sure I get where I'm trying to get so.

**THERAPIST 7:** Yeah, so you've got a sleep deficit going here too. (Yeah.) Yes? (Yeah.) Are you tired when you wake up in the morning or? (Skill 1: Engaging in a Therapeutic Inquiry—Clarification of Details)

**PATIENT 7:** I'm more like got to go, got to go, got to go.

**THERAPIST 8:** I see, so that energy. (Skill 1: Engaging in a Therapeutic Inquiry—Clarification of Details)

**PATIENT 8:** And it's heightened up, it's keyed up. So and then I noticed that I do wake up tired but then I notice a time and I'm done like you know got to go you know, there's no time to be tired. Just deal with it and go. So it's, it's stressful as my life usually is.

**THERAPIST 9:** Yeah, it's been like this not just recently but in the past too or? (Skill 1: Engaging in a Therapeutic Inquiry—Clarification of Details)

**PATIENT 9:** No, yeah, I, even when I was younger we were always, I was in like four or five different sports, I you know, we'd have school, then homework, basically we'd go wake up, school, get out early from school so you could go to practice, I did swim practice and then that was four hours and then come home, eat three bowls of cereal, do homework and go to bed. Because that's the only time I would eat would be when like lunch and then until then. So, that's been my life since I can even remember. So it's pretty . . . it's normal but lately the sleeping, usually I don't have that, that freak out of the three times waking up, that's been more recently. (I see.) So but the whole being on the go, it's kind of how I am. But the stress is just accumulating where I'm having a hard time dealing with it, I think.

**THERAPIST 10:** Right, so kind of characterologically you're always on the go. You've got high energy but right now it's turning more to anxiety. (Skill 1: Engaging in a Therapeutic Inquiry—Implications)

**PATIENT 10:** Right, it's, it's turning to something that I haven't really dealt with, at least, it's getting more hard to deal with so.

**THERAPIST 11:** And are there ways you've tried to deal with this anxiety? (Skill 1: Engaging in a Therapeutic Inquiry—Clarification of Details)

**PATIENT 11:** [*talking breathlessly, smiling*] Yeah. I do a lot of working out. I basically changed my eating patterns; I try and work out every day if I can. You know, I try for 5 days, just because it's something that you know, brings my stress level down and something and I find that when I'm working out I'm not really stressing. I'm thinking about the movements I'm making and it's very, it's therapeutic for me because you know, I'm not all keyed up. I'm thinking about what's going on in my life you know. (Right.) And how I can get myself stronger. So and I recently changed my eating patterns as I said. I'm on the Kellogg Diet. It's working, it's really, I like it. I mean I used you know, be the one that ate all the cheeseburgers and all that and now I just refrain from it. It's just not as important and I find myself craving better foods for myself because I have taken on this challenge so. So that's a positive in light of the stress, but that's a positive I think I've done for the coping. (Right.) And then I wanted to try and do some talk therapy. And that's why I'm really here today.

**THERAPIST 12:** [*smiling*] OK, well great. I think you've, you've kind of laid it all out there. (Yeah.) Very succinctly and straightforward there. I appreciate that and it's wonderful that you found exercise to be of help coping with anxiety. Because that's one of the ways that's really been proven to, to be extremely helpful. What kind of exercise do you do? (Skill 2: Being Aware of Countertransference Reactions—<u>I am pulled in two different directions; I have an urge to relax because she has such a pleasant, accommodating demeanor but also an urge to shake her and tell her to slow down and be real</u>.)

**PATIENT 12:** Well, I have like a ritual kind of things where I'll do the same thing. I'll go, I'll run for a bit but doing interval training because it's better for weight loss they say. And then I'll either do some arm workout or some leg work depending on you know, every other day you want to do every other so you don't need to do it every day. (Right.) And I'll try and do like ab work. Like on the floor do some crunches and stuff. At least three times a week so. (Yeah.) I like to mix it up. I like to get new ideas, so I'm always you know, looking for ideas.

**THERAPIST 13:** So you're what—about an hour working out? (Skill 1: Engaging in a Therapeutic Inquiry—Clarification of Details)

**PATIENT 13:** No.

**THERAPIST 14:** No? (Skill 1: Engaging in a Therapeutic Inquiry—Clarification of Details)

**PATIENT 14:** If I'm in my, if I've got to go it's an hour, but usually around an hour and a half to two, you know.

**THERAPIST 15:** You're really committed to it. (Skill 10: Case Formulation—Actions of the Self)

**PATIENT 15:** Yes. I commit. When I do something, I'm going to do it all the way or it's just not, it's just not worth my time, you know what I mean? It's just how I was raised. That's why I won't, that's probably why I won't stop at my masters, that's why I want to keep going. Because first of all, I know I won't go back and second of all, it's really what I want and I know that I want it. So I'm just going to deal with what I've got to do and get it done.

**THERAPIST 16:** Are you concerned about your weight? (Skill 1: Engaging in a Therapeutic Inquiry—Implications)

**PATIENT 16:** No, yes and no. My mom's a little worried about it. She thinks I'm a little anal about it, but I think it's better that I am concerned about it than not concerned about it. Because as soon as you slip off that slippery slope it's, it's going to come back and I've lost about 20 pounds from before I decided to you know, step up and do some exercising and I really don't want it to come back and I think I'm definitely have a fear about it coming back. So I could, some people would be like yeah you've got a problem. But it's just the way my mind works and I sound like I obsess, but it's always in my mind. Like with everything else. It's always right there and that's, I guess it's adding to what my stress levels at too so.

**THERAPIST 17:** Like to be mindful about exercising and what you're eating and (Yeah.) you don't want the weight to come back on. (Skill 10: Case Formulation—Introject)

**PATIENT 17:** Yeah, I know, that's a very scary thought is that the weight will come back. Not that I was heavy before, but that I just wasn't, I wasn't comfortable. You know, sometimes your pants are a little tighter and it just doesn't make anyone, at least personally I don't think it would make you feel to have to go buy new pants because you've gained 20 pounds. (Right, right.) So it feels great for me I guess, to be able to go and be like, oh I'm a size smaller. Like I haven't really had that before. So, it's a good feeling.

**THERAPIST 18:** Do you want to lose some more weight, or do you like the way you are now? (Skill 1: Engaging in a Therapeutic Inquiry—Implications; Skill 2: Being Aware of Countertransference Reactions—<u>I can feel myself getting concerned that Ann might have an eating disorder, which may have implications for her appropriateness for this demonstration video.</u>)

**PATIENT 18:** [*laughing*] I think, I probably would like to lose a little bit more weight, but not, not to the fact where you can see like bones. I want to be muscular. I want to be toned. That's my real goal. Is not to basically, not even lose weight but like to tone what I have. Because you have to have some body, a little bit of body fat on you to have muscle [*she demonstrates by showing her biceps.*] (Right, right.) So that's really my goal. (Right.) So I'm not really looking to lose weight as much as I'm looking to gain muscle which is important to me so.

**THERAPIST 19:** Sounds like feeling strong and comfortable in your own skin is very important to you right now. (Exercise 8: Using Metaphors) (Right, yeah.) So most of your life were you the 20 pounds heavier or have you gone up and down or?

**PATIENT 19:** It's been, when I was doing swimming competitively, I was always the heavier one. Not, just because I was so much heavier than everybody else. (I see.) There I was just a few pounds heavier and they were all like really skinny you know, if you seen a swim team. (Yeah.) So I really had the disadvantage because I was you know, I hit puberty and then I had started developing and gaining more weight. So I don't think I've had a weight problem but I've fluctuated. I mean sometimes you're at this point in your life and then you weigh this and then now I've just decided I'm going to take control of that. I'm not going to let, I'm going to take control over it. That was the big thing.

**THERAPIST 20:** It sounds like there are a number of areas in your life where you're kind of taking control. (Yes.) Is that right? (Skill 10: Case Formulation—Actions of the Self)

**PATIENT 20:** Yes. I guess others would say I'm a control freak.

**THERAPIST 21:** Oh really? (Skill 1: Engaging in a Therapeutic Inquiry—Clarification of Details)

**PATIENT 21:** Yes, if they put it, I like the things how I like them and it's not like if you don't do it my way I see it as a problem, but if I can kind of tell you why I do it my way and you can respect that I do it my way, then we're not going to have any problem. I mean I want to hear your way. Maybe I can fix my way. Maybe I can make improvement but it's just important for me to be able to be an overall strong person. That's and it's strong and independent and in all aspects.

**THERAPIST 22:** Where did you learn this? (Skill 10: Case Formulation—Acts of Others and Introject)

**PATIENT 22:** [*laughing*] I don't know I just, I guess I get it from my dad. He's very much you know, I want to get you the education, I want you to be able to support yourself. So I guess I just developed it from him.

**THERAPIST 23:** He's kind of a role model for you? (Skill 10: Case Formulation—Acts of Others and Introject)

**PATIENT 23:** Yes. Absolutely. He's, he's a great person. He works every day. He's a contractor, so I know, he gets up at 4 o'clock in the morning, works until 3 and then he coaches volleyball. Like my sister plays right now for her university She's, she's a great, great athlete. She is their star player. So my dad actually coaches a bunch of the kids around the neighborhood and then he does that until 9 o'clock and then he goes to bed. So I, my life is busy, but his life is crazy busy. Because then on the weekends you know, he's got tournaments with my sister and so you know, I guess I aspire to have that busy life. To never have a dull moment so.

**THERAPIST 24:** Wow. How does your mother cope with all that? (Skill 10: Case Formulation—Acts of Others and Introject)

**PATIENT 24:** She's as much a freak about volleyball as anybody so. (I see.) So, she gets involved. She goes to all the games. Never missed a tournament and she doesn't get involved in the coaching because you know, two heads butting there, they don't even get involved there. But she goes to the game, she participates, she's involved in all the activities and stuff.

**THERAPIST 25:** So she's another go, go, go person? (Skill 10: Case Formulation—Acts of Others and Introject)

**PATIENT 25:** Yes. Yeah, that's just, we just lucked out that everybody is like that.

**THERAPIST 26:** Sounds like there are some other siblings too? (Skill 1: Engaging in a Therapeutic Inquiry—Clarification of Details; Skill 10: Case Formulation—Acts of Others and Introject)

**PATIENT 26:** Yes, I have a sister and she, not so much a go, go, go girl. She's off, because this is her first semester. She, first year at her university and now she's home. So she's taking it slow and you know, practicing but sleeping in all the time. God, I wish I could have that but you know, at the same time I would be stir crazy. But she's, she's a great athlete and I respect her for what she's doing. It's a full-time job. Her during the school year also is like get up at 5, go work out, go to class, work out and do volleyball in the afternoon. It's just crazy and. She's got an amazing head on her shoulders to be able to do that as a freshman.

**THERAPIST 27:** Well, it sounds like an incredible family that you came from. Just really hardworking, high-energy people. (Skill 10: Case Formulation—Acts of Others and Introject)

**PATIENT 27:** Oh yeah. Well, we're all deficient in some ways, but I think we work well together, and I think that's important to be able to recognize your strengths and your weaknesses to be able to you know, deal with what you're doing and get where you want to go so.

**THERAPIST 28:** Was there anything about your childhood that you wish there would have been or been less of or is there anything looking back that? (Skill 10: Case Formulation—Actions of the Self)

**PATIENT 28:** Less of or more? (Yeah.) I wish I would have had more friends. Because we, we moved when I was younger. I had a lot of friends when I was like I don't know, second or third grade and then I moved and then it just got harder. Because you know, the cliques are already formed. (Yeah.) That's such, even that young age and even to be a new person in a new school is hard. (Right.) And then my life revolved around swimming. So I didn't have, when people were out playing, I was at the pool. So that would be and then you know, I struggled all through high school with you know, friends were difficult, a difficult area for me and but, now I think, I think now I have pretty much come to understand that I basically chose not to have any friends. Through, through sports and you know, it just was so hard for me I think.

**THERAPIST 29:** Hard you mention time wise. (Yes.) And so forth. But was it hard in other ways or just . . .? (Skill 1: Engaging in a Therapeutic Inquiry—Clarification of Details; Skill 10: Case Formulation—Introject)

**PATIENT 29:** I don't know. (You mentioned.) I just, sometimes the way I'm controlling and I try not to but you know, sometimes I guess I turn people off and I'll be very blunt with you. I'll tell you what I think and some people don't like that and I try and respect you know, my goal is to respect your boundaries but I want you to respect mine and understand that I have things I want to say and that I have a lot I want to do in my life and if you can't support me or if you can't understand that then maybe it's not meant to be. (Right. Right.) So my life is crazy enough as it is with as many friends as I have now. So I couldn't imagine having more.

**THERAPIST 30:** So, there are friends in your life now? (Skill 10: Case Formulation—Acts of Others)

**PATIENT 30:** Yes. Basically through my boyfriend. He is a very social person. He has, he's got different friends and oh, he's the most social person I know. And you know, I've just developed friendships through him. (All right.) And I'm happy about that. I mean, that, I don't need, I don't need any more than that. I mean we all go out and we all hang out and I don't need to you know, go out and look for friends anymore. I think I could have used it when I was in high school. So (Right, right.) even in college it was, it was a struggle there.

**THERAPIST 31:** [*slow, empathic voice*] It was, in college, a struggle to have friends. (Skill 3: Deepening Emotional Experience—Matching Tone to Underlying Emotion; Skill 10: Case Formulation—Actions of the Self and Acts of Others)

**PATIENT 31:** Yeah, I went away for my first semester to college, and that was, that was probably one of the worst years for me. I would stay in my room, basically I, what would happen was, my sleep pattern was completely reversed. I would stay up all night, go to class, sleep the rest of the day. It was completely backwards. I don't know how I managed to do that, but I did. But my roommate my first semester, she left after a month, so I was basically in there alone she left after a month, so I was basically in there alone and then my second semester, I knew the girl because I had joined, eventually I joined a cheerleading squad that they had there and that was a really, a great thing for me to do. Because it pulled me out of that a little bit, but I still had that pattern and that girl, she, she was just never there. She had, you know, she had her own friends and I didn't expect her to stay and she didn't expect me to want her to stay. So, my sleep pattern was completely reversed and it was crazy. But because I wasn't partying all night, I was just, I like to knit, so I was knitting and making things and I was on the computer playing games and doing homework. So, that was just a struggle for me and that's why I came home after that year and then I started at W. University.

**THERAPIST 32:** And it was a struggle because you were kind of more alone than you would have liked? (Skill 3: Deepening Emotional Experience—Vivid Language; Skill 10: Case Formulation—Actions of the Self and Acts of Others)

**PATIENT 32:** Absolutely. Yeah. Because the way that they had it set up it was like an L-shape or it was like, it was kind of like a C-shape I guess and I was on this end and everyone else was kind of you know, even like the dorm situation there were more girls that would get together on this side but I was left, you know, no one would even know I was there. Like I didn't know any of the girls' names. Not and it was probably partially my fault because when they would go out and do things I didn't want to or didn't know about them. Because I would seclude myself in there. So I guess that would be one of my bigger struggles. But when I came home it was much better. Not the friend situation because I'd stay at home and I would just commute to school. (I see.) But I, I think I liked it better being at home. I'm a very homebody person. That's just how I am.

**THERAPIST 33:** So now through your boyfriend you've got as many friends (I've got a lot of friends. Yeah.) as you need. (Skill 10: Case Formulation—Acts of Others and Actions of the Self)

**PATIENT 33:** Yeah, so I feel he's definitely helped me in that. Even just to open out of my shell. Because I've always been the kind of shy, shy person. You wouldn't think so because I can talk a lot, but I've been . . .

**THERAPIST 34:** But down deep . . . (Skill 5: Pointing Out Defenses)

**PATIENT 34:** But even around new people. Like even around new people I get really, I don't know what they're thinking, I don't know what's going on, so it just takes a little while for me to open up. I think it's just a defense mechanism for all the times that you know, you get hurt by people and it just.

**THERAPIST 35:** [*said softly and slowly while leaning forward and looking into Ann's eyes*] You've gotten hurt. (Skill 3: Deepening Emotional Experience—Matching Tone to Underlying Emotion)

**PATIENT 35:** Yeah. Well yeah, everyone, I think everyone has at least in some form.

**THERAPIST 36:** Is there an incident that kind of (Comes to mind?) comes to mind? About getting hurt and how you learned how to pull back a bit and check things out a bit more and also have a lot going on just in your own personal life. (Right.) Is there an incident that would kind of give me a sense about what that might have been like for you? (Skill 1: Engaging in a Therapeutic Inquiry—Clarification of Details)

**PATIENT 36:** Yeah absolutely. There are a few, but the one that really stands out, my best friends, OK, we moved three times but we moved into a new neighborhood and my best friends, I knew her for like 6 or 7 years and we just started growing apart at high school and I would keep trying to reconnect with her, but she would keep shutting me down and she ended up getting into drugs and things. So I was, I'm kind of glad that we ended up separating, but I was so close to her. I, you know, I was just, it was just really a strong connection. (Yeah.) But it just faded and that, that really hurt me. Because she didn't want, she didn't want to, she didn't want to connect with me.

**THERAPIST 37:** [*slowly and softly*] So that was painful because you kept going to her. (Yes.) You felt very close to her and you kept getting rejected and that. (Skill 3: Deepening Emotional Experience—Matching Tone to Underlying Emotion; Skill 10: Case Formulation—Actions of the Self and Acts of Others)

**PATIENT 37:** Yeah, absolutely. Yeah, she, she just wasn't having it. She was in a different place. I was all school, all like you know you can get your life around, but I didn't want to preach to her but I wanted to make sure that she knows that you know, there are better things out there than to go out and party and get drunk all the time. I mean, I just, I didn't have a drink until I was 21 personally. I just didn't want one. I was centered, I have always been focused like that, so I didn't understand her frame of mind. (Right.) Where she would need a drink. (Right.) But she, she was actually adopted, so I can now looking back I can be like wow, she obviously had some issues that I couldn't comprehend at the time. But it just still you know.

**THERAPIST 38:** And were you kind of blunt with her like you were telling me here without saying, you know, you can't keep doing this? (Skill 10: Case Formulation—Actions of the Self; Skill 2: Being Aware of Countertransference Reactions—earlier Ann had mentioned that she was an independent person who was blunt with others, which didn't ring true to me, given her pleasing presentation; so I questioned her behavior in light of the details of the situation.)

**PATIENT 38:** I don't think I was. Because with her I acted, I wanted her to be my friend. (I see.) So I would kind of just be, I guess I would tell her you know, do we really have to go out. Because I would go with her. I think I went with her a couple times and she was drinking because I would drive her home and I just, because I would drive her home and

I just, I tried to comfort her and you know, it just wasn't. She just kept pushing me away and that's what she did with everybody in her life so.

**THERAPIST 39:** [*slowly and softly while looking into Ann's eyes*] But that really hurt you. (Yeah.) And somewhere you kind of vowed, I'm not going to get myself in this kind of position over and over again. (Right.) Because it really hurt. (Skill 3: Deepening Emotional Experience—"I" Statements and Matching Tone to Underlying Emotion)

**PATIENT 39:** And plus I think it really hurt because I wasn't getting my needs met. She wasn't reciprocating, so I have a hard time with that. I think when I try and make friends now, I put all this effort into it you know. I will go out of my way. I'll find things or make ideas and suggestions or something. Thinking that if I'm putting all this effort, they'll give me something. But I'm just always on the defense. And I don't feel like, sometimes I don't feel like I'm getting anything back.

**THERAPIST 40:** Wow. (So . . .) That can also be very dismaying. (Skill 3: Deepening Emotional Experience—Vivid Language)

**PATIENT 40:** Yes. (Yeah.) It's frustrating because I want them to you know, you've got to meet somewhere and I feel like I'm always the one giving and it just is not, it's upsetting.

**THERAPIST 41:** And then does this get played out at all with your boyfriend? (Skill 10: Case Formulation—Expectations of Others and Acts of Others)

**PATIENT 41:** [*smiling*] Absolutely.

**THERAPIST 42:** Yeah? (Skill 1: Engaging in a Therapeutic Inquiry—Clarification of Details)

**PATIENT 42:** Yeah. Because I'm the one I guess, in the relationship that will go, I'll go every time to his house. (Oh.) Which is a good thing and a bad thing. I still live at home with my parents, so if he came up here, we really wouldn't have much to do. Because all of his friends are down there and you know we have mutual friends. I don't really have any friends up here. (Right.) So, we have more things to do if I'm at his house, then if he comes up to me. But I just wish that he would once in a while, take the initiative, come see me. When it's not convenient for him. (Right.) Because he'll come see me when he's, because he is in an apprenticeship and it's by my house, but he'll only come see me when they, on the days he goes to his apprenticeship. [*voice cracks, tearing up*] Which is kind of crappy because I'll come see him no matter what.

**THERAPIST 43:** [*slowly and softly*] So Ann, what's going on inside for you right now? I see something's going on. (Skill 3: Deepening Emotional Experience—Matching Tone to Underlying Emotion)

**PATIENT 43:** [*tearing up*] Just upsetting.

**THERAPIST 44:** [*softly, slowly, and reassuringly*] Yeah? Yeah, I can see that on your face. Yeah. (Skill 3: Deepening Emotional Experience—Matching Tone to Underlying Emotion)

**PATIENT 44:** [*sobbing*] I'm just frustrated. (OK.) Sorry.

**THERAPIST 45:** [*softly and slowly*] It's all right. No, this hurts. I can see that. It's like, "Why, why isn't he going out of his way for me? I go out of my way for him, why isn't he giving when it's not convenient?" This is of concern to you. (Skill 2: Being Aware of Counter-transference Reactions—<u>my countertransference has shifted from irritated/confused to deeply empathic and moved by her pain</u>; Skill 3: Deepening Emotional Experience—"I" Statements; Skill 10: Case Formulation—Actions of the Self and Acts of Others)

**PATIENT 45:** It's like what I said about the relationships with friends. [*sobbing deeply*] I give and I give and [*sounding angry*] I want something back.

**THERAPIST 46:** Yes. Does he know how much this hurts you? No. You've kind of kept that from him? (Skill 10: Case Formulation—Actions of the Self and Acts of Others)

**PATIENT 46:** I'm scared.

**THERAPIST 47:** Tell me about it. (Skill 1: Engaging in a Therapeutic Inquiry—Implications; Skill 10: Case Formulation—Actions of the Self)

**PATIENT 47:** I, I'm afraid he'll leave. I'll say my needs and he'll leave. It scares me because I just don't think I can find anyone else and I don't want to. It just terrifies me and I don't, I guess what I do which is bad, because I guess I enable. Because I don't, I don't bring it up. I don't show that it hurts me in real ways. Like tell him. I'm more subtle about it. (Yeah.) And I know that I can't expect him to read my mind, but at the same time I wish he would see you know, all the effort I put in and respect, respect it. I try really hard and that I love him and I want him to do the same. Just meet me halfway. Because I feel like I just give and I give and I have nothing left.

**THERAPIST 48:** [*softly*] Wow. Who would know that there's all this pain underneath going on for you. (Skill 3: Deepening Emotional Experience—Matching Tone to Underlying Emotion) I can really appreciate that you feel in such a bind. (Skill 3: Deepening Emotional Experience—Vivid Language)

**PATIENT 48:** [*nods*] I do and you know, I'm just struggling between telling him and not telling him and I want to tell him but I'm you know, I'm scared.

**THERAPIST 49:** You're scared. It sounds like somehow you don't believe it that you'd be enough. You know, that he really just loves the you that's the giving, giving, giving? (Skill 10: Case Formulation—Introject)

**PATIENT 49:** Yes. Absolutely. I think I'm not, I have to keep giving to make sure I'm enough for him. I absolutely feel that way and I think about that all the time and I'll cry and just cry about it and it's just frustrating because I know what to do. I'm a very, you know, goal-oriented person. (Yes.) I know what I have to do. I just don't know if I can do it and if I can, if it would, if he would leave.

**THERAPIST 50:** When you say you know what you have to do, what do you know? What is that? (Skill 1: Engaging in a Therapeutic Inquiry—Implications)

**PATIENT 50:** [*sadly*] I have to tell him. I have to tell him that it's really hurting me that he's doing this [*with resigned tone*] and he's not doing it on purpose, he just doesn't know. And you know, I understand, his life is just as stressful as mine, but I want him to know that I try really hard and I just want him to try hard too. And it doesn't mean buying me things. Like he'll sometimes say that, I don't buy you anything. [*heartfelt*] I don't want anything. I want you. (Right.) I want you to come you know, to help me, to understand what I'm going through [*angry*] and not always talk about you. I don't want to always talk about you! [*sadly*] I have things I want to say but I'm sometimes scared to say it because he doesn't like confrontation or you know, getting angry at each other or fighting and I don't blame him. I don't like fighting either but I think if you keep it inside it will make the fight even worse and I'll end up yelling at him for things that aren't what I'm really feeling. You know, to get out what I'm feeling through something else.

**THERAPIST 51:** Has that happened where you might end up in an argument about something that really isn't the issue because you're not talking about? (Skill 1: Engaging in a Therapeutic Inquiry—Implications)

**PATIENT 51:** [*interrupting*] Yes. I've noticed lately I've been very irritable with him. (Yeah.) Just in general. Like I just can't even be around him. I have a hard time being around him because I'm just whoa, I'm going to blow up or something. Not on purpose and I'm not mad at him, I'm just mad that I can't say it. I can't show him that I'm this upset. That his actions affect me in more ways that he can even imagine. And that he puts me on the back burner and that really hurts.

**THERAPIST 52:** Can you give me an example of like how he puts you on the back burner? I know you talked about when he comes and visits it's only when it's kind of convenient. (Skill 10: Case Formulation—Acts of Others)

**PATIENT 52:** Only when it's convenient.

**THERAPIST 53:** Are there other examples that kind of go along with this back burner business? (Skill 10: Case Formulation—Acts of Others)

**PATIENT 53:** Right, yeah. (Yeah.) Even I think last weekend, I stayed at his house and when I stay it's because I want to see him. And this has happened on multiple occasions. I left to go work out like I usually do and I came back and it was about like 2 o'clock and he usually does stuff around the house. Well he went to his friend's house and they have a farm and they work on cars and I understand that. He likes to work on cars. But he didn't come home until about 8 o'clock at night. (Oh, wow.) So I was there all by myself just watching TV. I didn't have anything to do. I wanted to see him. And that has happened on multiple occasions.

**THERAPIST 54:** On multiple occasions. So you're traveling an hour to see him and then you're alone there most of the day, and it's happened several times. (Skill 3: Deepening Emotional Experience—Vivid Language; Skill 10: Case Formulation—Actions of the Self and Acts of Others)

**PATIENT 54:** Yes. Oh, on more times than I can even count. I'll come over for a weekend and I'll see him for an hour.

**THERAPIST 55:** How do you understand this? How do you make sense of this? Because obviously you've thought a lot about it. (Skill 1: Engaging in a Therapeutic Inquiry—Comprehension)

**PATIENT 55:** Yes, I have. I make sense of it because I guess I rationalize his busy life and I say you know what, I know he's got stuff going on and I understand that you know, he wants to go hang out with the guys and I understand that and I guess I just accept it as me being selfless again. Me being putting up with it. (I see.) I drove an hour to see you, you don't want to see me evidently, so I guess I will give up my time and stay there and then you can leave.

**THERAPIST 56:** So, you see you rationalize his behavior. So, it makes it sound like you don't fully believe when you tell yourself that story. (Skill 5: Pointing Out Defenses)

**PATIENT 56:** I, no, not at all. (Yeah.) I, I mean there are some instances where he's working on a Saturday and I'm over there waiting for him, I understand that. You're making money. You're trying to pay off your house. I understand that. That's not a problem and I understood that going into it. I'll come over on the weekend knowing he has to work on

Saturday, I don't have a problem with that. My problem is that I come over to see you, you don't respect the fact that I drive an hour and I have to drive an hour back, sometimes at 5 o'clock in the morning to drive an hour back, sometimes at 5 o'clock in the morning so I can get to work on time and you don't respect that I want to spend time with you. Even if we're with friends, he just leaves me. There was one time, he was drunk and we were at his friend's house and he went with this other friend that I really do not like. Whole history with him and we're not taking that. But I bottom line is I really don't like him because he turns into a different person when he's with this guy. And I was at the friend's house. I don't drink all that often and wasn't drinking then. He left me to go to a bar. He just left me at the house and went to the bar and hung out with this guy. And he ironically, earlier in the night before he was completely drunk, he's like I would never leave you anywhere. I wouldn't do that to you. And so I went with them because you know, they'd been drinking and I had to drive. And so we went over to the house and then he proceeds to leave me. So I thought that was highly ironic and highly, it was funny but it was like hurt funny. Like I can't believe you told me this and then you go ahead and do that.

**THERAPIST 57:** So have you talked to him about this incident at all? (Skill 5: Pointing Out Defenses; Skill 10: Case Formulation—Actions of the Self)

**PATIENT 57:** [*nervously rubbing her lip*] I talked to him the next day, but he didn't remember it.

**THERAPIST 58:** What had happened? (Skill 1: Engaging in a Therapeutic Inquiry—Clarification of Details)

**PATIENT 58:** He didn't remember leaving me. I guess he thought we were going to meet him over there or something. So he just brushed it off. I cried that whole night because he was drunk the whole night. He basically passed out in the car. I cried the whole way, the way we went home.

**THERAPIST 59:** But he doesn't know that you're crying the whole night. He doesn't know how you're feeling so slighted by his behavior. He doesn't know this because (Doesn't know.) because you fear . . .? (Skill 3: Deepening Emotional Experience—Vivid Language; Skill 5: Pointing Out Defenses; Skill 10: Case Formulation—Actions of the Self and Expectations of Others)

**PATIENT 59:** Telling him.

**THERAPIST 60:** If you tell him he would say, "Who needs you. (Right.) If you're going to complain or if you need something from me, who needs you?" (Skill 10: Case Formulation—Acts of Others)

**PATIENT 60:** Yeah, right. He's blatantly said to me, "I don't need a clingy girlfriend" or things like that. Like I'm independent he says, you know, "I don't need a girlfriend." And I know the way he meant it was like you know, I need my space. [*voice trembling, on the verge of tears*] But the way he said it was just like, hurt so bad. Just because then why am I here if you don't want me to be here? [*starts crying*] I want to be here but if you don't want me to be here, I won't be here.

**THERAPIST 61:** [*concerned voice*] And this must be even more painful because you've led your life kind of being very into yourself and even when you, that painful time when you first went away to school, you crocheted, you were into the computer games and you remember back to that friend you know, that childhood child who then turned her back on you and. . . . (Skill 3: Deepening Emotional Experience—Vivid Language and Metaphor; Skill 10: Case Formulation—Actions of the Self and Acts of Others)

**PATIENT 61:**  And that's basically what he's saying.

**THERAPIST 62:**  Yeah, so I mean this must be like oh, here I've allowed myself to really get close, I've allowed myself to really attach to you and to care about you and to give to you and now this is particularly frightening because oh my goodness, now that I'm out on a limb. (Skill 3: Deepening Emotional Experience—"I" Statements and Vivid Language and Metaphor)

**PATIENT 62:**  Where am I going to go?

**THERAPIST 63:**  What will happen if you cut that limb down? (Skill 8: Using Metaphors)

**PATIENT 63:**  Right. (Yeah.) And I'm very independent but . . .

**THERAPIST 64:**  Right, I mean you're, you're kind of complex. (Yeah.) Right, there's that independent side of you. You work out and you're going to school and you're working at the real estate office and you're making your life and then there's this side of you that really wants to be connected and wants to be seen and appreciated for who she is and to be given to. And to have it kind of give and take, give and take. (Absolutely.) So, there are all those parts to you and here you are kind of, they're all kind of coming together all at once. (Skill 10: Case Formulation—Actions of the Self and Introject)

**PATIENT 64:**  And they're all taking a head there. It's frustrating.

**THERAPIST 65:**  Yeah, you're almost like right up against yourself. It's almost like you're right up against a pattern right, that you've established over your life. To kind of be OK. But now it's kind of . . . (Kind of OK.) Now it's not OK, that way of operating in the world. That giving, giving, giving, doing, doing, it's not OK right now. You want something more. (Yes.) But now it's like uh oh, if I dare ask for something more. (What's going to happen?) What's going to happen? Right, right. Well that's a you know, an important time for you. (Skill 5: Pointing Out Defenses; Skill 3: Deepening Emotional Experience—"I" Statements and Vivid Language; Skill 10: Case Formulation—Expectations of Others)

**PATIENT 65:**  Yes. Life changing.

**THERAPIST 66:**  Could be. (Skill 6: Introducing the Rationale for Treatment)

**PATIENT 66:**  I think so.

**THERAPIST 67:**  Could be. Sounds like there's some kind of self-esteem issue going on. Is that right? (Skill 10: Case Formulation—Introject)

**PATIENT 67:**  [*smiling and repeatedly nodding*] Yeah, always. (Always.) Since forever.

**THERAPIST 68:**  Forever. And here you are really dealing with it. (Skill 12: Providing a Corrective Emotional Experience)

**PATIENT 68:**  Finally, deal with it now.

**THERAPIST 69:**  So this is maybe part of why you're here? (Skill 6: Introducing the Rationale for Treatment)

**PATIENT 69:**  Yes, yes.

**THERAPIST 70:**  All right, so I think maybe I, I can see this is kind of staring me in the face right now. Maybe I can deal with this issue. Some of it has to do with my boyfriend, but some of it just has to do with me. (Absolutely.) What I feel I'm deserving of. Is that right? Yeah. (Skill 6: Introducing the Rationale for Treatment; Skill 3: Deepening Emotional Experience—"I" Statements; Skill 10: Case Formulation—Introject)

**PATIENT 70:** I definitely agree. And I am, I've always known it. You always have a feeling and I can, I can talk it out, but you know actually doing it is a completely different and that's with everything so. I think if I can make one change with the whole exercising and the, you know, eating right, I think I could make some more changes.

**THERAPIST 71:** [*smiles and nods*] Oh I see what you're saying. I see what you're saying. You're saying, "Look, I shifted this in my life." (Skill 3: Deepening Emotional Experience— "I" Statements; Skill 6: Introducing the Rationale for Treatment)

**PATIENT 71:** Maybe I can shift it again.

**THERAPIST 72:** I'm doing something healthy for myself. Maybe I can shift over here and do something healthy for myself. (Skill 6: Introducing the Rationale for Treatment; Skill 8: Using Metaphors)

**PATIENT 72:** That's what I want.

**THERAPIST 73:** That's what you want. [*pause*] So what's it feel like to hear yourself say that? (Skill 12: Providing a Corrective Emotional Experience)

**PATIENT 73:** It's a little nerve-racking. I'm a little anxious about it, but I know it's best. Because I can't keep it here; it's not helping me. I feel it and it's driving me crazy. It's not what I should be dealing with right now. I should be able to, I want a clean, smooth, I'm a very smooth . . . I want it to go well. These bumps, they're not helping. But I need to deal with them.

**THERAPIST 74:** It's almost like life is giving you the opportunity to become healthier. (Yes.) Right? (Skill 6: Introducing the Rationale for Treatment; Skill 12: Providing a Corrective Emotional Experience)

**PATIENT 74:** Different steps too. First in eating right and then through the exercise and now we can . . . [*trails off*] harder steps through you know.

**THERAPIST 75:** Harder steps because attachments are coming up about that and that's very close to the heart. [*touches her own heart*] (Skill 3: Deepening Emotional Experience— Vivid Language and Metaphor) (Right.) Right? (Yes.) I can appreciate that. You know, we're coming to the close of our time here today and if you'd like, we can continue (I'd love to) doing this. I think we have about five more sessions allocated and I can be here again in 2 weeks. (OK.) So we could meet again in 2 weeks? (That would be wonderful!) Well great. I think, I think you've been very forthcoming and really told your story in a way that I'm already getting a feel for what you're wrestling with. (Thank you.) It sounds like it was kind of a courageous act to come in. (Skill 7: Making Transference Interpretations— I am very aware here and throughout the session that it would be in keeping with Ann's style for her to attempt to please me by being the "good patient." At this point, I am aware of that likelihood but do not comment on it; Skill 11: Using Supervision to Recognize Reenactments—I might be pulled to respond to her pleasing presentation by joining her in being a superficially "pleasant" therapist; Skill 12: Providing a Corrective Emotional Experience)

**PATIENT 75:** Little bit. I've been wanting to. So, this is my opportunity. Even if it's on camera. I'm ready to do it.

**THERAPIST 76:** Indeed. Even if it's on camera. (Skill 6: Introducing the Rationale for Treatment)

**PATIENT 76:** Yeah.

**THERAPIST 77:** I'll look forward to seeing you in 2 weeks.

**PATIENT 77:** Yes, thank you so much, Hanna.

**THERAPIST 78:** OK. Bye-bye.

**PATIENT 78:** Bye.

## Annotated Psychodynamic Therapy Transcript 2: Session 5

**THERAPIST 1:** Well, good morning.

**PATIENT 1:** Morning.

**THERAPIST 2:** So this is our next-to-the-last session and we'll meet again next in 3 weeks.

**PATIENT 2:** Things are good, I think. Um, I've been doing a little bit of what we talked about, a little more meditation, and, um, I've started doing more journaling, just like I wanted to. So that's going really well.

**THERAPIST 3:** [*smiling broadly*] Is it?

**PATIENT 3:** Yes, I really like it. I miss it, because I used to do it when I was younger, but it's going really well, I think. And I started work this week, so, trying to get back in the swing of that.

**THERAPIST 4:** That's back at the real estate office?

**PATIENT 4:** Yeah, part time, so, about 20, 30 hours. I've been sleeping in till 9 or 10, because I can with summer vacation, so I'm trying to get back to being awake at 7:15. That's just normal, I guess, for being off for so long. So, it's going OK though, I think.

**THERAPIST 5:** OK. Did you have an agenda for today? (Skill 6: Introducing the Rationale for Treatment)

**PATIENT 5:** Um, not really. It was pretty much a really good week, nothing too drastically crazy happened. It was my boyfriend's birthday yesterday, so I actually got to see him, and we hung out with his family, and it was a lot of fun, and we went out to eat. He was doing really well. I got him some things for his birthday. And we hung out. So it was really laid back. But I definitely enjoyed it. Um, I don't know. I got my hair done, as you can tell. It was a challenge, too, because I never know what I'm going to do when I get in there. My stylist is really good, she'll throw out an idea and I'm like, "Oh, OK let's try that." And she's pretty good about it. So I'm a little nervous because I cut it, I don't usually cut it, I usually trim it. But I cut it. So, it made me a little nervous, but feeling a little better. It feels healthier, you know, after you cut it, it feels more "umphh."

**THERAPIST 6:** So you're pleased?

**PATIENT 6:** Yes, I'm very pleased. I really like it.

**THERAPIST 7:** Well, good, good. I think the health theme has been something that's been there from day 1. [*pause*] You know, I just had a thought. Your going to a good hair stylist and walking out with healthier hair reminds me in some ways of what's going on in our work together these past months—your coming here and leaving feeling healthier. (Skill 7: Making Transference Interpretations)

**PATIENT 7:** [*laughs with recognition*] Right, since we started, I've been getting healthier.

**THERAPIST 8:** [*smiling*] So some external changes and some internal ones. (Skill 8: Using Metaphors)

**PATIENT 8:** We've certainly been working on the internal ones.

**THERAPIST 9:** We have been. We have been. You know what? I think you've been very forthcoming in terms of trying to reflect on this theme, this pattern, that you have in your life, where sometimes you don't think about yourself versus others. You're more concerned about "where are they?" and how can you please them, and you've been very worried about how you might have to put up a wall to keep yourself, the real you, back here, safe, [*gesturing behind the wall formed by the therapist's hand*] so that this part [*gesturing in front of the wall*] won't be unacceptable to people; they might not see the real you, but they'll see this wall and this kind of other self that you throw out there. But that it's getting pretty tiring for you to keep doing. And we talked about how a part of you is screaming out to get free of that wall [*from the previous session where she said a part of her was screaming to tell her boyfriend that he is hurting her*]. (Skill 5: Pointing Out Defenses; Skill 8: Using Metaphors; Skill 10: Case Formulation—Actions of the Self)

**PATIENT 9:** Yeah, that was last time.

**THERAPIST 10:** Right. And I loved hearing last time about you on the diving board. [*In the last session, the patient talked about how she felt authentic when diving.*] (Skill 8: Using Metaphors)

**PATIENT 10:** Yeah, a whole different me, really.

**THERAPIST 11:** A whole different you. Yeah. So these have been some of the things I'm recollecting about our brief work together.

**PATIENT 11:** Yes, I definitely feel the same way. And I think one of the ways that it's really coming out is with my boyfriend. This wall is really . . . I try to tear down his walls. And you said last time maybe I should start with me. So I think that is one of the biggest parts of my life where it's really coming to a head. I think. Because school's going really well, work's work, but especially in that relationship, which I value so much, it's just, I don't, you know [*pause*] I can't be two people all the time. Especially when I see him all the time and we're so, you know, close; we're intimately close. I can't be that fake person and still be that close with someone. Because it's really bothering me, and I think I've thought of that this week.

**THERAPIST 12:** Yeah, did you have a chance to journal about that, was that part of the . . .

**PATIENT 12:** [*interrupting*] Yeah, I did journal; just thinking about how, like, I split the page in half, kind of like a pros and cons, but I did, like a me with the wall, and me without the wall. I just did like characteristics.

**THERAPIST 13:** Wow! (Skill 2: Being Aware of Countertransference Reactions—<u>I am impressed by her creativity and diligence</u>.)

**PATIENT 13:** So I don't know, I just got the pros and cons thing and I was like maybe I should try it this way. You know, me with the wall, I guess, I think I put something like always thinking about others, or like, I think I put it in context of me and my boyfriend; you know, always considering what *he* wants, pretty much doing whatever *he* asks whenever he asks. You know, and maybe sacrificing myself for him without him knowing. And then without the wall it's just, you know, wanting a mutual relationship, like we talked about, you know me coming forward and him coming forward. And maybe meeting each other at the inside. And just being myself, not having to pretend to be someone else. So, that was a very intense, intense journaling because, you saw things; you really think about it, but things that I really want to start addressing. And I think last time really helped with the feeling of the body that I think really helped. [*In the previous session, the therapist had Ann focus on her body, becoming aware of her somatic responses.*] You know, just to notice. Because I felt that tenseness, and I kind of knew what it was, but I'm kind of a little tense all the time, because I'm kind of an anxious type of person. But it's been getting, you know, stronger and stronger—so to be able to identify what it is, is just very empowering.

**THERAPIST 14:** Hmmm. So to identify what it is, and be aware of it, was empowering. (Skill 10: Case Formulation—Introject; Skill 12: Providing a Corrective Emotional Experience)

**PATIENT 14:** And to say it out loud, not just to think it, or to be like "Eh, maybe it's that, maybe it's not." But to really recognize it. And I don't want to rationalize, because that's what I do with everything. Trying to just, like you said, be in flow, and organic.

**THERAPIST 15:** Organic, right.

**PATIENT 15:** Be organic with it. So I think that's been really helpful. I like to process, and maybe just to let it be a feeling is a little different for me.

**THERAPIST 16:** Yeah, and in terms of our work, and our relationship, I've felt like we've been in flow. (Skill 3: Deepening Emotional Experience; Skill 8: Using Metaphors)

**PATIENT 16:** Oh, absolutely. I do too.

**THERAPIST 17:** So it's very interesting that you have participated in that flow in here because you didn't have to. (Skill 4: Making Process Comments; Skill 12: Providing a Corrective Emotional Experience)

**PATIENT 17:** No, no. Well, I think also it comes with . . . I want to have a relationship, I want to try and help myself. I think maybe if I was more close-minded to the situation I wouldn't be. And I think to some extent I kind of adapt to the way the person is, I try to at least. Like when I see how your personality is, or like how someone else's is, like my friends, I try to adapt [I see.] and be like, you know, maybe this will help them. See, I'm always thinking of others. But I think the flow has helped me even maybe not just adapting but to feel what that's like, because I've never really, in a relationship like this, had that experience. So I think it's been very helpful.

**THERAPIST 18:** OK. So maybe it started off more like how could you do a good job here with the cameras and the lights and the help trainees that might be looking at this tape, how can you help me. (Skill 7: Making Transference Interpretations; Skill 11: Using Supervision to Recognize Reenactments)

**PATIENT 18:** Make your job a little easier. Yes.

**THERAPIST 19:** Make my job easier. (Skill 4: Making Process Comments; Skill 7: Making Transference Interpretations)

**PATIENT 19:** But it's definitely changed.

**THERAPIST 20:** It's changed . . .

**PATIENT 20:** [*interrupting*] Dramatically. From the first session that was kind of what I was, you know, I was trying to be helpful. But I just kind of let it flow and it just kind of just took over. It's not like that now.

**THERAPIST 21:** [*agreeing*] It's not. It just kind of took over, you're not kind of processing, well, what can I say next. (Skill 10: Case Formulation—Actions of the Self)

**PATIENT 21:** Not at all.

**THERAPIST 22:** Not at all.

**PATIENT 22:** It's just kind of been flowing. (Wow!) So it feels great. Because I'm not over-analyzing anything, really. When I go home, I analyze it, but not in the moment.

**THERAPIST 23:** Not in the moment; there's like a trust that it'll be OK. And yet, it isn't like it's been all, you know, fun and games in here. (Skill 4: Making Process Comments)

**PATIENT 23:** No, no, not really at all. It's hard work.

**THERAPIST 24:** It *is* hard work. And even in that, you've had trust in the process and not been overanalyzing or thinking "what can I say or do now that will please Hanna?" (Skill 4: Making Process Comments; Skill 7: Making Transference Interpretations; Skill 10: Case Formulation—Actions of the Self)

**PATIENT 24:** Yes, "what can I do to help all this." But I think the trust thing is one of my bigger issues also. Just to be able to do this, it does take a level of trust, and I didn't really think of it that way. But that might be why I'm not able to do it with other people—to be able to be vulnerable, to put myself out there.

**THERAPIST 25:** Be vulnerable. (Skill 12: Providing a Corrective Emotional Experience)

**PATIENT 25:** Yeah, like we've said before. With me, you know, taking down the wall. I think I've kind of done that here in a way to learn from what's going on.

**THERAPIST 26:** Yes, you have. And then you've also done it outside of here. (Skill 12: Providing a Corrective Emotional Experience)

**PATIENT 26:** Yes, with my friend, yes. [*In a previous session, the therapist gave her home-work to try paying attention to her own needs while in relationship to someone else.*]

**THERAPIST 27:** With your friend and also the journaling, putting it down, saying it, it already becomes different. (Skill 5: Pointing Out [absence of] Defenses)

**PATIENT 27:** Yeah, I don't know why, but definitely, especially when you feel this way about a person, and actually say it to that person, it changes everything. And that's . . . me and change, usually don't go together very well.

**THERAPIST 28:** [*teasing tone*] Well, look at your hair! (Skill 8: Using Metaphors)

**PATIENT 28:** Well, interpersonally, I'm still terrified to create it . . . to bring that up with my boyfriend, especially. Because I don't . . .

**THERAPIST 29:** [*interrupting*] Are you terrified of having a deeper level of intimacy with him? (Skill 5: Pointing Out Defenses)

**PATIENT 29:** Maybe. I think that could be a very good reason, because, well you know, like I said before, he's said some flippant things about me where he's like, "You know, I can take you or leave you." And to be that intimate with someone, and then to have them say that to you, what do you expect me to do? I might want to go to that level, but I don't know if you [boyfriend] want to go to that level. So that's where I'm very uneasy about that, because you know, I just don't want to put myself in that position, and you don't want to be in that position with me, you know what I mean. So at times I think he does, and then there's times when I'm like, "I don't know."

**THERAPIST 30:** What about you? Do you want to go to that level? (Skill 1: Engaging in a Therapeutic Inquiry; Skill 12: Providing a Corrective Emotional Experience)

**PATIENT 30:** I think I'm pretty much almost at that level, but not the way I want to be. Like I'm at that level with the wall, I think. I'm not at that level with me—like you know what I mean? Like not with the real "this is Ann take it or leave it." I'm more at that level with "this is Ann; this is how I think you want me to be." You know what I mean? But I think I need to get to the [*pause*] the first step is to talk to him and you know tell him how I've been feeling.

**THERAPIST 31:** You know, maybe there's something in between "this is Ann take it or leave it," and "this is Ann the way I think you want her." (Skill 10: Case Formulation—Actions of the Self and Introject)

**PATIENT 31:** Like a happy medium?

**THERAPIST 32:** A more balanced place because it sounds like both are kind of distant. "This is Ann, take it or leave it," that's not how you are with this guy. It's not like, you know, have a coffee or don't have a coffee, I mean, you're really into him. (Absolutely.) So that would be pretty false to say "take it or leave it," right? But here, "This is Ann the way I think you want her," is also false. (Absolutely.) It's not really you. I think what both of these have in common is they're not really you. (Skill 10: Case Formulation—Actions of the Self; Skill 12: Providing a Corrective Emotional Experience)

**PATIENT 32:** Right. Neither of them. You know, balance, as you've been saying, is hard, because I'm more of a black-and-white thinker. I'm more hard on myself I think.

**THERAPIST 33:** You are more hard on yourself. (Skill 10: Case Formulation—Introject) You know I don't experience you as a black-and-white thinker. (Oh, really?) (Skill 4: Making Process Comments) Yeah, really. I don't. I think you keep [*pause*], I was going to say a balancing act; there's so much like balancing that you do, "Should I step a little this way, or that way, or will this be OK?" And then you're also very aware of what you're feeling. Like it was so poignant last session when you said this part of you is screaming to "Tell him already!" Right? (Skill 3: Deepening Emotional Experience)

**PATIENT 33:** Maybe I just think I am. That's interesting. I don't . . .

**THERAPIST 34:** [*interrupting*] I was wondering if maybe the home that you grew up in was more black-and-white.

**PATIENT 34:** Yeah, very black and white. You know, you give your best or you don't do it at all.

**THERAPIST 35:** Yeah. Right. You, fix it, don't cry! It's like there are these boxes, you know, you need to fit into and I see you as someone who now kind of has more flow than boxes.

**PATIENT 35:** I can feel that now. I think before we even began talking, I thought of myself as more here, here, [*gesturing as if pointing to separate boxes*] separate issues, separate things. You know what I mean? (Right.) But I don't think everybody's like that, I don't think everybody can be. As you said before, it makes you standoffish, it makes you [*pause*] you can't be intimate. You can't be close, you're more off-putting. So I've definitely learned a lot about myself, that I can be less of a black-and-white thinker, maybe not even think of myself as a black-and-white thinker. Maybe just flow with it, which I've never, you know, really done. You go to school and you don't really learn anything about emotions, and then when you have these emotions, it's hard to deal with them. So you deal with them in ways you deal with any problem, you put it in a box. (Right.) And emotions can't be solved unless you do some thinking about it and sometimes you just want to solve them right away, but it just takes time.

**THERAPIST 36:** Yeah, it's really important to reflect on those emotions.

**PATIENT 36:** And why. I know why, but I don't know why . . . like I know what causes it, but I don't know the why. You know, the "why" is it impacting me so much. Especially with my boyfriend, because I think with most other guys I've dated, I haven't let it bother me so much.

**THERAPIST 37:** The "it"? (Skill 1: Engaging in a Therapeutic Inquiry)

**PATIENT 37:** Just, um, if things have gone bad or if they've hurt me. I haven't let it bother me.

**THERAPIST 38:** The "take it or leave it" Ann.

**PATIENT 38:** It's very different with him, I don't know why, I just feel differently, I guess. So when he does things, and it hurts me; I put it up with it. And that's the wall, I guess.

**THERAPIST 39:** Right, right. So you know how to say "goodbye, I'm not going to take this." You've done that in other relationships. And you know how to contort yourself to be the way your boyfriend wants you to be. But what you want practice doing is how can I take some of those bricks down—not scare myself to death—but take some bricks down. Peer out, let him see me, and see if what I get back is as bad as I think it is. (Skill 8: Using Metaphors; Skill 10: Case Formulation—Expectations of Others; Skill 12: Providing a Corrective Emotional Experience)

**PATIENT 39:** Right, that's exactly what I want to do. But I think throughout, I've come to the realization that I *need* to. Because this is not working for where it is right now, it's causing me way too much internal pain that I just haven't expressed to him. I've expressed to myself, I've expressed in my journal, but you know where it counts, I'm not doing it.

**THERAPIST 40:** You know what it sounds to me like, Ann? It sounds like for the first time in your life, maybe for the first time in your life with your boyfriend, you are experiencing a yearning for true intimacy.

**PATIENT 40:** Absolutely. I think so. Without the walls, without the . . .

**THERAPIST 41:** [*interrupting*] Without the protection of "this isn't important to me, who cares, I'll just do this, I'll just do that." It's like, no, this feels different to you inside. (Skill 5: Pointing Out Defenses)

**PATIENT 41:** Yeah. It feels different. And it makes me want to try something different than what I've done before. So . . .

**THERAPIST 42:** [*interrupting*] But it's scary because it's so different from what you've done before, you know? I mean those walls weren't constructed for no good reason. You've had to protect yourself in a family where you were sometimes the mother to your mother, and your father was demanding compliance. (Skill 5: Pointing Out Defenses; Skill 10: Case Formulation—Putting It All Together)

**PATIENT 42:** Yeah, very much.

**THERAPIST 43:** Like, "OK, you want me to do this, I'll do this." (Skill 3: Deepening Emotional Experience—Using "I" Statements) So, you know those walls weren't constructed for no reason. They had value back then. (Skill 5: Pointing Out Defenses)

**PATIENT 43:** I needed them back then.

**THERAPIST 44:** You probably did. Very much. I mean how else would a 10-year-old girl deal with what a 10-year-old girl had to deal with (Skill 5: Pointing Out Defenses)

**PATIENT 44:** Right. I don't know, probably couldn't. I think if I didn't have those walls, I wouldn't be the person I am today either. Which is a value that I think is important to be able to recognize that you are who you are because of what you've done and the relationships you've had in your past. And it doesn't make you a bad person, or wrong, it just makes you the person you are, and if you want to change, you have to recognize that there are things you need to change.

**THERAPIST 45:** So, can I have you say something?

**PATIENT 45:** Um hum.

**THERAPIST 46:** And as you say it, I want you to like own it. (OK.) And I want you to see how your body feels as you say it. "I am a valuable person." (Skill 3: Deepening Emotional Experience; Skill 10: Case Formulation—Introject; Skill 12: Providing a Corrective Emotional Experience)

**PATIENT 46:** [*meekly*] I am a valuable person.

**THERAPIST 47:** Say it again. (Skill 3: Deepening Emotional Experience)

**PATIENT 47:** [*bottom lip is trembling; tearing up*] I am a valuable person.

**THERAPIST 48:** What's coming up? (Skill 3: Deepening Emotional Experience)

**PATIENT 48:** Tears.

**THERAPIST 49:** [*gentle voice, said softly and slowly*] And what do those tears say? If those tears could talk, what would they say? (Skill 3: Deepening Emotional Experience; Skill 8: Using Metaphors)

**PATIENT 49:** "No, you're not."

**THERAPIST 50:** [*nodding head, speaking very softly*] Right. So this is a very private, internal battle. (Skill 8: Using Metaphors; Skill 10: Case Formulation—Introject)

**PATIENT 50:** Oh, yeah. It's just so hard, I don't know why that would affect me so. Like, just saying that, I can hardly say it.

**THERAPIST 51:** Is that right?

**PATIENT 51:** Because it doesn't feel real.

**THERAPIST 52:** Yes. You can't own it. (Skill 10: Case Formulation—Introject)

**PATIENT 52:** No, I can't.

**THERAPIST 53:** You can't own it yet. (Skill 12: Providing a Corrective Emotional Experience)

**PATIENT 53:** No. And that's awful. It feels awful. Something so simple, just . . . [*trails off*]

**THERAPIST 54:** So some of what you're wrestling here on the other side of the wall is not only the feared response from that person; it's not only your boyfriend saying "no you're not a valuable person to me," but it's *you* believing that. (Skill 5: Pointing Out Defenses; Skill 8: Using Metaphors; Skill 10: Case Formulation—Introject)

**PATIENT 54:** Right, oh yeah. Very much.

**THERAPIST 55:** Very much.

**PATIENT 55:** But it's hard for me to bring down those walls when I don't think I necessarily, you know, should. Or, like I'm valuable enough to do so.

**THERAPIST 56:** Right. That I'm entitled to do so. (Skill 3: Deepening Emotional Experience—Using "I" Statements; Skill 10: Case Formulation—Introject)

**PATIENT 56:** Right.

**THERAPIST 57:** "Look world, here I am." You can't fully get behind that yet. (Skill 3: Deepening Emotional Experience; Skill 10: Case Formulation—Introject)

**PATIENT 57:** I never have.

**THERAPIST 58:** [*sad*] Yeah. And that's part of this whole puzzle, part of this whole puzzle. (Skill 2: Being Aware of Countertransference Reactions—<u>I am feeling very sad to hear this</u>; Skill 8: Using Metaphors; Skill 10: Case Formulation—Introject)

**PATIENT 58:** I don't know why, I mean. That's what scares me, I usually can rationalize. But that, just saying that hurt me so much. And I don't really know why, you know.

**THERAPIST 59:** [*said slowly and softly*] Why would you not value you? (Skill 3: Deepening Emotional Experience; Skill 5: Pointing Out Defenses)

**PATIENT 59:** Right, it doesn't make any sense. But, I don't . . . I just . . . that's how it feels. That it feels wrong, it feels like I'm lying.

**THERAPIST 60:** So someway that message got in and you started owning it, right? (Right!) You weren't born this way. So somewhere that message, somehow you picked up messages from the outside saying "you're not valuable," or "you're not good enough," or "you don't measure up enough." Somehow those messages were there and you started owning them like they were real. Do you have any idea about those messages when you were really young? Is there anything that will help you understand how that got presented to you as a reality? I don't mean maybe directly, like anyone said to you "You don't measure up," but the message got sent. Do you have a sense about that? (Skill 8: Using Metaphors; Skill 10: Case Formulation—Acts of Others and Introject)

**PATIENT 60:** I think it had more to do with me making friends than anything. As I've told you before, I've had a hard time trying to make friends, even when I was young. We moved, I had a lot of friends when I was little, like from first grade to third grade. And then we moved, and then you know even that young, because by fourth grade, your friends are friends you'll have until high school. I didn't have that, I was the new kid. And I just remember eating lunch alone, you know, and just having a hard time.

**THERAPIST 61:** So do you think somehow that alone time and not having friends and not having people say "come and play with me" somehow you started interpreting that as there's something wrong with you? (Skill 10: Case Formulation—Introject)

**PATIENT 61:** Absolutely. You know, "what did I do wrong?"

**THERAPIST 62:** Right. As kids will, because kids always try to find meaning, and one of the ways they try to find meaning, as you know, is they blame themselves. Right? So maybe at that developmental level you started blaming you. Even though, as you say it, it had to do a lot more with things like moving and ending up in a school where there's already cliques. Right. But as a child you wouldn't have that ability to see that, have that perspective. (Skill 10: Case Formulation—Introject)

**PATIENT 62:** That was probably a big part of it, you know. And then as I got older with sports, I wasn't always the best, but in my family you have to be the best, it's kind of what's expected. So I just, I guess I interpreted that as a failure of myself.

**THERAPIST 63:** Oh, because you weren't good enough in the sports? So maybe there's another link there, maybe somehow because sports is so valued in your family, you got the idea "I'm not valuable. I'm not as valuable as like my sister who's the athlete," right? (Skill 10: Case Formulation—Introject)

**PATIENT 63:** Yes, I think that's really why, one of the reasons why I quit volleyball; I couldn't compete with her. And she's 3 years younger than me, and I couldn't compete with her. And when I didn't make varsity my freshman year, that was it . . . I was done. I couldn't deal with it anymore. I said you know what I've had enough of it, I was having fights . . . I wasn't causing the fights, but the girls were making fun of me for . . . I don't know, because we used to be best friends. I had three girls that we were good friends until high school, and then we had a falling out, and then they proceeded to make fun of me on the team. And just laughing at me when I'd make a mistake, so I just couldn't. Because they were on the freshman team, and I was on the freshman team. If I was on the varsity team, I wouldn't have had to deal with that. So I was just done. And then my sister was doing really well and I just couldn't, I couldn't compete. So I had enough, I was done. I was . . . I haven't picked up a volleyball since. Won't.

**THERAPIST 64:** And oftentimes when kids get wounded in that way about not making the team or whatever they go home and their parents convey to them that they're so worthwhile, and this is a small thing, and who cares. But it sounds like in your family . . . [*trails off*] (Skill 10: Case Formulation—Acts of Others)

**PATIENT 64:** It wasn't as bad as I think I make it sound, honestly. It wasn't that I didn't make varsity and my dad was mad at me, I was more mad at myself for not making varsity. And you know having to deal with those stupid girls. And I don't think . . . he would never come out and say "that's awful" or anything like that.

**THERAPIST 65:** But maybe you felt like you were letting him down. (Skill 10: Case Formulation—Acts of Others)

**PATIENT 65:** Yeah. I felt that way. It didn't mean he would tell me I was no good or anything like that, I just felt I was better and I could have made the team but, you know, it didn't work out that way. And I was just, I was done with it. And I could tell how upset he was when I decided to quit. It really . . . it hurt him because we were doing volleyball all the time, since I was like 11. And it was like one of the things that we did together. And like me my sister and dad would go practice and all that.

**THERAPIST 66:** It was a way to be with him. (Skill 3: Deepening Emotional Experience; Skill 10: Case Formulation—Acts of Others)

**PATIENT 66:** Right. It wasn't a pleasant experience, but it was a way to be together.

**THERAPIST 67:** It wasn't pleasant? (Skill 10: Case Formulation—Acts of Others)

**PATIENT 67:** No, not really. Very harsh, like making mistakes. So . . . you can't.

**THERAPIST 68:** I see. Really put down. (Skill 10: Case Formulation—Acts of Others)

**PATIENT 68:** Yeah. So it was a way to be together, and sometimes it was nice, but there was a lot of yelling involved. You know, because that's just the way that he thought that we would learn. But he's definitely changed—he's not like that with my sister anymore. He coaches a lot of other kids, and it's just a totally different, a whole different atmosphere.

**THERAPIST 69:** But again, kids taking in those messages very seriously when they're young. Maybe there was a message here about "I'm not good enough, I'm not trying enough, I'm failing. I can't even compete with my sister who's younger. You know, I'm getting messages from people around me and in my home that somehow maybe I'm . . ." (Skill 10: Case Formulation—Acts of Others and Introject)

**PATIENT 69:** [*interrupting*] I'm deficient.

**THERAPIST 70:** "I'm deficient." (Skill 3: Deepening Emotional Experience)

**PATIENT 70:** It's especially hard now since she's so good. I've been to maybe three games since I could drive. I just I can't.

**THERAPIST 71:** [*said softly*] It's hard for you to be there. (Skill 3: Deepening Emotional Experience)

**PATIENT 71:** It's very hard.

**THERAPIST 72:** What happens? (Skill 1: Engaging in a Therapeutic Inquiry)

**PATIENT 72:** Well, sometimes I would go to a game, and I would just pretend that I was my sister. That I was the one out there making all the great plays. You know I just, I just wished that could be me, you know in a way. That you know I could have been that good.

**THERAPIST 73:** So your daydream would take you out of your feeling deficient, and bring you closer to your Dad. You could just bypass all that pain for those moments. (Skill 9: Exploring Fantasy)

**PATIENT 73:** So when I go it's just, you know, reliving memories that I really don't want to. I don't want to remember when we used to spend three hours at the volleyball court after school and practice certain moves, and do stupid stuff like that. I don't want to remember that. When I watch her play and she's so good I remember we used to do the same things, so why I couldn't, you know, why couldn't I get myself together. Why couldn't I be that good?

**THERAPIST 74:** Right. Can you hear yourself giving yourself messages like you must have gotten or given yourself when you were a little kid? (Skill 10: Case Formulation—Introject)

**PATIENT 74:** Uh huh, I hear it. I've always known that something like that screwed me up a little bit. That you know, with my self-esteem. But, you know, if you don't think about it, you don't think about it.

**THERAPIST 75:** Yeah. So maybe we're starting to get at some of the reasons for why when you say "I'm a valuable person" it hurts and you can't own it. And the tears come up and they tell you "No, you're not." Maybe it goes all the way back. (Oh, yeah.) It goes back to that move, it goes back to those messages you got in your family. There's a *New Yorker* cartoon, it's one of my favorite *New Yorker* cartoons, and it's a dog looking in a mirror with lots of torn paper all around, and he looks in the mirror and he sees his reflection and he says, "Bad dog." (Skill 8: Using Metaphors; Skill 10: Case Formulation—Introject)

**PATIENT 75:** [*smiling*] That's funny. Oh wow. That's pretty much the same thing.

**THERAPIST 76:** Yeah. The messages we tell ourselves about ourselves got in there from out there. (Skill 10: Case Formulation—Introject) (Right.) And then we start owning them like they're true as opposed to just messages that were more about where were at developmentally or because something traumatic happened. Now as an adult we have that perspective, but as the kid we owned it. [*slowly*] And then we kept telling ourselves that year after year, year after year until we just believed it. (Skill 10: Case Formulation—Introject)

**PATIENT 76:** Right. Until it just became a part of me, not a message anymore.

**THERAPIST 77:** That's right. I like the way you say that; it became a part of you, not a message. (Skill 10: Case Formulation—Introject)

**PATIENT 77:** Because after a while you hear it all the time . . .

**THERAPIST 78:** [*interrupting*] Well, you're telling yourself 24/7. (Skill 10: Case Formulation—Introject) (Yeah.) You hear it all the time because you're telling yourself. And then you fear if you let down the wall everyone else will see it. What you're feeling. You're negative self-evaluation. As opposed to "this is just a message," and unfortunately [*said slowly and with emphasis*], you've been owning it too long. (Skill 3: Deepening Emotional Experience; Skill 5: Pointing Out Defenses; Skill 10: Case Formulation—Introject)

**PATIENT 78:** And then I guess with that, it's just the fear that the message with be confirmed, you know?

**THERAPIST 79:** And, in a strange way, since you don't let people see who you really are, it is being confirmed. It can never be disproven, right? So in a way, it is a self-fulfilling prophecy. Right? (Skill 5: Pointing Out Defenses)

**PATIENT 79:** Right. Because there's no one to say "no."

**THERAPIST 80:** That's right. There's no one to say, "No, I love you, for who you are, and thank you for letting me see who you are." (Skill 3: Deepening Emotional Experience; Skill 12: Providing a Corrective Emotional Experience)

**PATIENT 80:** I don't want anyone to get the chance.

**THERAPIST 81:** [*nodding*] To disconfirm. Do you get the sense in here, of any disconfirmation? (Skill 4: Making Process Comments)

**PATIENT 81:** No, like, I feel very comfortable and I feel more valuable than any other place, than any other relationship, just because you haven't, you know, confirmed that I'm an unvaluable person or anything like that.

**THERAPIST 82:** So let me ask you, because I feel like you've really taken down your wall here, right? (Skill 5: Pointing Out [absence of] Defenses) Do you feel like it's just because I'm a therapist, and this is my position, and even though privately I'm making all kinds of judgments, I couldn't possibly let you know that, and I'm just kind of being fake here. Or do you get the sense that down deep now that you've let me really see you, I really *do* think you're a valuable person? Do you have a sense about that? (Skill 4: Making Process Comments; Skill 12: Providing a Corrective Emotional Experience)

**PATIENT 82:** [*immediately replying*] Yes. I think it's not fake at all. I don't think you'd be that way; you don't seem the type. You know, to say something to your face, and then say something else to someone else. So no, I feel like we have a really trusting connection, that you would, if you felt something like that, you would tell me. You know what I mean?

**THERAPIST 83:** I'd find a way to tell you. (Skill 4: Making Process Comments; Skill 12: Providing a Corrective Emotional Experience)

**PATIENT 83:** Right, in a more appropriate way. And there's been some challenges you've given me and things like that so I can see that, you know, we're very connected, and we flow, and that what you're saying, you really mean it.

**THERAPIST 84:** Good, I'm so glad. I'm so glad you can feel it because I feel it inside, but sometimes you don't know if the other person's feeling it too. (Skill 2: Being Aware of Countertransference Reactions—I am moved by her recognition of my presence; Skill 4: Making Process Comments; Skill 12: Providing a Corrective Emotional Experience)

**PATIENT 84:** No, I feel it. Absolutely.

**THERAPIST 85:** So this has been an important experience. You've let down the wall, and although we've only known each other a short time, you've done an amazing amount of work in here, that you're also taking outside of here. And the sense you get back is, "I get the sense she doesn't think I'm a mess. She actually seems to value me." (Skill 12: Providing a Corrective Emotional Experience)

**PATIENT 85:** I agree.

**THERAPIST 86:** So that's a new experience. (Skill 12: Providing a Corrective Emotional Experience)

**PATIENT 86:** Yes. I've never brought down the wall. (That's right.) I think the reason, you know, in the beginning with the therapeutic relationship, I understand that you're not going to devalue me to begin with—you know you're not supposed to. But I think that helped me bring down the wall easier in such a short period of time but that the outside relationships take much longer.

**THERAPIST 87:** That's right. That's right. But you didn't get here overnight.

**PATIENT 87:** Right, no, not at all.

**THERAPIST 88:** And you're not going to change it overnight, but I think of that thing they say, "A journey of a thousand steps begins with one step." I think you're already down that path. You've already started on that path. You know I'm aware we're going to have to end soon for today, and we will have one more time to meet. But I see that you're on that journey. (Skill 6: Introducing the Rationale for Treatment) A little scary, right? It's a new path, but you have a sense it's a healthier path. (Skill 12: Providing a Corrective Emotional Experience)

**PATIENT 88:** I feel more me.

**THERAPIST 89:** [*smiling, looking into Ann's eyes*] I feel more you. I'll very much look forward to seeing you in our last session. (Skill 12: Providing a Corrective Emotional Experience)

**PATIENT 89:** Me too, I always do.

**THERAPIST 90:** Bye. (Thank you.) You're welcome.

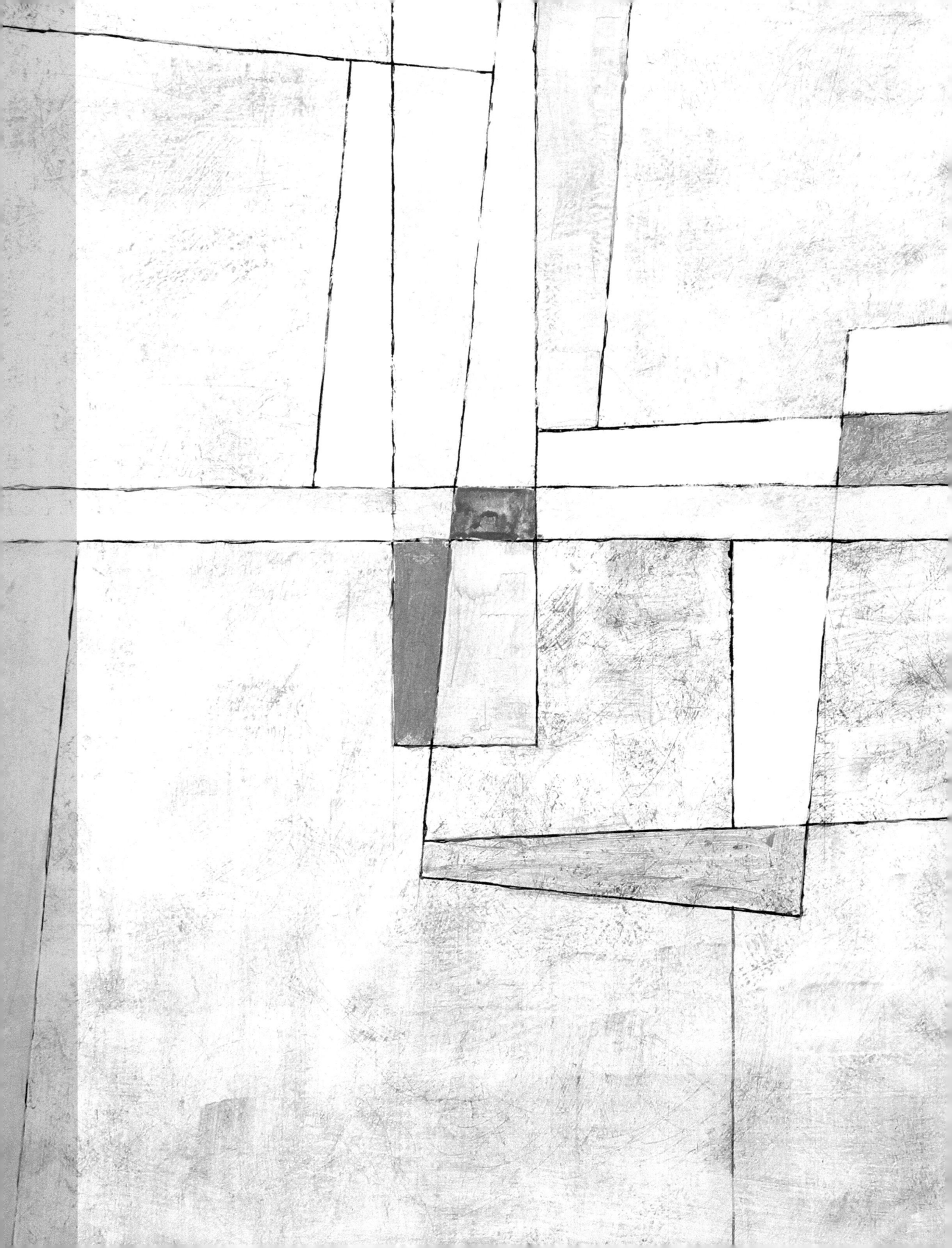

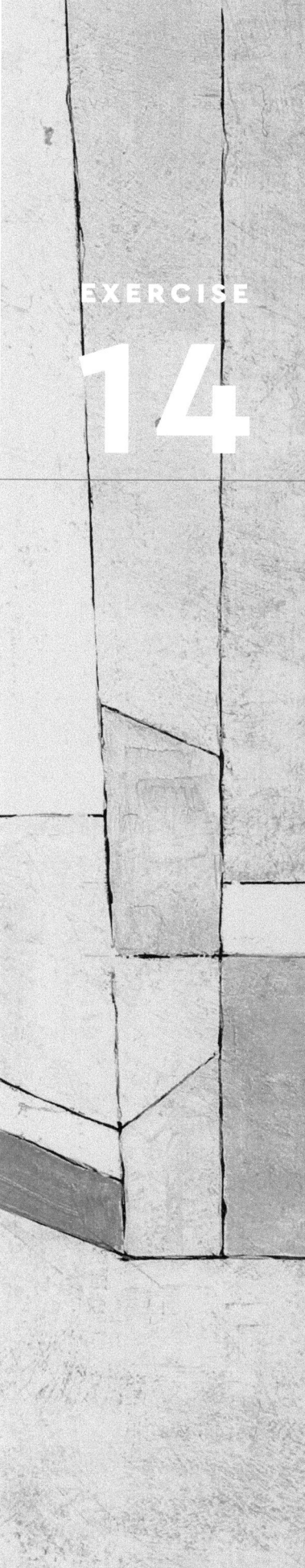

# Mock Psychodynamic Therapy Sessions

In contrast to highly structured and repetitive deliberate practice exercises, a mock psychodynamic session is an unstructured and improvised role-play therapy session. Like a jazz rehearsal, mock sessions let you practice the art and science of *appropriate responsiveness* (Hatcher, 2015; Stiles & Horvath, 2017), putting your psychotherapy skills together in a way that is helpful to your mock patient. This exercise outlines the procedure for conducting a mock psychodynamic session. It offers different patient profiles you may adopt when taking the patient role. The final recommendation gives you the option to play yourself, a choice we have found to be highly rewarding.

Mock sessions are also an opportunity for trainees to practice the following:

- using psychotherapy skills responsively
- navigating challenging choice-points in therapy
- choosing which interventions to use
- tracking the arc of a therapy session and the overall big-picture therapy treatment
- guiding treatment in the context of the patient's preferences
- determining realistic goals for therapy in the context of the patient's capacities
- knowing how to proceed when the therapist is unsure, lost, or confused
- recognizing and recovering from therapeutic errors
- discovering your personal therapeutic style
- building endurance for working with real patients

## Mock Psychodynamic Session Overview

For the mock session, **you will perform a role-play of an initial therapy session.** As is true with the exercises to build individual skills, the role-play involves two to three people: One trainee role-plays the therapist, another trainee role-plays the patient, and (if available) a trainer (a professor or a supervisor) observes and provides feedback. This is an open-ended role-play, as is commonly done in training. However, this differs in two important ways from the role-plays used in traditional training. First, the trainee

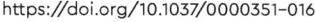

https://doi.org/10.1037/0000351–016

*Deliberate Practice in Psychodynamic Psychotherapy*, by H. Levenson, V. Gay, and J. L. Binder

therapist will use a hand gesture to indicate how difficult the role-play feels. Second, the trainee patient will attempt to make the role-play easier or harder to ensure the therapist is practicing at the right difficulty level.

## Preparation

1. Download the Deliberate Practice Reaction Form and the Deliberate Practice Diary Form from the "Clinician and Practitioner Resources" tab at https://www.apa.org/pubs/books/deliberate-practice-psychodynamic-psychotherapy (also available in Appendixes A and B, respectively). Every student will need their own copy of the Deliberate Practice Reaction Form on a separate piece of paper so they can access it quickly.

2. Designate one student to role-play the therapist and one student to role-play the patient. The trainer will observe and provide corrective feedback.

## Mock Psychodynamic Session Procedure

1. The trainees will role-play an initial (first) therapy session. The trainee role-playing the patient selects a patient profile from the end of this exercise.

2. Before beginning the role-play, the therapist raises a hand at the level of the chair seat (see Figure E14.1). The therapist will use this hand gesture throughout the whole role-play to indicate how challenging it feels to help the patient. The starting hand level

**FIGURE E14.1. Ongoing Difficulty Assessment Through Hand Level**

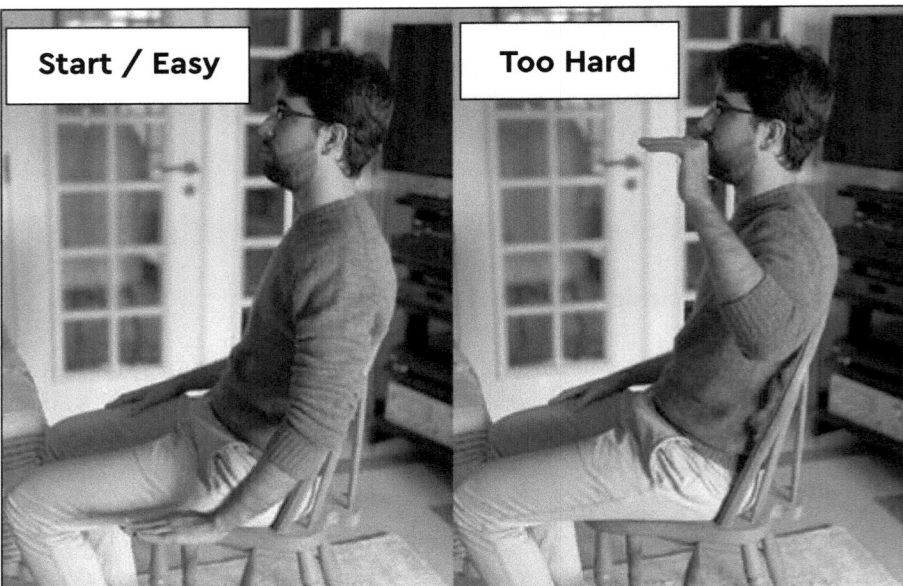

*Note.* Left: Start of role-play. Right: Role-play is too difficult. From *Deliberate Practice in Emotion-Focused Therapy* (p. 156), by R. N. Goldman, A. Vaz, and T. Rousmaniere, 2021, American Psychological Association (https://doi.org/10.1037/0000227-000). Copyright 2021 by the American Psychological Association.

(chair seat) indicates that the role-play feels easy. By raising the hand, the therapist indicates that the difficulty is rising. If the hand rises above neck level, it indicates that the role-play is too difficult.

3. The therapist begins the role-play. The therapist and patient should engage in the role-play in an improvised manner, as they would engage in a real therapy session. The therapist keeps their hand by their side throughout this process. (This may feel strange at first!)

4. Whenever the therapist feels that the difficulty of the role-play has changed significantly, they should move their hand up if it feels more difficult and down if it feels easier. If the therapist's hand drops below the seat of the chair, the patient should make the role-play more challenging; if the therapist's hand rises above neck level, the patient should make the role-play easier. Instructions for adjusting the difficulty of the role-play are described in the "Varying the Level of Challenge" section later in the exercise.

**Note to Therapists**

Remember to be aware of your vocal quality. Match your tone to the patient's presentation. Thus, if the patient presents in a vulnerable manner with soft emotions, soften your tone to be soothing and calm. If the patient, on the other hand, is aggressive and angry, match your tone to be firm and solid (but not angry). If you choose responses that are prompting patient exploration, such as gathering the data for the cyclical maladaptive pattern, remember to adopt a more querying, exploratory tone of voice.

5. The role-play continues for at least 15 minutes. The trainer may provide corrective feedback during this process if the therapist gets significantly offtrack. However, trainers should exercise restraint and keep feedback as short and tight as possible because this will permit the therapist to have more time for experiential training.

6. After the role-play is finished, the therapist and patient switch roles and begin a new mock session.

7. After both trainees have completed the mock session as a therapist, the trainer provides an evaluation, the trainees do a self-evaluation, and the three discuss the experience.

## Varying the Level of Challenge

If the therapist indicates that the mock session is too easy, the person enacting the role of the patient can use the following modifications to make it more challenging (see also Appendix A):

- The patient can improvise with topics that are more evocative or make the therapist uncomfortable, such as expressing currently held strong feelings (see Figure A.2).
- The patient can use a distressed voice (e.g., angry, sad, sarcastic) or unpleasant facial expression. This increases the emotional tone.

- Blend complex mixtures of opposing feelings (e.g., love and rage).
- Become confrontational, questioning the purpose of therapy or the therapist's fitness for the role.
- Be vague as to what the patient is feeling or do not use any feeling words.

If the therapist indicates that the mock session is too hard, the patient can try the following modifications:

- The patient can be guided by Figure A.2 to
  - present topics that are less evocative,
  - present material on any topic but without expressing strong feelings, or
  - present material concerning the future or the past or events outside therapy.

- The patient can ask the questions in a soft voice or with a smile. This softens the emotional stimulus.

- The therapist can take short breaks during the role-play.

- The trainer can expand the "feedback phase" by discussing psychodynamic or psychotherapy theory.

## Mock Session Patient Profiles

Following are six patient profiles for trainees to use during mock sessions, presented in order of difficulty. Following these six profiles is an advanced profile, where trainees have the option of playing themselves. The choice of patient profile may be determined by the trainee playing the therapist, the trainee playing the patient, or by the trainer.

The most important aspect of role-plays is for trainees to convey the emotional tone indicated by the patient profile (e.g., "angry" or "sad"). Trainees may adjust a patient profile to be one they are more comfortable role-playing. For example, a trainee may change the patient profile from female to male or from 45 to 22 years old. On the other hand, stretching to play a particular patient profile can pay off in terms of increased empathy and understanding.

### Beginner Profile: Processing Grief With a Receptive Patient

Helen is a 35-year-old, second-generation, Chinese American woman who does freelance office work. She sought therapy when a close friend, Sandra, found her crying uncontrollably in the bathroom during a birthday party for Sandra's 10-year-old daughter. Helen confided in her that she had miscarried a child in the fifth month of pregnancy when she was 25. Although she had two healthy children, ages 6 and 8, she felt like she never grieved her unborn child. Her friend, who had had good experiences in therapy, urged Helen to seek therapy.

- **Symptoms:** Helen is fairly symptom free except for this sudden onset of sobbing and feelings of intense loss while at the birthday party. Usually a very private person, she was embarrassed that she had "broken down" in such a public way.

- **Patient's goals for therapy:** Helen wants to explore her feelings and the reason she had gone a decade without grieving her loss.

- **Attitude toward therapy:** Helen enters treatment curious and relieved to be there. She is also somewhat ashamed and frightened by her sobbing.

- **Strengths:** Helen has a long-lasting and loving marriage. She is a good mother and enjoys her children. Helen is sincere and intelligent and has learned to trust some people, such as her close friends after they have proven themselves.

### Beginner Profile: A Young Patient Who Is Conflicted

Marie, an 18-year-old, is the middle child in her home with an older and a younger brother. Her family immigrated from Mexico when she was 5 years old. Her mother was recently diagnosed with stomach cancer; her father is a caring man who works hard as a manager of an apartment complex to keep the family sheltered and fed. Marie was accepted to start at a 4-year college 250 miles from home in a couple of months, but her mother would like her to live at home to help take care of her. Marie's friends think she should go to college. Marie has been a responsible daughter and has done well in school and has many friends. She earned a coveted work-study scholarship at the college and was set to go until her mother's diagnosis. Her parents value family above all else but are also very proud of their daughter's accomplishments.

- **Symptoms:** Marie is starting to drink alcohol, and her senior grades are slipping. She feels misunderstood by her parents and her friends. She feels very conflicted. If she goes to college, she fears she will feel guilty, especially if her mother's health worsens; if she stays, she fears she will be depriving herself of this opportunity and that she will feel resentful, especially toward her mother. She is also concerned her friends might be angry with her.

- **Patient's goals for therapy:** Marie wants to figure out what to do.

- **Attitude toward therapy:** Friends have told Marie good things about therapy, but her parents are somewhat tentative about her doing it. She hopes that she will learn what she needs to learn.

- **Strengths:** Marie is smart, loves her family, and has good friends.

### Intermediate Profile: The Patient Whose Life Is Perfect[1]

Donna, a 49-year-old, married woman with two grown children, was referred for outpatient treatment by her primary care physician who thought she might be depressed. Donna is cooperative in giving short answers to the therapist's questions but repeatedly reassures the therapist that she is "fine"—in fact, "better than fine." She has a responsible job as an administrative assistant in a company where her duties range from getting coffee for the sales team to organizing large meetings. In her words, "I have two great sons, a great husband, a nice home, and a really good life. My doctor thinks I might be depressed, but I don't think that's the case at all. Since the beginning of fall, I've seen him for headaches, and sometimes I don't sleep through the night, but I really don't have anything to complain about." Donna was raised "to be seen and not heard." Her parents impressed on her that she should be thankful for what she has. Her mother was particularly critical of Donna growing up. Donna's younger brother was born blind, and Donna "always realized how much easier I had it than he did. I really shouldn't need anything else to feel happy."

- **Symptoms:** Donna has headaches, stomachaches, and insomnia that are somatic expressions of her feeling worthless and depressed now that her sons are away at college, and she did not get an expected promotion at work.

---

1. There is a video portrayal of Donna and a written description of her dynamics, time-limited dynamic therapy, and intervention (Levenson, 2018).

- **Patient's goals for therapy:** Donna is unsure if she has any goals for therapy.

- **Attitude toward therapy:** Although Donna does not think she needs therapy, she is willing to come at the request of her trusted physician, whom she's seen for years.

- **Strengths:** Donna is a hardworking, dedicated person who has been "a good mother, a good wife, and a good employee."

### Intermediate Profile: The Patient Who Keeps Others at Arm's Length

Mrs. Follette is a 59-year-old, African American widow with three grown daughters. She had initially come to outpatient therapy because she was having some "memory problems." However, after coming to three sessions, these memory problems faded and were "no longer bothering me." She works as a supervisor in the human relations department for a large company. She reported, "I try to keep to myself, which is a good thing because my five sisters are an uncaring bunch. And my three daughters, while they live nearby, each has her own family and is very busy." She went on to explain, "I get nervous when other people get too close. I prefer to be by myself. You never know what some people have in the back of their minds. It's best not to depend on anyone. If I don't take care of myself, who will?" When the therapist tried to get a history, Mrs. Follette stated that she was taken advantage of by her sisters and her aunt. She acknowledged that her stepfather also took advantage of her, but she didn't want to go into more detail. Later in therapy, she revealed that this stepfather ("who was like a father to me") had raped her when she was 21 years old. She did not tell anyone, not even her mother, but "somehow I think she knew." Mrs. Follette also has been very hurt and traumatized by systemic racism and discrimination, socially and in the workplace.

- **Symptoms:** Mrs. Follette has suppressed anger at her mother and has expressed anger toward her sisters, aunt, and father as well as ambivalence about not getting close to her daughters and their children.

- **Patient's goals for therapy:** Mrs. Follette would like to be more open with her relatives but feels like there is "too much bad history" between her and them. She does not want to talk about the rape and the effect that it might have had on her. Her mother is currently rather feeble, and she wonders if she will need to be the one to take care of her.

- **Attitude toward therapy:** Mrs. Follette went to therapy when her husband died 20 years ago, but she had a bad experience: When she told her therapist about how her sisters and aunt were not there for her while she was grieving, she felt the therapist blamed her for pushing them away. She never did tell the therapist about the rape.

- **Strengths:** Mrs. Follette is extremely resilient. She has strong convictions about fairness and social justice. She successfully raised three daughters largely on her own and is a valued employee.

### Advanced Profile: The Patient With the Diet Doctor Father Who Eats Compulsively[2]

Lydia Ludlow is a 45-year-old woman who came to this country from Argentina when she was 13. She is recently separated from her husband. Ms. Ludlow's previous therapist

---

2. A written description of Ms. Ludlow, including her dynamics, time-limited dynamic therapy formulation and intervention, and follow-up, is available (Levenson, 1995).

recently increased her fee, so she came to a low-fee clinic to be seen by a trainee-therapist. Her presenting problems are marital difficulties, compulsive eating, and financial problems. She comes across in a naïve, almost childlike, demanding, way. "My parents have been trying to fix me my whole life, if I let them. My father is a doctor specializing in weight control and my mother is a size 4. They have concentrated on my physical defects. They just want to fix me! And now my husband is getting ready to leave me because I am not the perfect little wife."

- **Symptoms:** Lydia has mood lability, feels she has a special status, and engages in compulsive eating.

- **Patient's goals for therapy:** Lydia wants to find stability in herself and her relationships. She believes that the therapist will be able to help her.

- **Attitude towards therapy:** Lydia has been in therapy before. She feels her previous therapist abandoned her when the therapist raised her fee, and so she quit that therapy and sought out a new therapist (you) at a low-fee clinic. Lydia is worried that you may betray or abandon her. She wants to come two or three times a week "because you have probably never seen anyone quite like me before!"

- **Strengths:** Lydia can be very open to what the therapist says (when she feels safe in the therapy).

### Advanced Profile: The Patient Looking for a Fight

"Colt" Charles Pettigrew is a White male, rookie police officer sent for mandatory counseling to help with his "anger issues." His superiors required him to get psychotherapy for what they called his "excessive drinking and violent behavior" while off-duty. As Colt saw it, his problems were that "sometimes guys get smart with you, and I have to show them." He also felt that what he did on his own time was his business. "Colt" is a nickname his father gave him because he was a spritely, active child. Later on, Colt was diagnosed with attention-deficit disorder. For a long time, it was his dream to become a police officer. "Look, I know how to handle myself since I was 8. My old man made me fight my cousin, Bobby. Well Bobby was 12 and pretty big. At first, I was scared, but then I got really angry. So, I beat him good! Bobby was a bleeding mess when I was done with him. Dad was real happy with me, that day. Of course, later he punched me a few times for talking back to him. But that kind of thing happened in my family. And it made me the man I am today, I can tell you."

- **Symptoms:** Colt is belligerent and quick to have his anger turn to physical acts of pushing or punching. Alcohol abuse is likely.

- **Patient's goals for therapy:** Initially, Colt announced, "So, look, let's get through this! I don't need anything more than your signature letting me go back to work." Eventually, he acknowledged that he sometimes loses control but denied that this was ever on the job.

- **Attitude towards therapy:** Colt is angry about being sent for therapy. He does not see any reason for talking with someone: "So, I came here because they made me. Let's get this over with!"

### Advanced Profile: Play Yourself

The last example is for trainees who would like to play themselves. This follows in the tradition of psychodynamic training that strongly encourages (and sometimes requires) trainees to be in their own therapy. From a relational, psychodynamic perspective, this is the most productive way to learn to be a psychodynamic therapist. Being in the patient role, one learns an immense amount about what it is like to be vulnerable, on the downside of power in an important relationship. In addition, being a patient yourself might give you greater empathy for your own patients because you have walked in their shoes, so to speak. As a patient, you can explore your own experience in a productive manner. In her widely used textbook *Psychoanalytic Psychotherapy*, Nancy McWilliams (2004) lauded the usefulness of therapist's own therapy:

> Personal treatment may not inoculate us with "objectivity," but it can vastly increase our capacity to observe and make good use of the dynamics that inevitably get stirred up in our work. With all its hazards and limitations, personal treatment seems to me the best route to mature, empathic listening. (p. 63)

Being the patient and able to have genuine thoughts and feelings in response to the interventions of the trainee seated across from you will benefit your peer therapist. They will be able to see the impact of what they say and evaluate from moment-to-moment whether they are being helpful by watching your authentic responses. The psychodynamic therapist wishes to create new emotional experiences and foster insight, and thus your peer therapist can decide which interventions (using what skills) might deepen your emotional experiencing and prove helpful.

### Note to Trainees

The person playing the patient should choose a personal issue or topic that feels comfortable to explore and deepen. Throughout the exercise, the trainee–patient needs to self-monitor and choose how much to self-disclose factually and emotionally (i.e., how vulnerable to become and how much feels safe to reveal). Finally, when the trainee–patient plays themselves, we do not recommend that the therapist use a hand gesture to indicate difficulty level because that may distract the patient and prevent exploration. In addition, the trainee–therapist must be aware and self-monitor their own comfort level (just like a real therapist). If the content or emotional tone of the session becomes uncomfortable, the therapist can choose less provocative interventions or invite the patient to step back and talk about their experience rather than feel it. Changing the subject to a less "hot" topic might also be helpful. If either trainee starts to feel too deeply immersed in the role-play, asking for the supervisor's help to make the experience more didactic than emotional (e.g., to elucidate the teaching points in the mock session) could be beneficial.

### Instructions

Work in pairs. One trainee playing the patient chooses a personal issue to discuss that feels comfortable to explore in the training setting. Trainees may choose an issue that they have been struggling with recently and want to talk over, problem solve, or gain insight into. If you are playing yourself as patient, you may want to think over in advance (a) what relational problems or issues, symptoms, or behaviors you wish to discuss; (b) what your goal for the session might be (exploration as a goal is valid!); and (c) what attitude toward your therapy you wish to convey (such as curiosity about your own experience).

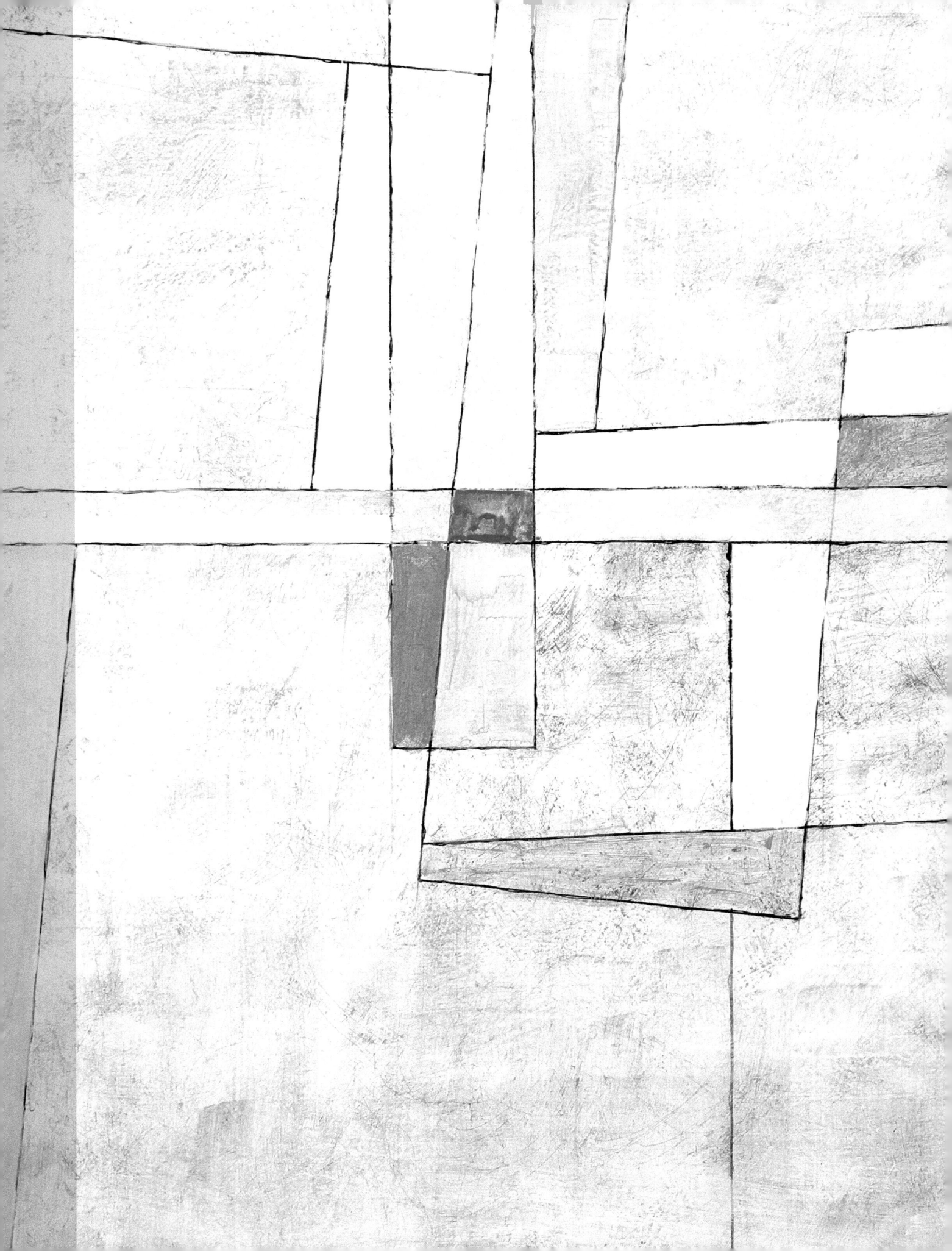

# Strategies for Enhancing the Deliberate Practice Exercises

Part III consists of one chapter, Chapter 3, that provides additional advice and instructions for trainers and trainees so that they can reap more benefits from the deliberate practice exercises in Part II. Chapter 3 offers seven key points for getting the most out of deliberate practice, guidelines for practicing appropriately responsive treatment, evaluation strategies, methods for ensuring trainee well-being and respecting their privacy, and advice for monitoring the trainer–trainee relationship.

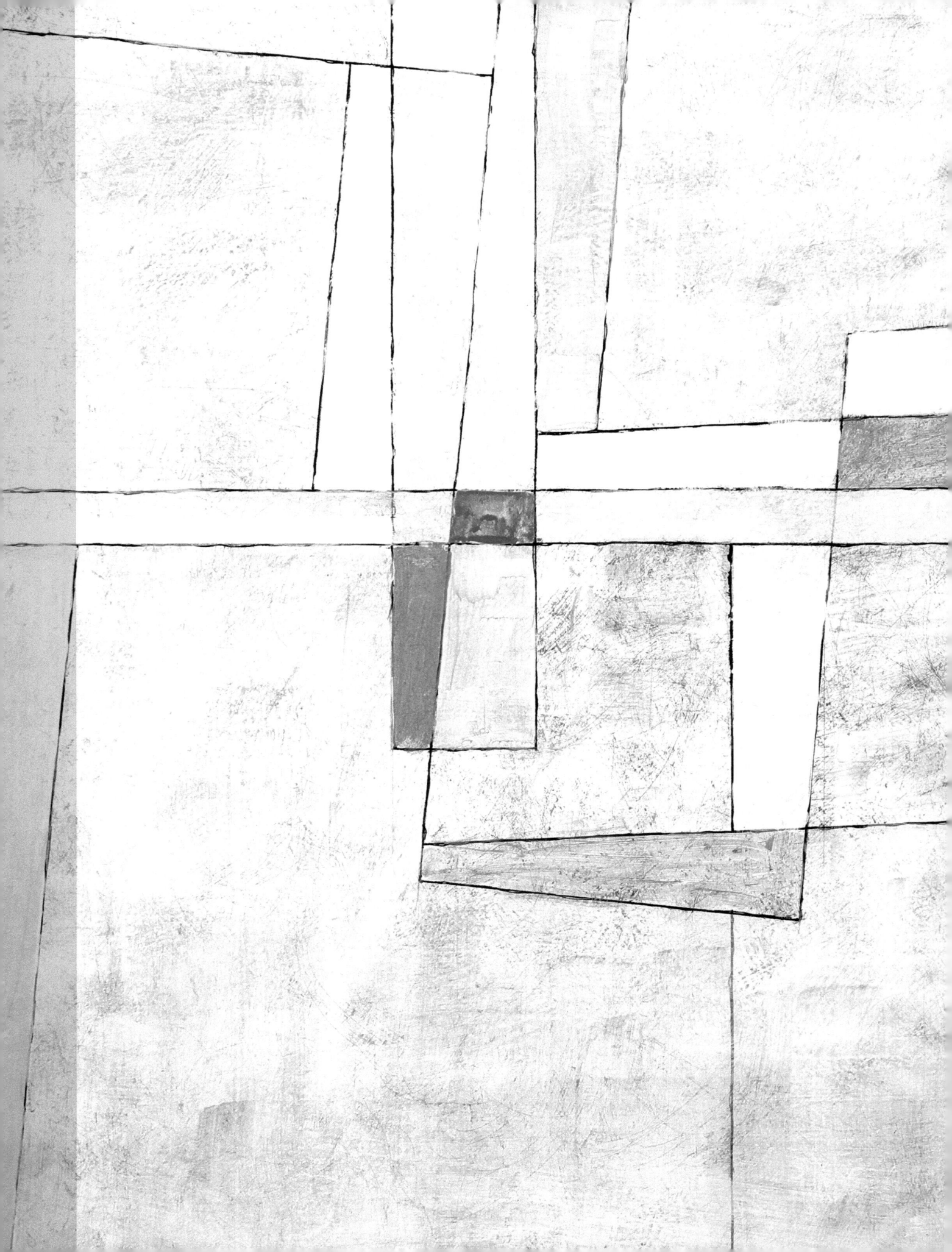

# How to Get the Most Out of Deliberate Practice for Dynamic Psychotherapy: Additional Guidance for Trainers and Trainees

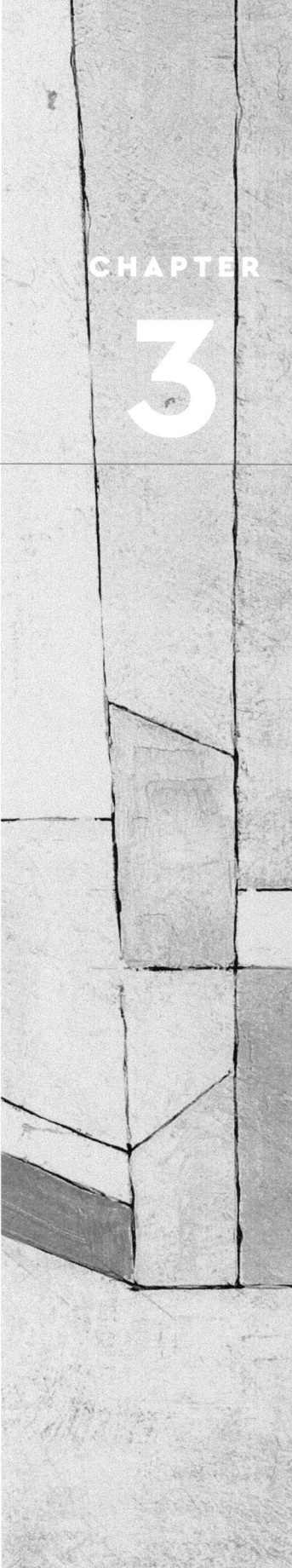

In this book, we have proposed that dynamic psychotherapy instructors and supervisors can incorporate deliberate practice methods into their curricula and supervision—not as a replacement of something, but as an addition—a missing ingredient.

Louis Pasteur, the 19th-century bacteriologist, had it right when he said, "The more prepared or knowledgeable you are, the more likely you will be able to make the most of chance opportunities and observations." Pasteur uttered those words in 1854 when he welcomed students to a new training institute devoted to teaching applied sciences. We value both learning to apply theory (models of the mind, models of psychopathology) and learning to engage in the intimate, sometimes scary work of trying to help people who suffer. The laboratories we use in this book are the classroom, supervision sessions, and students' extracurricular reflections. The equipment we use is our current dynamic theory, the discipline of deliberate practice, and 12 graduated exercises. We hope to provoke just the right amount of arousal (excitement, trepidation, and challenge) in students who can discover in their turn the utility and value of dynamic psychotherapy.

In Chapter 2, and in the exercises themselves, we provided instructions for completing these deliberate practice exercises. This chapter provides guidance to trainers on big-picture topics that trainers will need to integrate deliberate practice successfully into their training program. This guidance is based on research findings in deliberate practice and the responses from trainers at more than a dozen psychotherapy training programs who tested the deliberate practice exercises in this book. We cover topics including evaluation, getting the most from deliberate practice, trainee well-being, respecting trainee privacy, trainer self-evaluation, responsive treatment, and the trainee–trainer alliance. We show how to personalize the patient context for your particular setting and patient population.

https://doi.org/10.1037/0000351-017

*Deliberate Practice in Psychodynamic Psychotherapy*, by H. Levenson, V. Gay, and J. L. Binder

## Seven Points for Getting the Most From Deliberate Practice

### Point 1: Discover How to Be in a Psychodynamic Frame of Mind

Doing psychodynamic therapy (PDT) is a way of both being with and working with patients. Although many of the exercises in this text focus on the technical aspects of PDT and rehearsing specific PDT skills, **the stance of the psychodynamic therapist is critical.** PDT requires an openness of mind and heart. The therapist needs to build empathy for the patient, reflect on the possible meanings of the patient's statements, and explore what the patient's world might be like. Doing PDT is complex. A single patient statement might represent a vast array of meanings, emotions, and connections with personal values, goals, and identities. Above all, a PDT sensibility involves listening that is both intently focused and intuitively free-floating. There is a comfort with "not knowing" and allowing the process to evolve. One of us (H. L.) jokes with her students that she gets paid more for what she doesn't say to patients than what she does say—which means that the psychodynamic therapist senses, feels, and thinks a great deal but might share only a fraction of this with patients. Perhaps the therapist's thoughts and feelings will not be appreciated by the patient if offered directly, perhaps the timing is not right, perhaps the therapist is unsure, or perhaps the patient is on the edge of providing their own associations.

### Point 2: Use Deliberate Practice Exercises as a Map, Not the Territory

Although the deliberate practice exercises in this book are intended to build skills helpful to trainees in actual sessions with real patients, **the exercises themselves should not be thought of as templates merely to be inserted into sessions.** Many of the skills in this book can be thought of as "inner skills" (Rousmaniere, 2019) that can help the therapist-in-training understand, recognize, and become more aware. For example, a person learning to play basketball might stand a precise distance from the hoop and practice shooting baskets over and over. However, that repetitive behavior will never happen in a real game, and the player may rarely shoot a basket from that exact spot. Nonetheless, the procedural memory of how to shoot a basket will be invaluable when the opportunity arises. Similarly, although you may never give a transference interpretation that sounds as succinct as those in Exercise 7 or a dream interpretation that is as simple and direct as those in Exercise 9, your practicing how to recognize transference phenomena and see conflict resolution in dreams will help you respond in more subtle and nuanced ways when the therapeutic situation calls for it.

### Point 3: Create Realistic Emotional Stimuli

A key component of deliberate practice is using stimuli that provoke reactions in trainees that match real-life settings. For example, pilots train with flight simulators that present mechanical failures and dangerous weather conditions; surgeons practice with surgical simulators that present medical complications with only seconds to respond. In the same way, using challenging stimuli increases trainees' capacity to perform therapy effectively under stress with challenging patients. The stimuli used for dynamic psychotherapy deliberate practice exercises are role-plays with challenging patient statements. **It is important that the trainee who is role-playing the patient perform the script with appropriate emotional expression and maintain eye contact with the therapist. Both enhance the realism and therefore value of the exercise.** For example, if the patient statement calls for sad emotion, the trainee should try to express sadness eye-to-eye with the therapist. We offer four suggestions regarding emotional expressiveness:

1. The emotional tone of the role-play matters more than the exact words of the script. Trainees role-playing the patient should feel free to improvise if that helps them be more emotionally expressive. Trainees need not stick exactly to the script. In fact, to literally read the script during the exercise can sound flat and prohibit eye contact. Rather, trainees in the patient role should first read the patient statement silently, then, when ready, say it in an emotional manner while looking directly at the trainee playing the therapist. This will help the experience feel more real and engaging for the therapist.

2. Trainees whose first language is not English may benefit from reviewing and changing the words in the patient statement script before each role-play. The goal is to find words that feel congruent to the trainee–patient and that facilitate emotional expression.

3. Trainees role-playing the patient should try to use tonal and nonverbal expressions of feelings. For example, if a script calls for anger, the trainee could speak with an angry voice and make fists; if a script calls for shame or guilt, the trainee could hunch over and wince; if a script calls for sadness, the trainee could speak in a soft or deflated voice. Sometimes the script indicates that the patient is crying. We do not expect trainees to be able to cry on demand; do your best to convey the emotion that matches your capacities and inclinations.

4. If trainees have persistent difficulty acting believably when following a particular script in the role of patient, it may help to first do a "demo round" by reading directly from paper and then, immediately after, dropping the paper to make eye contact and repeating the same patient statement from memory. Some trainees reported that this helped them "become available as a real patient" and made the role-play feel less artificial. Some trainees did three or four "demo rounds" to get into their role as a patient.

## Point 4: Customize the Exercises to Fit Your Setting and Context for Training

We have written the patient examples for the 12 initial exercises to be largely nameless and gender-inclusive (gender-neutral). We have done this not to keep the patient variables "vague" but rather to allow the trainers and trainees the option of using names and other identifiers that would be more appropriate given their culture, country, and clinical setting. For example, trainees could change the patient's gender to align with their own gender identity or insert patient names to better reflect their own ethnicity or culture. Of course, some changes (e.g., the emotional tone of the patient's statements) might completely change the emotional response of the therapist. But deliberate practice is more about using training *principles* than about specific content. As long as the skill criteria are followed, the exercise (even with major changes) will remain relevant.

The exercises may be altered by trainers given different training contexts. For example, trainees may be working in a primary care clinic or a prison setting. We encourage you to adapt the exercises and terms for your training circumstances. Furthermore, all trainers have an individual teaching style and all trainees their individual learning process. We urge trainees and trainers to adjust exercises to optimize their practice. In our experience with many trainers and trainees, we found that most spontaneously customized the exercises for their training circumstances.

### Point 5: Discover Your Personal Therapeutic Style

Deliberate practice in psychotherapy is like learning to play jazz. Jazz musicians pride themselves in their skillful improvisations. "Finding your own voice" is a prerequisite for expertise in jazz musicianship. Yet improvisations are not a collection of random notes. They are the culmination of extensive deliberate practice over time. Indeed, the ability to improvise is built on many hours of dedicated practice of scales, melodies, harmonies, and so on. As we noted in Chapter 1, Miles Davis, arguably one of the best-known American jazz musicians, once said, "Sometimes you have to play a long time to be able to play like yourself" (Cook, 2005, p. 34). He could have been talking to a room full of therapists. In the same way, we encourage trainees to experience the scripted interventions in this book not as ends in themselves but as ways to develop skill in a systematic fashion. Dedicated practice in these therapeutic "scales" and "melodies" provides a foundation for therapeutic creativity and individual style. It may take *you* a long time to sound authentically like yourself.

### Point 6: Continually Adjust Difficulty

A crucial element of deliberate practice is training at an optimal difficulty level: neither too easy nor too hard. To achieve this, carry out difficulty assessments and adjustments using the Deliberate Practice Reaction Form in Appendix A. **Do not skip this step!** If trainees don't feel any of the "good challenge" reactions at the bottom of the Deliberate Practice Reaction Form, then the exercise is probably too easy; if they feel any of the "too hard" reactions, then the exercise could be too difficult for the trainee. Advanced trainees and therapists may find all the patient statements too easy. If so, they should follow the instructions in Appendix A on making patient statements harder and to make the role-plays sufficiently challenging.

### Point 7: Extend Your Deliberate Practice Beyond These Exercises

The 12 skill-focused exercises in this book are only a beginning—both in terms of the scope of practice and intensity. The mock sessions (Exercise 14) provide an opportunity to practice integrating the 12 PDT skills in a single session. They benefit trainees by providing greater contextualization of the individual therapy responses associated with each skill and showing how to integrate the disparate pieces of training in a coherent manner. You might also try setting intentional practice goals for work with real patients. Ideally these practice and real sessions can be recorded for later self-observation or for observation and feedback by a supervisor. In addition to watching your own videos, viewing videos of experienced PDT therapists is invaluable, especially if you try to identify the skills they are using and what characterizes those skills. Exercise 13 contains annotated transcripts of two sessions from a six-session PDT (time-limited dynamic psychotherapy). A commercially available video of these two sessions (or all six sessions) is available from the American Psychological Association (APA; Levenson & Carlson, 2010; Levenson & Friedlander, in production). The two-session version contains an interview with the first author (H. L.) about the use of deliberate practice exercises in PDT.

## Responsive Treatment

The exercises in this book are designed to help trainees to not only acquire the specific skills of PDT but also to use them in ways that are responsive to each individual patient (Binder, 2004; Binder & Betan, 2013; Levenson, 2021; Silberschatz, 2021; Tishby, 2021). Because contemporary, relational dynamic psychotherapy is by its very nature a two-person psychology where interventions should always be context dependent, PDT requires therapist responsiveness—"doing the right thing, in the right way, at the right time" (Levenson, 2021). The basis for these choices in PDT largely comes from the therapist's *facilitative interpersonal skills* (Anderson et al., 1999, 2009, 2016, 2020), implicit relational knowing (Lyons-Ruth et al., 1999; Stern et al., 1998), and theoretical and technical expertise wherein therapists exercise flexible judgment, based on their perceptiveness of their patients' emotional state, needs, and goals, and integrate techniques and other relevant expertise in pursuit of optimal patient outcomes. The effective therapist responds to the emerging context. As Stiles and Horvath (2017) suggested, therapists are effective when they are appropriately responsive to patients' distinctiveness. Or as Binder (2004) proposed, "The skillful use of therapeutic techniques is ultimately based on an ability to *flexibly* adapt them to immediate contextual circumstances" (p. 8). In PDT, doing the "right thing" is always seen as different strokes for different folks. Thus, from the beginning PDT therapists learn to provide patients with responses individually tailored to them (e.g., their attachment style), at that particular point in time (e.g., what is the nature of the alliance), while tracking what occurs between therapist and patient (e.g., enactments). Using this set of skills is complex achievement—which is part of the reason that writing this deliberate practice book for psychodynamic trainees was so challenging!

Appropriate responsiveness counters a misconception that deliberate practice rehearsal is designed to promote robotic repetition of therapy techniques. On the one hand, psychotherapy researchers have shown that over-adherence to a particular model while neglecting patient preferences reduces therapy effectiveness (e.g., Castonguay et al., 1996; Henry et al., 1993; Owen & Hilsenroth, 2014). On the other hand, therapist flexibility improves outcomes (e.g., Bugatti & Boswell, 2016; Kendall & Beidas, 2007; Kendall & Frank, 2018). It is important, therefore, that trainees practice their newly learned skills in a manner that is flexible and responsive to the needs of a diverse range of patients (Hatcher, 2015; Hill & Knox, 2013). It is crucial for trainees to develop perceptual skills to observe what the patient is experiencing in the moment. (This is similar to the Deliberate Practice Reaction Form in Appendix A: We ask ourselves is our intervention too challenging or too easy.) By assessing their interventions based on the patient's reactions in a moment-by-moment context, therapists increase their effectiveness.

Supervisors must help their supervisees to attune themselves to the specific needs of the patients during sessions. Process supervision (Greenberg & Tomescu, 2017; Levenson, 1995; Levenson & Strupp, 1999), the practice of supervisor and supervisee listening to recorded sessions, stopping at poignant moments, and considering patient's feelings and meanings, lends itself to teaching appropriate responsiveness. The supervisor can stop the recording, ask the supervisee to reflect on the patient's feelings and meanings, and help the supervisee consider which response would be best in that moment. By enacting responsiveness with the supervisee, the supervisor demonstrates its value and makes it explicit. These methods demonstrate the essential "melody" of appropriate responsiveness. By doing that, the trainee and supervisor help the trainee master not just the techniques, but how the trainee can foster therapeutic growth. Helping trainees to keep this overarching goal in mind while reviewing their therapy process is a valuable feature of supervision that is difficult to obtain otherwise (Hatcher, 2015).

It is also important that deliberate practice occur within a context of wider dynamic psychotherapy learning. As noted in Chapter 1, training should be combined with supervision of actual therapy recordings, theoretical learning, observation of competent PDT clinicians, as well as personal therapeutic work. When the trainer or trainee determine that the trainee is having difficulty acquiring dynamic psychotherapy skills, it is important to assess what is missing. Assessment should then lead to the appropriate remedy, as the trainer and trainee collaboratively determine what is needed.

## Making Use of the Psychotherapy of Everyday Life: The Psychodynamic Emphasis on Fantasy and Entertainment

One of the ways students can get the most out of deliberate practice from a psychodynamic viewpoint is to make use of patients' abundant references to fantasy and entertainment. Sigmund Freud (1856–1939), the founder of psychoanalysis and its many offspring, was immersed in cultural studies, the critique of religion, and the exploration of fantasy. Freud applied his clinical theorems to dramas, novels, myths, and fairy tales—in ways that were unusual for a serious physician. He did so because he wished to construct a *general psychology* of human emotions, suffering, and repair. Those phenomena appear continuously in popular culture and popular religion going as far back as the early Greeks around the ninth century bce.

Pursuing his ambition, Freud wrote dozens of essays and books on cultural artifacts, especially religion because it seemed to be the chief competitor of psychoanalytic psychotherapy. Freud himself created cultural forces that extend to our times. He shaped how novelists, poets, and TV writers—and especially originators of online role-playing games (beginning with Dungeons & Dragons)—conceive of their work.

All deliberate practice manuals in this APA series share common goals and techniques regarding classroom instruction and practice. However, dynamic psychotherapy makes use of additional sources of information and practice. Students can get the most out of psychodynamic deliberate practice by focusing on their patients' fantasies and sources of entertainment. Those are the worlds of culture, TV shows, movies, daydreams, song lyrics, advertisements, and social media. Unique to our book is our claim that exploring a patient's fantasy life (daydreams, dreams, and the like) helps in "grokking" (i.e., to understand intuitively or by empathy) that person's wishes, fears, hopes, and aspirations. For example, patients fascinated by stories about alternate timelines are often wrestling with similar themes in their daily lives. Yearning to go back in time and do it better is common to our species.

In his best-selling novel *The Midnight Library*, Matt Haig (2020) portrays Nora, a young woman driven by multiple catastrophes to suicidal despair. After trying to kill herself, Nora wakes up in a magical library whose custodian lets her explore different life paths. In the novel's front matter, Haig cites Sylvia Plath's comments, "I can never be all the people I want and live all the lives I want. . . . I want to live and feel all the shades, tones, and variations of mental and physical experiences possible in my life" (unnumbered page). That Sylvia Plath, a brilliant poet, killed herself out of suicidal despair adds grimness to this passage.

Imagine that your patient enthusiastically describes her fascination with Sylvia Plath and with *The Midnight Library*. Using the deliberate practice skills "deepening affect" and "inquiry" you would first acknowledge her feeling (fascination) and second inquire about both topics—Plath and *The Midnight Library*. You need not know the details of either subject. "Inquiry" (Exercise 1) gives you permission to learn from your patient about each topic—in as much depth as needed—and about her fascination with them. Depending on her answers, one might investigate a possible parallel between the patient's fascination with the topics and the patient's own desires. For example, you might ask if she has contemplated self-harm or self-destruction.

Another patient of yours—say, a young man—might also talk excitedly about *The Midnight Library*. Using the deliberate practice exercise on inquiry, you learn that he's yearning for the power to redo his life's choices, to "do it again" and get it right. He does not focus on the Plath citation or on Nora's suicide attempt that initiates the story. In this instance, we would have little reason to ask him about suicide. However, we might explore the patient's yearning for magical solutions to his emotional problems. The deliberate practice skill "pointing out defenses" (Exercise 5) would help us learn why the patient gravitated to magical devices.

The themes of interpersonal and intrapsychic struggles and striving appear in abundance. Each narrative, whether it be in a novel, movie, poem, or online role-playing game, portrays human beings whom we can better understand using the ideas and skills expanded in this book.

Another way students can get the most out of deliberate practice is by using movie clips and one's own recordings of clinical sessions as stimuli. Visual stimuli often arouse strong affects, and thus movie clips or portions of clinical sessions with patients can be watched by students (and more advanced therapists) wishing to achieve self-awareness of internal states. Tony Rousmaniere (2019), one of the editors of the Deliberate Practice Series, has written a book titled *Mastering the Inner Skills of Psychotherapy: A Deliberate Practice Manual*. In this text, Rousmaniere recommended selecting a video clip 3 to 5 minutes long:

> The ideal video for this exercise is a session of your work as a therapist that you found very challenging. . . . If you don't have a video of your work as a therapist, then you can use a video clip from a movie, television show, news report, documentary, political debate, or any other media that you find very evocative. (p. 52)

The next step is to watch the video while observing your reactions. You can use the Deliberate Practice Reaction Form (see Appendix A), trying to notice at least five different reactions. The best video will feel challenging but not too hard; the goal is to build one's psychological capacity. The author reassuringly stated that over time, the therapist will begin to discern which reactions are helpful in therapy and which are not. Rousmaniere described various ways to use visual stimuli to improve the therapist's attention, emotional downregulation, and self-recovery. In a useful appendix to his book, he listed a set of provocative movie clips (with links to YouTube).

## Being Mindful of Trainee Well-Being

Although negative effects that some patients experience in psychotherapy have been well documented (Barlow, 2010), negative effects of training and supervision on trainees have received less attention (Ellis et al., 2014). PDT has a strong tradition of creating and sustaining safety in training and supervision (McWilliams, 2021; Sarnat, 2016), building on the supervisory alliance where the supervisor is attentive to the feelings and needs of the trainee. Collaboration of goals and tasks of training and supervision is founded upon such core relational conditions.

To support self-efficacy, deliberate practice trainers must ensure that trainees are practicing at a correct difficulty level. The exercises in this book suggest frequently assessing and adjusting the difficulty level so that trainees can rehearse at a level that targets their personal skill threshold. Trainers and supervisors must provide an appropriate challenge. One risk to trainees that is particularly pertinent to this book occurs when using role-plays that are too difficult. The Deliberate Practice Reaction Form in Appendix A will help trainers ensure that role-plays are done at an appropriate challenge level. Trainers or trainees may be tempted to skip the difficulty assessments and adjustments, out of their motivation to focus on rehearsal to make faster progress and quickly acquire skills. However, across all our test sites, we found that skipping the difficulty assessments and adjustments caused more problems and hindered skill acquisition more than any other error. Thus, trainers are advised to remember that **one of their most important responsibilities is to remind trainees to do the difficulty assessments and adjustments.**

Additionally, the Deliberate Practice Reaction Form serves a dual purpose of helping trainees develop the important skills of self-monitoring and self-awareness (Bennett-Levy, 2019). This will help trainees adopt a positive and empowered stance regarding their self-care and will facilitate career-long professional development.

## Respecting Trainee Privacy

The deliberate practice exercises in this book may produce complex or uncomfortable personal reactions within trainees, including memories of past traumas. Exploring psychological and emotional reactions may make some trainees feel vulnerable. (Therapists at every career stage, from trainees to seasoned therapists with decades of experience, commonly experience shame, embarrassment, and self-doubt in this process.) Although these experiences may help build trainees' self-awareness, training should remain focused on professional skill development and not merge into personal therapy (e.g., Ellis et al., 2014). Therefore, trainers should remind trainees to maintain appropriate boundaries for themselves.

Trainees have the final say about what to disclose or not disclose to their trainer. Trainees should keep in mind that the goal is to expand their self-awareness and psychological capacity to stay active and helpful while experiencing uncomfortable reactions. The trainer does not need to know specific details about the trainee's inner world for this to happen.

Trainees should be instructed to share only personal information that they feel comfortable sharing. The Deliberate Practice Reaction Form and difficulty assessment process help trainees build self-awareness while retaining control over their privacy. Remind trainees that the goal is for them to learn about their inner world. They do not have to share that information with trainers or peers (Bennett-Levy & Finlay-Jones, 2018). Likewise, trainees should respect the confidentiality of their peers.

## Trainer Self-Evaluation

We tested these exercises at a range of training sites around the world, including graduate courses, practicum sites, and private practice offices. Although trainers reported that the exercises were highly effective, some were disoriented by how different deliberate practice felt compared with traditional methods of clinical education. Many felt comfortable evaluating their trainees' performance but were less sure about their performance as trainers.

The most common concern from trainers was, "My trainees are doing great, but I'm not sure if I am doing this correctly!" To address this concern, we recommend trainers perform periodic self-evaluations using the following five criteria:

1. Observe trainees' work performance.
2. Provide continual corrective feedback.
3. Ensure that sufficient time is spent on skill rehearsal.
4. Ensure that the trainee is practicing at the right difficulty level (neither too easy nor too challenging).
5. Continuously assess trainee performance with real patients.

### Criterion 1: Observe Trainees' Work Performance

Determining how well we are doing as trainers means having valid information about how well trainees are responding to training. To provide corrective feedback and evaluation we must observe trainees practicing skills. One risk of deliberate practice is that trainees gain competence in performing therapy skills in role-plays, but those skills do not transfer to trainees' work with real patients. Thus, trainers will ideally observe samples of trainees' work with real patients, either live or via recorded video. Supervisors and consultants rely heavily—and, too often, exclusively—on supervisees and consultee narratives of their work with patients (Goodyear & Nelson, 1997). Haggerty and Hilsenroth (2011) described this challenge:

> Suppose a loved one has to undergo surgery and you need to choose between two surgeons, one of whom has never been directly observed by an experienced surgeon while performing any surgery. He or she would perform the surgery and return to his or her attending physician and try to recall, sometimes incompletely or inaccurately, the intricate steps of the surgery they just performed. It is hard to imagine that anyone, given a choice, would prefer this over a professional who has been routinely observed in the practice of their craft. (p. 193)

### Criterion 2: Provide Continual Corrective Feedback

Trainees need corrective feedback to learn what they are doing well, what they are doing poorly, and how to improve their skills. Feedback should be as specific and incremental as possible. Examples of specific feedback are "Your voice sounds rushed. Try slowing down by pausing for a few seconds between your statements to the patient" and "You are making excellent eye contact with the patient." Examples of vague and nonspecific feedback are "Try to build better rapport with the patient" and "Try to be more open to the patient's feelings."

### Criterion 3: Ensure That Sufficient Time Is Spent on Skill Rehearsal

Deliberate practice emphasizes skill acquisition via behavioral rehearsal. Trainers should resist getting caught up in patient conceptualization at the expense of focusing on skills. For many trainers, this requires self-restraint. It is often more enjoyable to talk *about* psychotherapy (e.g., case conceptualization, treatment planning, nuances of psychotherapy models, similar cases the supervisor has had) than to watch trainees rehearse skills. Trainees have many questions and supervisors have an abundance of experience; the allotted supervision time can easily be filled sharing conceptual knowledge. The supervisor enjoys teaching, while the trainee doesn't have to struggle with acquiring new and challenging skills. While answering questions is important, trainees' intellectual knowledge about psychotherapy can quickly surpass their procedural ability to perform psychotherapy, particularly with patients they find difficult. Here's a simple rule of thumb: The trainer provides the knowledge, but the behavioral rehearsal provides the skill (Rousmaniere, 2019).

### Criterion 4: Practice at the Right Difficulty Level—Neither Too Easy nor Too Challenging (Zone of Proximal Development)

Deliberate practice involves *optimal strain*: practicing skills just beyond the trainee's current skill threshold so they can learn incrementally without becoming overwhelmed or insufficiently challenged (Ericsson, 2006).

Trainers should use difficulty assessments and adjustments throughout deliberate practice to ensure that trainees are practicing at the right difficulty level. Note that some trainees are surprised by their unpleasant reactions to exercises (e.g., disassociation, nausea, blanking out) and may be tempted to "push through" exercises that are too hard. This can happen out of fear of failing a course, fear of being judged as incompetent, or negative self-impressions by the trainee (e.g., "This shouldn't be so hard"). On the other hand, if trainees are not struggling a bit, then they are not straining those muscles to become stronger. Trainers should normalize the fact that there will be wide variation in perceived difficulty of the exercises and encourage trainees to respect their own personal training process.

### Criterion 5: Continuously Assess Trainee Performance With Real Patients

The goal of deliberately practicing psychotherapy skills is to improve trainees' effectiveness at helping real patients. One of the risks in deliberate practice training is that its benefits will not generalize: Trainees' acquired competence in specific skills may not translate into work with real patients. Thus, it is important that trainers assess the impact of deliberate practice on trainees' work with real patients. Ideally, this is done through triangulation of multiple data points:

1. patient data (verbal self-report, routine outcome monitoring data, live supervision, use of videos of sessions)
2. supervisor's report
3. trainee's self-report

If the trainee's effectiveness with real patients does not improve after deliberate practice, the trainer should carefully assess difficulty levels. If the trainer feels it is a skill acquisition issues, the trainer can change the deliberate practice routine to better suit the trainee's learning needs and style.

Therapists have traditionally been evaluated from a lens of *process accountability* (Markman & Tetlock, 2000; see also Goodyear, 2015), which focuses on demonstrating specific behaviors (e.g., fidelity to a treatment model) without regard to the impact on patients. We propose that clinical effectiveness is better assessed through a lens tightly focused on patient outcomes and that learning objectives shift from performing behaviors that experts have decided are effective (i.e., the competence model) to highly individualized behavioral goals tailored to each trainee's zone of proximal development and performance feedback. This model of assessment has been termed *outcome accountability* (Goodyear, 2015) and focuses on patient changes, rather than therapist competence, independent of how the therapist might be performing expected tasks.

## Guidance for Trainees

The central theme of this book is that skill rehearsal is not automatically helpful. Deliberate practice must be done well for trainees to benefit (Ericsson & Pool, 2016). In this chapter, we offer guidance for effective deliberate practice. We also provide additional advice for trainees. That advice is drawn from what we have learned at our volunteer deliberate practice test sites. We discuss how to discover your own training process, active effort, and playfulness, taking breaks during deliberate practice, your right to control self-disclosure to trainers, monitoring training results, monitoring complex reactions toward the trainer, and your personal therapy.

### Individualized Psychodynamic Training: Finding Your Zone of Proximal Development

Deliberate practice works best when training targets each trainee's personal skill thresholds. Also called the *zone of proximal development*, a term first coined by Vygotsky in reference to developmental learning theory (Zaretskii, 2009), this is the area just beyond the trainee's current ability but that is possible to reach with the assistance of a teacher or coach (Wass & Golding, 2014). **If a deliberate practice exercise is either too easy or too hard, the trainee will not benefit.** To maximize training productivity, elite performers follow a "challenging but not overwhelming" principle: Tasks that are too far beyond their capacity will prove ineffective and even harmful, but it is equally true that mindlessly repeating what they can already do confidently will prove fruitless. Because of this, deliberate practice requires ongoing assessment of the trainee's current skill and concurrent difficulty adjustment to target a "good enough" challenge.

### Active Effort

It is important for trainees to maintain an active and sustained effort while doing the deliberate practice exercises in this book. This is best achieved when trainees take ownership of their practice by guiding their training partners to adjust roleplays to be as high on the difficulty scale as possible without harming themselves. This will look different for every trainee. Although it can feel uncomfortable or even frightening, this is the zone of proximal development where the most gains can be made. Simply reading and repeating the written scripts will provide little or no benefit. These efforts should lead to more confidence and comfort in session with real patients.

### Stay the Course: Effort Versus Flow

Deliberate practice works only if trainees push themselves hard enough to break out of their old patterns of performance, which then permits growth of new skills (Ericsson & Pool, 2016). Because deliberate practice constantly focuses on the edge of one's performance capacity, it is inevitably a strenuous endeavor. Indeed, professionals are unlikely to make lasting performance improvements unless there is sufficient engagement in tasks that are just at the edge of their current capacity (Ericsson, 2003, 2006). From athletics or fitness training, many of us are familiar with this process of being pushed out of our comfort zones followed by adaptation. The same process applies to our mental and emotional abilities.

Many trainees are surprised to learn that deliberate practice for dynamic psychotherapy feels harder than psychotherapy with real patients. This may be because when working with a real patient a therapist can get into a state of *flow* (Csikszentmihalyi, 1997), where work feels effortless. In such cases, therapists may want to move back to offering response formats with which they are more familiar and feel more proficient, and use those for a short time, in part to increase a sense of confidence and mastery.

### Discover Your Own Training Process

The effectiveness of deliberate practice is directly related to the effort and ownership trainees exert while doing the exercises. Trainers can provide guidance, but it is important for trainees to learn about their idiosyncratic training processes over time. The following are a few examples of personal training processes that trainees discovered while engaging in deliberate practice:

- One trainee noticed that she is good at persisting while an exercise is challenging but that she requires more rehearsal than other trainees to feel comfortable with a new skill. This trainee focused on developing patience with her pace of progress.

- One trainee noticed that he could acquire new skills quickly, with only a few repetitions. However, he also noticed that his reactions to evocative patient statements jumped quickly and unpredictably from the "good challenge" to "too hard" categories. So he needed to attend to his reactions listed in the Deliberate Practice Reaction Form.

- One trainee described herself as "perfectionistic" and felt a strong urge to "push through" an exercise even when she had anxiety reactions, such as nausea and disassociation, in the "too hard" category. This caused the trainee not to benefit from the exercises and to risk becoming demoralized. This trainee focused on going slower, developing self-compassion regarding her anxiety, and asking her training partners to make role-plays less challenging.

Trainees are encouraged to reflect on their experiences using the exercises to learn about themselves and their personal learning processes.

### Being Playful and Taking Breaks

Psychotherapy is serious work that often involves painful feelings. However, practicing psychotherapy can be playful and fun. Trainees should remember that one of the main goals of deliberate practice is to experiment with different approaches and styles of therapy. If deliberate practice feels rote, boring, or routine, it probably isn't going to help improve trainees' skill. In this case, trainees should try to liven it up. A good way to do this is introduce a playful atmosphere. For example, trainees can try the following:

- Use different vocal tones, speech pacing, body gestures, or other languages. This can expand trainees' communication range.
- Practice while removing visual cues (e.g., with a blindfold). Watch videos without the sound. This can increase sensitivity in the other sensory modes.
- Practice nonverbal communication by not using any words.
- Practice while standing up or walking around outside. This can help trainees get new perspectives on the process of therapy.

Supervisors might ask trainees if they would like to take a 5- to 10-minute break between questions, particularly if the trainees are dealing with difficult emotions and feeling stressed out.

## Monitoring Training Results

While trainers evaluate trainees using a competency-focused model, trainees are also encouraged to look for results of deliberate practice within themselves. Trainees should experience the results of deliberate practice within a few training sessions. A lack of results can be demoralizing and cause trainees to lose focus on deliberate practice. Trainees who are not seeing results should discuss this problem with their trainers and experiment with adjusting their deliberate practice process. Measurements of results can include patient outcomes and improving the trainee's own work as a therapist, the trainee's personal development, and the trainee's general training.

## Patient Outcomes

The most important result of deliberate practice is an improvement in trainees' patient outcomes. This can be evaluated using routine outcome measurement (Lambert, 2010; Prescott et al., 2017), qualitative data (McLeod, 2017), and informal discussions with patients. However, trainees should note that an improvement in patient outcome due to deliberate practice can sometimes be challenging to achieve quickly, given that the largest amount of variance in patient outcome is due to patient variables (Bohart & Wade, 2013). For example, a patient with severe, chronic symptoms may not respond quickly to any treatment, regardless of how effectively a trainee practices. For some patients, an increase in patience and self-compassion regarding their symptoms may signify progress, even when there is no decrease in symptoms. Thus, trainees should keep their expectations for patient change realistic in the context of their patient's symptoms, history, and presentation. Trainees should not force their patients to improve in therapy for trainees to feel that they are making progress in training (Rousmaniere, 2016). The judgment whether a particular patient is being helped is especially difficult in PDT where it is expected that sometimes patients' symptoms get worse before they get better (Levenson et al., 2002). For example, a patient who has been denying how important the early loss of a parent was on their development may, through the PDT, start grieving and report feeling sadder than when therapy began. Exercise 6 on explaining the PDT rationale and what to expect in a PDT may be helpful so the patients themselves can appreciate that they are not deteriorating but rather improving by facing affects they have been avoiding for much of their life.

## Trainees' Work as a Therapist

One important result of deliberate practice is how trainees assess what it feels like to do therapy. For example, trainees at test sites reported feeling more comfortable sitting with evocative patients, more confident addressing uncomfortable topics in therapy, and more responsive to a broader range of patients.

## Trainees' Personal Development

Another important result of deliberate practice is the trainee's personal growth. For example, trainees at test sites reported becoming more in touch with their own feelings, having increased self-compassion, and experiencing enhanced motivation to work with a broader range of patients.

### Trainees' Training Process

Another valuable result of deliberate practice is improvement in the trainees' learning process. Trainees at test sites reported becoming more aware of their personal training style, preferences, strengths, and challenges. Over time, trainees should grow to feel more ownership of their training process. We also emphasize that training to be a psychotherapist is a complex process that occurs over many years. Experienced, expert therapists continue to grow well beyond their graduate school years (Orlinsky et al., 2005). As pointed out in Chapter 1, the authors of this book collectively have more than 150 years of experience doing therapy, yet each of us feels he or she is continually being stretched personally and professionally in the work we do. Every week, we have sessions that puzzle us and patients who trigger us, teach us, or both.

### The Trainee–Trainer Alliance: Monitoring Complex Reactions Toward the Trainer

Trainees who engage in difficult deliberate practice often report experiencing complex feelings toward their trainers. For example, one student said, "I know this is helping, but I also don't look forward to it!" Another trainee reported simultaneously feeling both appreciation and frustration toward her trainer. Trainees are advised to recall intensive training they have done in other fields, such as athletics or music. When a coach pushes trainees to the edge of their ability, it is common for trainees to have complex reactions toward the coach.

This does not necessarily mean that the trainer is doing something wrong. In fact, intensive training inevitably stirs up reactions toward the trainer, such as frustration, annoyance, disappointment, or anger that coexist with the appreciation of the trainer. If trainees do not experience complex reactions, it is worth wondering if the deliberate practice is sufficiently challenging. What we asserted earlier about rights to privacy applies here as well. Because professional mental health training is hierarchical and evaluative, trainers should not require or even expect trainees to share complex reactions they may experience toward them. Trainers should stay open to trainees sharing their reactions, but the choice always remains with the trainee.

### Trainee's Own Therapy

When engaging in deliberate practice, many trainees discover aspects of their inner world that may benefit from doing their own psychotherapy. For example, one trainee discovered that her patients' anger stirred up painful memories of abuse; another found himself disassociating while practicing empathy skills; and another trainee experienced overwhelming shame and self-judgment when she couldn't master skills after just a few repetitions.

While these discoveries were unnerving at first, they were ultimately beneficial because they motivated the trainees to seek out their own therapy. In earlier generations, personal therapy was mandatory for all trainees in PDT. Although it is no longer required, many PDT supervisors strongly encourage students to take part in their own therapy. Doing so can give trainees an irreplaceable experience of confronting their personal straggles. In turn, they become better attuned to their patients' trepidations about entering PDT (McWilliams, 2013).

Many contemporary therapists have sought out their own therapy. In fact, Norcross and Guy (2005) found in their review of 17 studies that approximately 75% of the more than 8,000 therapist participants had sought their own therapy. Orlinsky et al. (2005) found that more than 90% of therapists who sought therapy for themselves reported it to be helpful.

---

### QUESTIONS FOR TRAINEES

1. Are you balancing the effort to improve your skills with patience and self-compassion for your learning process?
2. Are you attending to any shame or self-judgments that arise from training?
3. Are you mindful of your personal boundaries and respecting any complex feelings you may have toward your trainers?
4. Are you acquainted with how well-respected PDT therapists have dealt with their personal and professional challenges at various points in their careers?

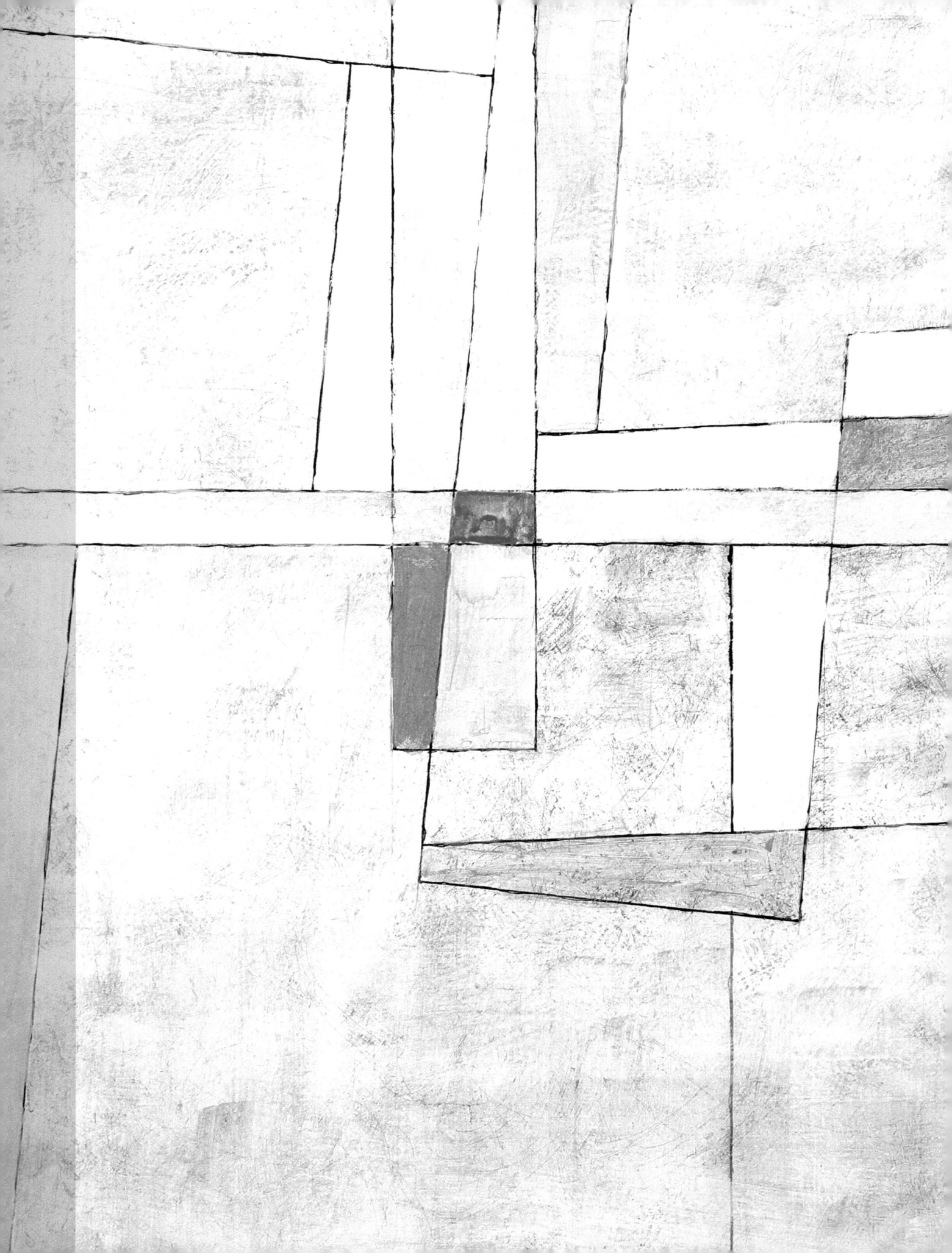

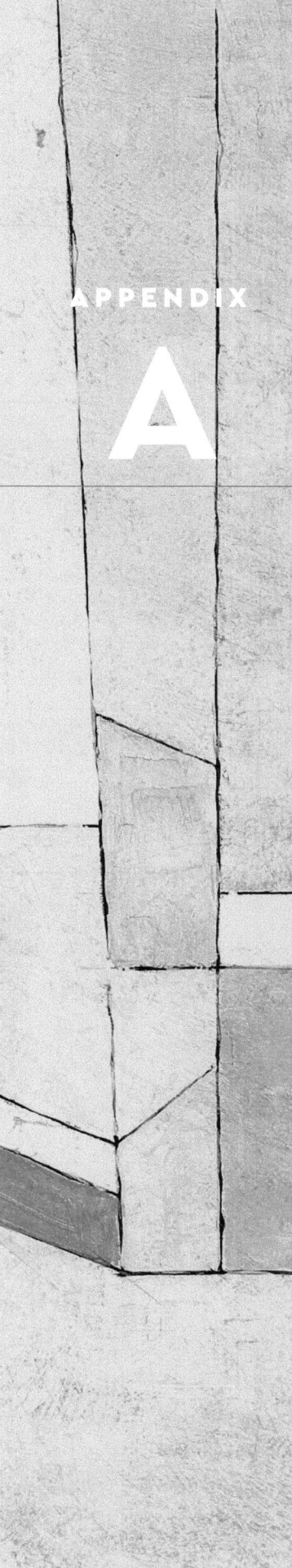

# Difficulty Assessments and Adjustments

Deliberate practice works best if the exercises are performed at a good challenge that is neither too hard nor too easy. To ensure that they are practicing at the correct difficulty, trainees should do a difficulty assessment and adjustment after each level of patient statement is completed (beginner, intermediate, and advanced). To do this, use the following instructions and the Deliberate Practice Reaction Form (see Figure A.1), which is also available in the "Clinician and Practitioner Resources" tab online (https://www.apa.org/pubs/books/deliberate-practice-psychodynamic-psychotherapy). **Do not skip this process!**

## How to Assess Difficulty

The therapist completes the Deliberate Practice Reaction Form (Figure A.1). If they

- rate the difficulty of the exercise above an 8 or had any of the reactions in the "Too Hard" column, follow the instructions to make the exercise easier;

- rate the difficulty of the exercise below a 4 or didn't have any of the reactions in the "Good Challenge" column, proceed to the next level of harder patient statements or follow the instructions to make exercise harder; or

- rate the difficulty of the exercise between 4 and 8 and have at least one reaction in the "Good Challenge" column, do not proceed to the harder patient statements but rather repeat the same level.

## Making Patient Statements Easier

If the therapist ever rates the difficulty of the exercise above an 8 or has any of the reactions in the "Too Hard" column, use the next level easier patient statements (e.g., if you were using advanced patient statements, switch to intermediate). But if you already were using beginner patient statements, use the following methods to make the patient statements even easier:

- The person playing the patient can use the same beginner patient statements but this time in a softer, calmer voice and with a smile. This softens the emotional tone.

**FIGURE A.1.  Deliberate Practice Reaction Form**

| **Question 1: How challenging was it to fulfill the skill criteria for this exercise?** |
| --- |

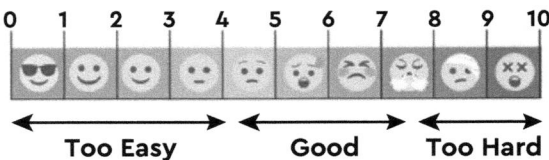

**Too Easy**          **Good**          **Too Hard**

| **Question 2: Did you have any reactions in "good challenge" or "too hard" categories? (yes/no)** | | | | | |
| --- | --- | --- | --- | --- | --- |
| **Good Challenge** | | | **Too Hard** | | |
| **Emotions and Thoughts** | **Body Reactions** | **Urges** | **Emotions and Thoughts** | **Body Reactions** | **Urges** |
| Manageable shame, self-judgment, irritation, anger, sadness, etc. | Body tension, sighs, shallow breathing, increased heart rate, warmth, dry mouth | Looking away, withdrawing, changing focus | Severe or overwhelming shame, self-judgment, rage, grief, guilt, etc. | Migraines, dizziness, foggy thinking, diarrhea, disassociation, numbness, blanking out, nausea, etc. | Shutting down, giving up |

| **Too Easy** ⬇ Proceed to next difficulty level | **Good Challenge** ⬇ Repeat the same difficulty level | **Too Hard** ⬇ Go back to previous difficulty level |
| --- | --- | --- |

*Note.* From *Deliberate Practice in Emotion-Focused Therapy* (p. 180), by R. N. Goldman, A. Vaz, and T. Rousmaniere, 2021, American Psychological Association (https://doi.org/10.1037/0000227-000). Copyright 2021 by the American Psychological Association.

- The patient can improvise with topics that are less evocative or make the therapist more comfortable, such as talking about topics without expressing strong feelings, the future/past (avoiding the here and now), or any topic outside therapy (see Figure A.2).

- The therapist can take a short break (5–10 minutes) between questions.

- The trainer can expand the "feedback phase" by discussing psychodynamic therapy or psychotherapy theory and research. This should shift the trainees' focus toward more detached or intellectual topics and reduce the emotional intensity.

## Making Patient Statements Harder

If the therapist rates the difficulty of the exercise below a 4 or didn't have any of the reactions in the "Good Challenge" column, proceed to next level harder patient statements. If you were already using the advanced patient statements, the patient should make the exercise even harder, using the following guidelines:

- The person playing the patient can use the advanced patient statements again with a more distressed voice (e.g., very angry, sad, sarcastic) or unpleasant facial expression. This should increase the emotional tone.

**FIGURE A.2. How to Make Client Statements Easier or Harder in Role-Plays**

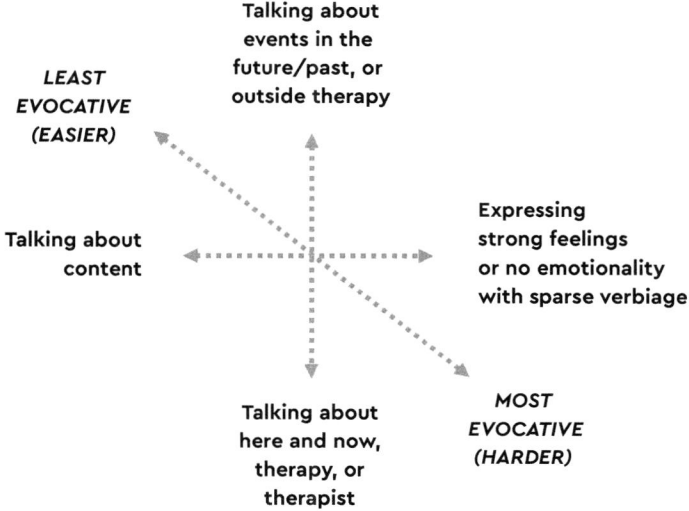

*Note.* Adapted from figure created by Jason Whipple, PhD.

- The patient can improvise new patient statements with topics that are more evocative or make the therapist uncomfortable, such as expressing strong feelings or talking about the here and now, therapy, or the therapist (see Figure A.2).

- Also, the patient can give minimal emotional signals and sparse verbiage. Sometimes these less-than-forthcoming patients are the most difficult to engage.

*Note.* The purpose of a deliberate practice session is not to get through all the patient statements and therapist responses but rather to spend as much time as possible practicing at the correct difficulty level. This may mean that trainees repeat the same statements or responses many times, which is OK, as long as the difficulty remains at the "good challenge" level.

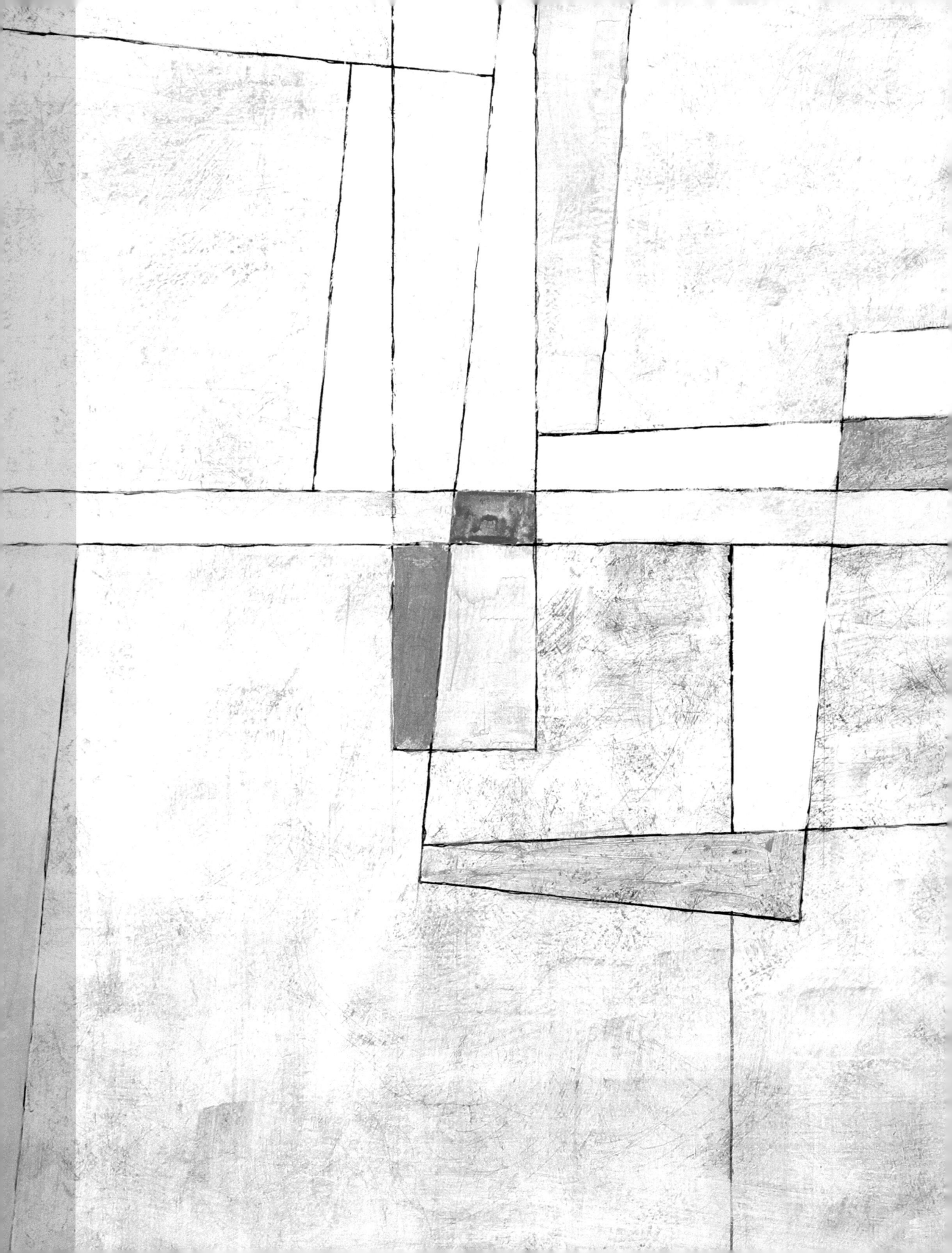

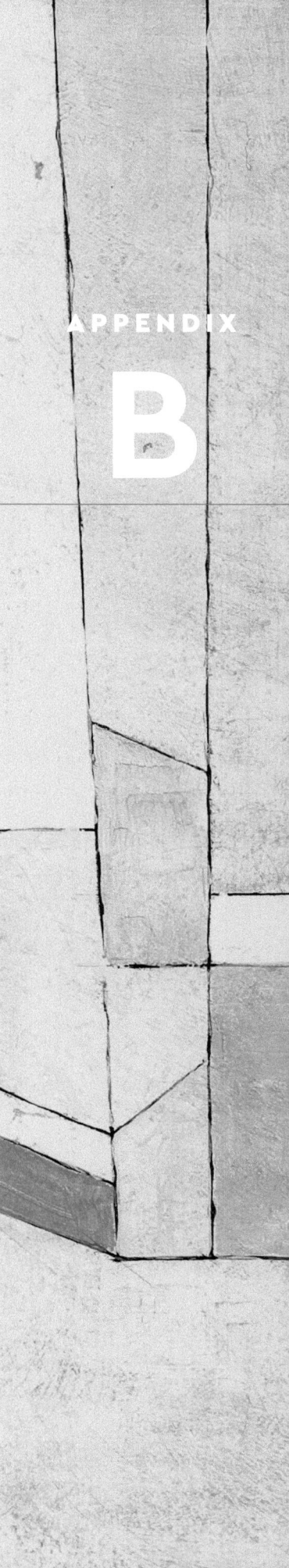

# Deliberate Practice Diary Form

To optimize the quality of the deliberate practice, we have developed a Deliberate Practice Diary Form that can also be downloaded from the "Clinician and Practitioner Resources" tab (https://www.apa.org/pubs/books/deliberate-practice-psychodynamic-psychotherapy). This form provides a template for the trainee to record their experience of the deliberate practice activity and, ideally, will aid in the consolidation of learning. This form is not intended to be used as part of the evaluation process with the supervisor.

## Deliberate Practice Diary Form

Use this form to consolidate learnings from the deliberate practice exercises. Please protect your personal boundaries by only sharing information that you are comfortable disclosing.

Name: _____ Date: _____
Exercise: _____

Question 1. What was helpful or worked well this deliberate practice session? In what way?

Question 2. What was unhelpful or didn't go well this deliberate practice session? In what way?

Question 3. What did you learn about yourself, your current skills, and skills you'd like to keep improving? Feel free to share any details, but only those you are comfortable disclosing.

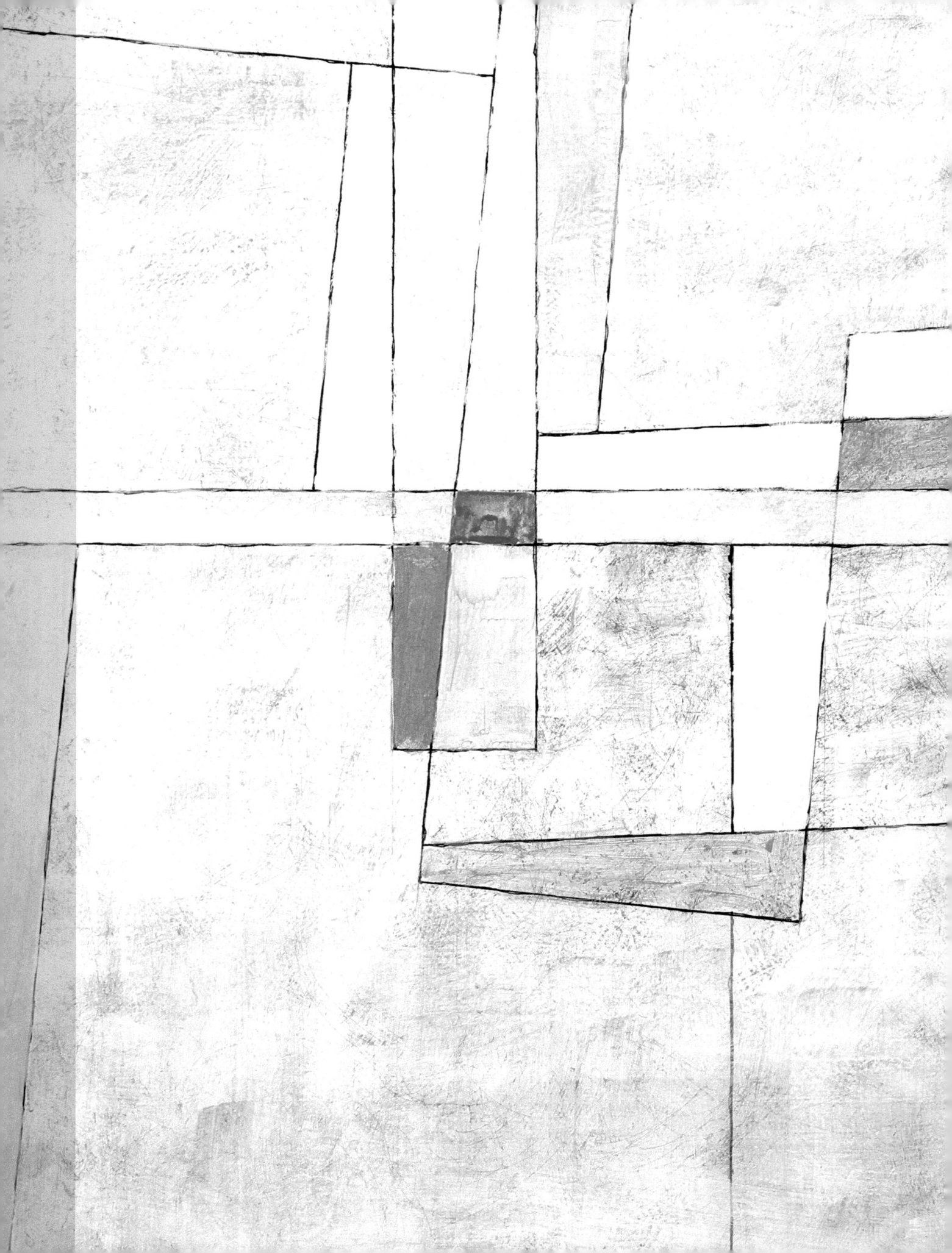

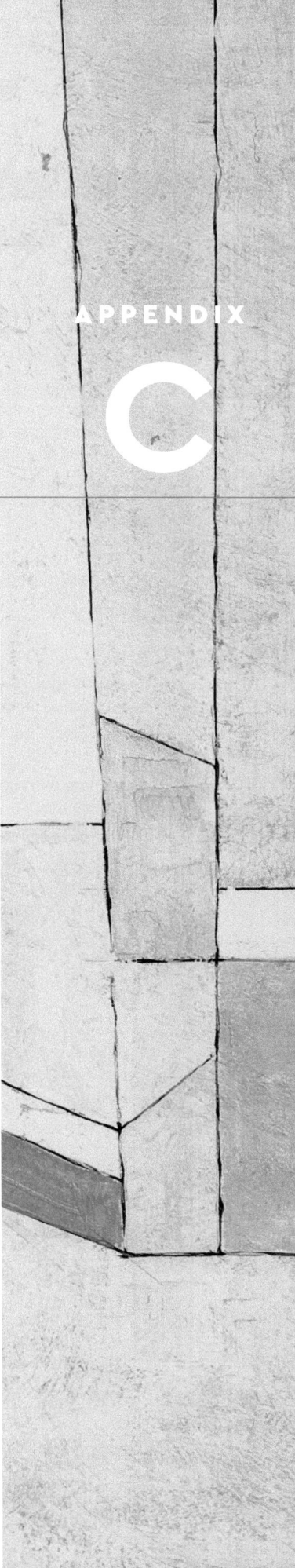

# Sample Psychodynamic Therapy Syllabus With Embedded Deliberate Practice Exercises

This appendix provides a sample one-semester, three-unit course dedicated to teaching psychodynamic psychotherapy. This course is appropriate for graduate students (master's and doctoral) at all levels of training, including first-year students who have not yet worked with patients. We present it as a model that can be adopted to a specific program's contexts and needs. For example, instructors may borrow portions of it to use in other courses, in practica, in didactic training events at externships and internships, in workshops, and in continuing education for postgraduate therapists. We have included a range of possible readings for the homework assignments. Instructors therefore have a choice of materials from which to select.

**Course Title:** Relational Psychodynamic Psychotherapy: Formulation and Intervention Using Deliberate Practice

## Course Description

This course teaches the theory, principles, and core skills of a relational psychodynamic psychotherapy. As a course with both didactic and practicum elements, it will review the theory and research on formulation, discuss strategies of intervention, illustrate psychotherapy change processes, and foster the use of deliberate practice to enable students to acquire relevant skills.

## Course Objectives

Students who complete this course will be able to do the following:

1. Describe the core theory, process, research, and skills of psychodynamic psychotherapy
2. Apply the principles of deliberate practice for career-long clinical skill development
3. Demonstrate key psychodynamic skills
4. Evaluate how they can integrate psychodynamic skills into their developing therapeutic framework
5. Employ psychodynamic approaches with patients from diverse cultural backgrounds
6. Describe the ways in which modern (two-person) psychodynamic psychotherapy differs from older (one-person) psychodynamic approaches
7. Understand how the central tenets of psychodynamic psychotherapy are part of an evidenced-based practice
8. Maintain self-awareness while being present in the relationship with the patient

| Date | Lecture and Discussion | Skills Lab | Relevant Readings and Videos |
|---|---|---|---|
| Week 1 | Introduction to psychodynamic therapy (PDT) theory, history, and research<br>Principles of deliberate practice | Find your way around the Sentio University site: https://sentio.org/ | Blagys & Hilsenroth (2000); Levenson (2017, Chapter 2); Levy et al. (2019); Shedler (2022); Wachtel (2011, Chapter 1); Wolitzky (2011) |
| Week 2 | Maintaining a curious stance<br>Types of questions and when to use<br>Listening with the third ear | Exercise 1: Engaging in a therapeutic inquiry | Binder (2004, Chapter 5); Hill (2020, Chapter 9) |
| Week 3 | The therapeutic relationship<br>Transference and countertransference<br>The real relationship | Exercise 2: Being aware of countertransference reactions | Eubanks et al. (2018); Fauth & Williams (2005); Gelso et al. (2005); Hayes et al. (2011); Hill (2020, Chapter 3); Levenson (1995, Chapter 3) |
| Week 4 | Accessing, deepening, and expressing emotion | Exercise 3: Deepening emotional experience | Geller (2017); Goldman et al. (2021); Levenson (2020); Schore & Schore (2008). Video: Geller (2015) |
| Week 5 | Working with the process<br>Immediacy in the session | Exercise 4: Making process comments | Hill (2020, Chapter 13); Teyber & Teyber (2014) |
| Week 6 | Defenses | Exercise 5: Pointing out defenses and inquiring about underlying fear | Howard (2017, Chapter 11); McCullough et al. (2003, Chapter 5) |
| Week 7 | Developing a working alliance<br>Providing a treatment rationale<br>Concepts/processes of PDT | Exercise 6: Introducing the rationale for treatment | Levenson (2017, Chapter 3); McWilliams (2004, Chapter 4); Shedler (2022). Video: Levenson (2018) |
| Week 8 | Working in the here and now | Exercise 7: Making Transference interpretations | Høglend et al. (2006); Levy & Scalia (2012) |
| Week 9 | Gaining entrance to the patient's inner world | Exercise 8: Using metaphors | Angus & Rennie (1989); Lloyd (2017); Malkomsen et al. (2021); Sims (2003) |
| Week 10 | The power of the unconscious | Exercise 9: Exploring fantasy | Cabaniss et al. (2011, Chapter 24); Glausiusz (2014); Levin (1996) |
| Week 11 | Formulation in PDT | Exercise 10: Case formulation: gathering data for the cyclical maladaptive pattern | Binder & Betan (2022); Inderbitzin & Levy (1990); Levenson (2017, Chapter 4); McWilliams (1999, Chapter 8). Video: Levenson & Carlson (2010, Brief Dynamic Therapy Over Time [transcript is provided in Exercise 13]) |
| Week 12 | Reenactments in PDT<br>Parallel process<br>Use of supervision | Exercise 11: Using supervision to recognize reenactments | Levenson (2013); Safran & Kraus (2014); Sarnat (2016). Video: Levenson (1999, Time-Limited Dynamic Therapy) |
| Week 13 | Corrective emotional experiences<br>Primary change mechanisms | Exercise 12: Providing a corrective emotional experience | Christian et al. (2012); Levenson et al. (2020); Sharpless & Barber (2012). Video: Levenson & Carlson (2010, Brief Dynamic Therapy Over Time [transcript is provided in Exercise 13]) |
| Week 14 | Working with real sessions | Exercise 13: Annotated interpersonal–psychodynamic therapy session transcripts | Friedlander et al. (2018); Wachtel (2011) |
| Week 15 | Putting it all together:<br>Self-evaluation<br>Skill coaching<br>Mutual feedback | Exercise 14: Mock psychodynamic therapy sessions | Paper: design a psychodynamic deliberate practice exercise **or** identify psychodynamic skills in a trainee's therapy session |

**Format of Class**

Classes are 3 hours long. Course time is divided into three parts: learning psychodynamic principles, observing video demonstrations, and practicing psychodynamic skills.

*Lecture/Discussion Class:* Each week, there will be one lecture/discussion class for 1.5 hours focusing on psychodynamic theory and related research.

*Psychodynamic Skills Lab:* Each week there will be one psychodynamic skills lab for 1.5 hours. Skills labs are for practicing psychodynamic skills using the exercises in this book. The exercises use therapy simulations (role-plays) with the following goals:

1. Build trainees' skill and confidence for using psychodynamic skills with real patients
2. Provide a safe space for experimenting with different therapeutic interventions, without fear of making mistakes
3. Provide plenty of opportunity to explore and "try on" different styles of therapy, so that eventually trainees can discover their own personal, unique therapy style

*Annotated Session Transcript:* Toward the end of the semester (Week 14), trainees could do the Annotated Interpersonal–Psychodynamic Therapy Session Transcripts (Exercise 13). The repeated readings of the transcripts under various instructions will facilitate the trainees in seeing how all 12 psychodynamic exercises in this book might appear in the context of real sessions. If they haven't done so already, the students could watch a video of the actual sessions being conducted by the first author (H. L.) and gain yet another level of context—that of the nonverbal and paralinguistic. There are also four published studies using these transcripts and accompanying video (Friedlander et al. 2018, 2020; Levenson, 2020; Levenson et al., 2020). Reading these studies could provide yet another layer of information—ways researchers identify various skills and processes in real sessions.

*Mock Therapy Sessions:* For the last class, a Mock Psychodynamic Therapy Session (Exercise 14) is assigned. In contrast to the highly structured and repetitive deliberate practice exercises, a psychotherapy mock session is an unstructured and improvised role-played therapy session. Mock sessions let trainees

1. practice using psychodynamic skills responsively,
2. experiment with clinical decision making in an unscripted context,
3. discover their personal therapeutic style, and
4. build endurance for working with real patients.

**Homework**

Homework will be assigned each week and will include reading, 1 hour of skills practice with an assigned practice partner, and occasional writing assignments. For the skills practice homework, trainees will repeat the exercise they did for that week's skills lab. Because the instructor will not be there to evaluate performance, trainees should instead complete the Deliberate Practice Reaction Form, as well as the Deliberate Practice Diary Form, for themselves as a self-evaluation.

**Writing Assignments**

Students could be assigned a writing assignment. Some possible topics for the papers are as follows:

• Using a partial transcript of one of the trainees' therapy cases with a real patient, the trainee names where each of the 12 psychodynamic skills was used, and in other places where one of the 12 skills could have (more effectively) replaced what the trainee did say.

- Write a deliberate practice exercise delineating another psychodynamic skill that was not one of the 12 skills used in this book, using the format used in this book.

## Multicultural Orientation

This course is taught in a *multicultural context*, defined as "how the cultural worldviews, values, and beliefs of the patient and therapist interact and influence one another to co-create a relational experience that is in the spirit of healing" (Davis et al., 2018, p. 3). Multicultural competencies are included in accreditation requirements and American Psychological Association's (APA's; 2017b) *Multicultural Guidelines: An Ecological Approach to Context, Identity, and Intersectionality*. These include multicultural awareness, knowledge, and skills. Core features of the multicultural orientation include cultural comfort, humility, and responding to cultural opportunities (or previously missed opportunities). Throughout this course, students are encouraged to reflect on their own cultural identity and improve their ability to attune with their patients' cultural identities (Hook et al., 2017). For further guidance on this topic and deliberate practice exercises to improve multicultural skills, see the book *Deliberate Practice in Multicultural Therapy* (Harris et al., in press).

## Vulnerability, Privacy, and Boundaries

This course is aimed at developing therapy skills, self-awareness, and interpersonal skills in an experiential framework and as relevant to clinical work. This course is not psychotherapy or a substitute for psychotherapy. Using psychodynamic psychotherapy with patients requires balancing emotional vulnerability, openness, and presence while simultaneously maintaining appropriate personal boundaries and the psychotherapeutic frame. Students should interact at a level of self-disclosure that is personally comfortable and helpful to their own learning. Although becoming aware of internal emotional and psychological processes is necessary for a therapist's development, it is not necessary to reveal all that information to the trainer. It is important for students to sense their own level of safety and privacy. Students are not evaluated on the level of material that they choose to reveal in the class.

In accordance with APA's (2017a) *Ethical Principles of Psychologists and Code of Conduct*, students are **not required to disclose personal information.** Because this class is about developing both interpersonal and psychodynamic competence, the following are some important points for students to consider as they make choices to self-disclose:

- Students choose how much, when, and what to disclose. Students are not penalized for the choice not to share personal information.

- The learning environment is susceptible to group dynamics much like any other group space, and therefore students may be asked to share their observations and experiences of the class environment with the singular goal of fostering a more inclusive and productive learning environment.

## Confidentiality

Due to the nature of the material covered in class, there are many occasions when personal life experience (self, friends, or family) may be pertinent for the learning environment. While it cannot be required to share personal experiences, some trainees may be inclined to do so. Additionally, the content of patient case material is sensitive and demands ethical consideration. To create a safe learning environment that is respectful of patient and therapist information and of diversity, and to foster open and vulnerable conversation in class, class members are required to maintain strict confidentiality within and outside of the instruction setting.

## Evaluation

*Self-Evaluation:* At the end of the semester (Week 15), trainees will perform a self-evaluation. This will help trainees track their progress and identify areas for further development. The "Guidance for Trainees" section in Chapter 3 of this book highlights potential areas of focus for self-evaluation.

## Grading Criteria

As designed, students would be accountable for the level and quality of their performance in

- the readings and discussion in class,
- the skills lab (exercises, transcripted and mock sessions),
- homework, and
- the final paper.

## Required Readings and Other Media

Angus, L. E., & Rennie, D. L. (1989). Envisioning the representational world: The client's experience of metaphoric expression in psychotherapy. *Psychotherapy: Theory, Research, Practice, Training, 26*(3), 372–379. https://doi.org/10.1037/h0085448

Binder, J. L. (2004). *Key competencies in brief dynamic psychotherapy: Clinical practice beyond the manual.* Guilford Press.

Binder, J. L., & Betan, E. J. (2022). The cyclical maladaptive pattern. In T. D. Eells (Ed.), *Handbook of psychotherapy case formulation* (3rd ed., pp. 113–143). Guilford Press.

Blagys, M. D., & Hilsenroth, M. J. (2000). Distinctive features of short-term psychodynamic-interpersonal psychotherapy: A review of the comparative psychotherapy process literature. *Clinical Psychology: Science and Practice, 7*(2), 167–188. https://doi.org/10.1093/clipsy.7.2.167

Cabaniss, D. L., Cherry, S., Douglas, C. J., & Schwartz, A. (2011). *Psychodynamic psychotherapy: A clinical manual.* John Wiley & Sons.

Christian C., Safran, J. D., & Muran J. C. (2012). The corrective emotional experience: A relational perspective and critique. In L. G. Castonguay & C. E. Hill (Eds.), *Transformation in psychotherapy: Corrective experiences across cognitive behavioral, humanistic, and psychodynamic approaches* (pp. 51–67). American Psychological Association. https://doi.org/10.1037/13747-004

Eubanks, C. F., Muran, J. C., & Safran, J. D. (2018). Repairing alliance ruptures. In J. C. Norcross & B. E. Wampold (Eds.), *Psychotherapy relationships that work: Evidence-based responsiveness* (3rd ed., pp. 549–579). Oxford University Press.

Fauth, J., & Williams, E. N. (2005). The in-session self-awareness of therapist-trainees: Hindering or helpful? *Journal of Counseling Psychology, 52*(3), 443–447. https://doi.org/10.1037/0022-0167.52.3.443

Friedlander, M. L., Angus, L., Wright, S. T., Günther, C., Austin, C. L., Kangos, K., Barbaro, L., Macaulay, C., Carpenter, N., & Khattra, J. (2018). "If those tears could talk, what would they say?" Multi-method analysis of a corrective experience in brief dynamic therapy. *Psychotherapy Research, 28*(2), 217–234. https://doi.org/10.1080/10503307.2016.1184350

Geller, S. (2015). *Presence in psychotherapy* [Video]. https://www.youtube.com/watch?v=sShXDGjcjV0

Geller, S. (2017). *A practical guide to cultivating therapeutic presence.* American Psychological Association. https://doi.org/10.1037/0000025-000

Gelso, C. J., Kelley, F. A., Fuertes, J. N., Marmarosh, C., Holmes, S. E., Costa, C., & Hancock, G. R. (2005). Measuring the real relationship in psychotherapy: Initial validation of the therapist form. *Journal of Counseling Psychology, 52*(4), 640–649. https://doi.org/10.1037/0022-0167.52.4.640

Glausiusz, J. (2014). Living in an imaginary world. *Scientific American Mind, 23*(1). https://www.scientificamerican.com/article/living-in-an-imaginary-world/

Goldman, R. N., Vaz, A., & Rousmaniere, T. (2021). *Deliberate practice in emotion-focused therapy.* American Psychological Association. https://doi.org/10.1037/0000227-000

Hayes, J. A., Gelso, C., & Hummel, A. (2011). Managing countertransference. In J. C. Norcross (Ed.), *Psychotherapy relationships that work: Evidence-based responsiveness* (2nd ed., pp. 239–258). Oxford University Press. https://doi.org/10.1093/acprof:oso/9780199737208.003.0012

Hill, C. E. (2020). *Helping skills: Facilitating exploration, insight, and action* (5th ed.). American Psychological Association. https://doi.org/10.1037/0000147-000

Høglend, P., Amlo, S., Marble, A., Bøgwald, K.-P., Sørbye, O., Sjaastad, M. C., & Heyerdahl, O. (2006). Analysis of the patient–therapist relationship in dynamic psychotherapy: An experimental study of transference interpretations. *American Journal of Psychiatry, 163*(10), 1739–1746. https://doi.org/10.1176/ajp.2006.163.10.1739

Howard, S. (2017). *Skills in psychodynamic counselling and psychotherapy* (2nd ed.). Sage Publications.

Inderbitzin, L. B., & Levy, S. T. (1990). Unconscious fantasy: A reconsideration of the concept. *Journal of the American Psychoanalytic Association, 38*(1), 113–130. https://doi.org/10.1177/000306519003800107

Levenson, H. (1995). *Time-limited dynamic psychotherapy: A guide to clinical practice.* Basic Books.

Levenson, H. (1999). *Time limited dynamic psychotherapy* [Film; educational DVD]. Pychotherapy.net. https://www.psychotherapy.net/video/time-limited-dynamic-psychotherapy

Levenson, H. (2013). Time-limited dynamic psychotherapy: Working with reactions to chronically depressed clients. In A. W. Wolf, M. R. Goldfried, & J. C. Muran (Eds.), *Transforming negative reactions to clients: From frustration to compassion* (pp. 193–219). American Psychological Association. https://doi.org/10.1037/13940-009

Levenson, H. (2017). *Brief dynamic psychotherapy* (2nd ed.). American Psychological Association. https://doi.org/10.1037/0000043-000

Levenson, H. (2018). *Time-limited dynamic psychotherapy: An integrative perspective* [includes video]. In M. J. Dewan, B. N. Steenbarger, & R. P. Greenberg (Eds.), *The art and science of brief psychotherapies: An illustrated guide* (3rd ed.). American Psychiatric Association Publishing. https://www.appi.org/Products/Psychotherapy/Art-and-Science-of-Brief-Psychotherapies-Third-Edi?SearchText=levenson,%20han&sku=37079

Levenson, H. (2020). Enlivening psychodynamic brief therapy with emotion-focused interventions: An integrative therapist's approach. *Clinical Social Work Journal, 48*(3), 267–278. https://doi.org/10.1007/s10615-020-00762-z

Levenson, H., Angus, L., & Pool, E. (2020). Viewing psychodynamic/interpersonal theory and practice through the lens of memory reconsolidation. In R. D. Lane & L. Nadel (Eds.), *Neuroscience of enduring change: Implications for psychotherapy* (pp. 296–323). Oxford University Press. https://doi.org/10.1093/oso/9780190881511.003.0012

Levenson, H. (Guest Expert), & Carlson, J. (Host). (2010). *Brief dynamic therapy over time* [Film; educational DVD]. American Psychological Association. https://www.apa.org/pubs/videos/4310871

Levin, K. (1996). Unconscious phantasy in psychotherapy. *American Journal of Psychotherapy, 50*(2), 137–153.

Levy, K. N., Keefe, J. R., & Ehrenthal, J. C. (2019). Research support for psychodynamic constructs. In D. Kealy & J. S. Ogrodniczuk (Eds.), *Evolving clinical practice* (pp. 89–106). Elsevier.

Levy, K. N., & Scala, J. W. (2012). Transference, transference interpretations, and transference-focused psychotherapies. *Psychotherapy*, *49*(3), 391–403. https://doi.org/10.1037/a0029371

Lloyd, J. (2017). Therapeutic use of metaphor: Cultural connectivity. *Journal of Experiential Psychotherapy*, *20*(2), 3–10.

Malkomsen, A., Røssberg, J. I., Dammen, T., Wilberg, T., Løvgren, A., Ulberg, R., & Evensen, J. (2021). Digging down or scratching the surface: How patients use metaphors to describe their experiences of psychotherapy. *BMC Psychiatry*, *21*, Article 533. https://doi.org/10.1186/s12888-021-03551-1

McCullough, L., Kuhn, N., Andrews, S., Kaplan, A., Wolf, J., & Hurley, C. L. (2003). *Treating affect phobia: A manual for short-term dynamic psychotherapy*. Guilford Press.

McWilliams, N. (1999). *Psychoanalytic case formulation*. Guilford Press.

McWilliams, N. (2004). *Psychoanalytic psychotherapy: A practitioner's guide*. Guilford Press.

Safran, J. D., & Kraus, J. (2014). Alliance ruptures, impasses, and enactments: A relational perspective. *Psychotherapy*, *51*(3), 381–387. https://doi.org/10.1037/a0036815

Sarnat, J. E. (2016). *Supervision essentials for psychodynamic psychotherapies*. American Psychological Association. https://doi.org/10.1037/14802-000

Schore, J. R., & Schore, A. N. (2008). Modern attachment theory: The central role of affect regulation in development and treatment. *Clinical Social Work Journal*, *36*(1), 9–20. https://doi.org/10.1007/s10615-007-0111-7

Sharpless, B. A., & Barber, J. P. (2012). Corrective emotional experiences from a psychodynamic perspective. In L. G. Castonguay & C. E. Hill (Eds.), *Transformation in psychotherapy: Corrective experiences across cognitive behavioral, humanistic, and psychodynamic approaches* (pp. 31–49). American Psychological Association. https://doi.org/10.1037/13747-003

Shedler, J. (2022). That was then, this is now: Psychoanalytic psychotherapy for the rest of us. *Contemporary Psychoanalysis*, *58*(2–3), 405–437. https://doi.org/10.1080/00107530.2022.2149038

Sims, P. A. (2003). Working with metaphor. *American Journal of Psychotherapy*, *57*(4), 528–536. https://doi.org/10.1176/appi.psychotherapy.2003.57.4.528

Teyber, E., & Teyber F. M. (2014). Working with the process dimension in relational therapies: Guidelines for clinical training. *Psychotherapy*, *51*(3), 334–341. https://doi.org/10.1037/a0036579

Wachtel, P. L. (2011). *Inside the session: What really happens in psychotherapy*. American Psychological Association. https://doi.org/10.1037/12321-000

Wolitzky, D. L. (2011). Psychoanalytic theories of psychotherapy. In J. C. Norcross, G. R. VanderBos, & D. K. Freedheim (Eds.), *History of psychotherapy: Continuity and change* (pp. 65–100). American Psychological Association. https://doi.org/10.1037/12353-003

## Supplemental Readings

Alexander, F., & French, T. M. (1946). *Psychoanalytic therapy: Principles and application*. Ronald Press.

Barber, J. P., Khalsa, S.-R., & Sharpless, B. A. (2010). The validity of the alliance as a predictor of psychotherapy outcome. In J. C. Muran & J. P. Barber (Eds.), *The therapeutic alliance: An evidence-based guide to practice* (pp. 29–43). Guilford Press.

Curtis, J. T., Silberschatz, G., Sampson, H., & Weiss, J. (1994). The Plan Formulation Method. *Psychotherapy Research*, *4*(3–4), 197–207. https://doi.org/10.1080/10503309412331334032

Davis, D. E., DeBlaere, C., Owen, J., Hook, J. N., Rivera, D. P., Choe, E., Van Tongeren, D. R., Worthington, E. L., & Placeres, V. (2018). The multicultural orientation framework: A narrative review. *Psychotherapy*, *55*(1), 89–100. https://doi.org/10.1037/pst0000160

Gill, M. M. (1954). Psychoanalysis and exploratory psychotherapy. *Journal of the American Psychoanalytic Association*, *2*(4), 771–797. https://doi.org/10.1177/000306515400200413

Goodwin, B. J., Coyne, A. E., & Constantino, M. J. (2018). Extending the context-responsive psychotherapy integration framework to cultural processes in psychotherapy. *Psychotherapy, 55*(1), 3–8. https://doi.org/10.1037/pst0000143

Hook, J. N., Davis, D. E., Owen, J., & DeBlaere, C. (2017). *Cultural humility: Engaging diverse identities in therapy.* American Psychological Association. https://doi.org/10.1037/0000037-000

Kiesler, D. J. (1988). *Therapeutic metacommunication: Therapist impact disclosure as feedback in psychotherapy.* Consulting Psychologists Press.

Kohut, H. (1977). *The restoration of the self.* International Universities Press.

Levenson, H. (2003). Time-limited dynamic psychotherapy: An integrationist perspective. *Journal of Psychotherapy Integration, 13*(3–4), 300–333. https://doi.org/10.1037/1053-0479.13.3-4.300

Levy, K. N., Johnson, B. N., Cooch, C. V., & Kivity, Y. (2019). Attachment style. In J. C. Norcross & B. E. Wampold (Eds.), *Psychotherapy relationships that work: Vol. 2. Evidence-based therapist responsiveness* (3rd ed., pp. 15–55). Oxford University Press.

Malan, D. (1995). *Individual psychotherapy and the science of psychodynamics* (2nd ed.). Butterworth-Heinemann.

Norcross, J. C., & Wampold, B. E. (Eds.). (2019). *Psychotherapy relationships that work* (Vols. 1–2, 3rd ed.). Oxford University Press.

Osimo, F., & Stein, M. J. (2012). *Theory and practice of experiential dynamic psychotherapy.* Karnac.

Safran, J. D. (2012). *Psychoanalysis and psychoanalytic therapies.* American Psychological Association.

Safran, J. D., & Muran, J. C. (2000). *Negotiating the therapeutic alliance: A relational treatment guide.* Guilford Press.

Shedler, J. (2010). The efficacy of psychodynamic psychotherapy. *American Psychologist, 65*(2), 90–109. https://doi.org/10.1037/a0018378

Siegelman, E. Y. (1990). *Metaphor and meaning in psychotherapy.* Guilford Press.

Wachtel, P. L. (2008). *Relational theory and the practice of psychotherapy.* Guilford Press.

Westra, H. A., Norouzian, N., Poulin, L., Coyne, A. E., Constantino, M. J., Hara, K., Olson, D., & Antony, M. M. (2021). Testing a deliberate practice workshop for developing appropriate responsivity to resistance markers. *Psychotherapy, 58*(2), 175–185. https://doi.org/10.1037/pst0000311

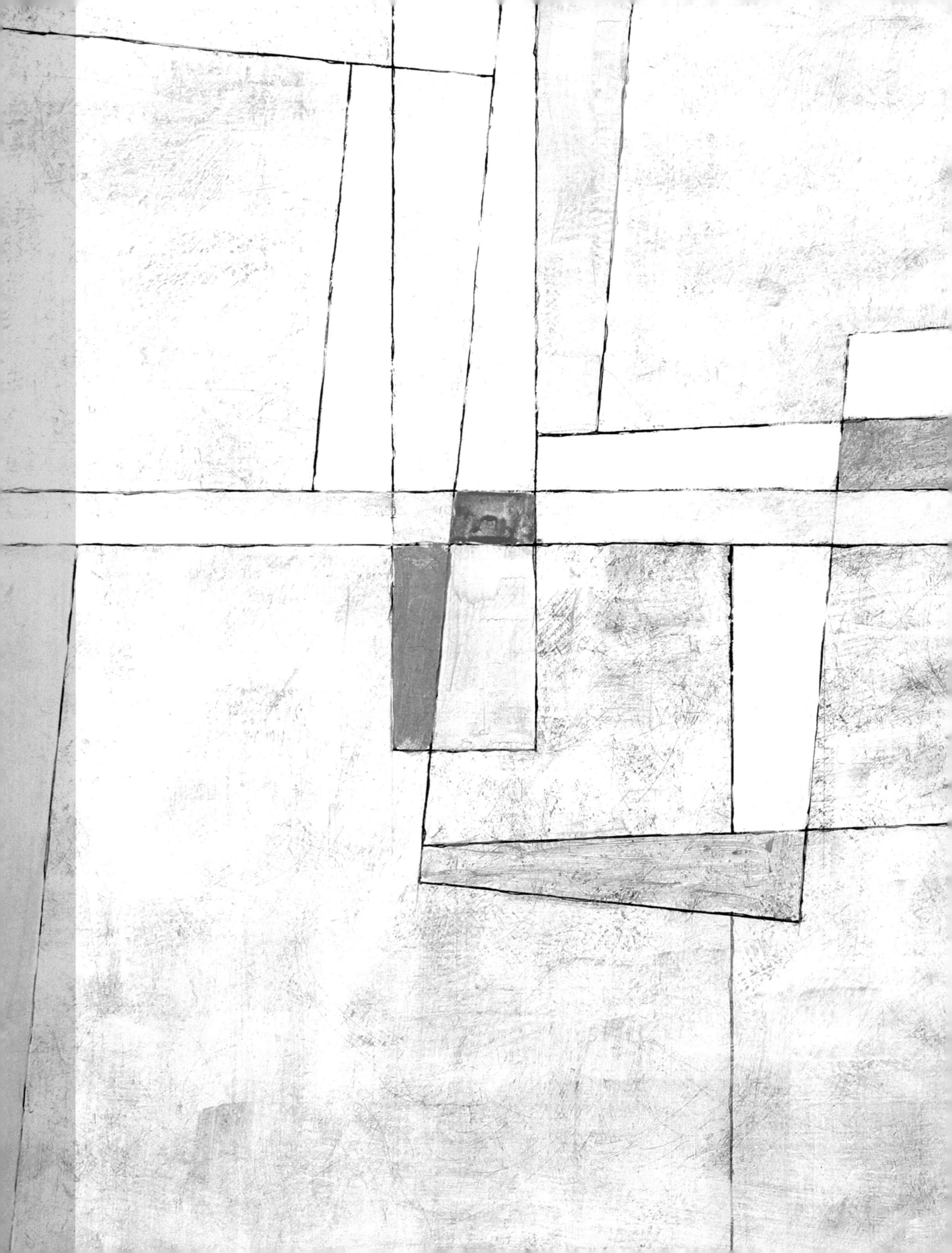

# References

Alexander, F., & French, T. M. (1946). *Psychoanalytic therapy: Principles and application.* Ronald Press.

American Psychological Association. (2017a). *Ethical principles of psychologists and code of conduct* (2002, amended June 1, 2010, and January 1, 2017). https://www.apa.org/ethics/code

American Psychological Association. (2017b). *Multicultural guidelines: An ecological approach to context, identity, and intersectionality.* https://www.apa.org/about/policy/multicultural-guidelines.pdf

Anderson, T., Crowley, M. E., Himawan, L., Holmberg, J. K., & Uhlin, B. D. (2016). Therapist facilitative interpersonal skills and training status: A randomized clinical trial on alliance and outcome. *Psychotherapy Research, 26*(5), 511–529. https://doi.org/10.1080/10503307.2015.1049671

Anderson, T., Finkelstein, D., & Horvath, S. A. (2020). The facilitative interpersonal skills method: Difficult psychotherapy moments and appropriate therapist responsiveness. *Counselling & Psychotherapy Research, 20*(3), 463–469. https://doi.org/10.1002/capr.12302

Anderson, T., Ogles, B. M., Patterson, C. L., Lambert, M. J., & Vermeersch, D. A. (2009). Therapist effects: Facilitative interpersonal skills as a predictor of therapist success. *Journal of Clinical Psychology, 65*(7), 755–768. https://doi.org/10.1002/jclp.20583

Anderson, T., Ogles, B. M., & Weis, A. (1999). Creative use of interpersonal skills in building a therapeutic alliance. *Journal of Constructivist Psychology, 12*, 313–330. https://doi.org/10.1080/107205399266037

Angus, L. E., & Rennie, D. L. (1989). Envisioning the representational world: The client's experience of metaphoric expression in psychotherapy. *Psychotherapy: Theory, Research, Practice, Training, 26*(3), 372–379. https://doi.org/10.1037/h0085448

Arlow, J. A. (1979). Metaphor and the psychoanalytic situation. *The Psychoanalytic Quarterly, 48*(3), 363–385. https://doi.org/10.1080/21674086.1979.11926882

Bailey, R. J., & Ogles, B. M. (2019, August 1). Common factors as a therapeutic approach: What is required? *Practice Innovations, 4*(4), 241–254. https://doi.org/10.1037/pri0000100

Barber, J. P., Khalsa, S.-R., & Sharpless, B. A. (2010). The validity of the alliance as a predictor of psychotherapy outcome. In J. C. Muran & J. P. Barber (Eds.), *The therapeutic alliance: An evidence-based guide to practice and training* (pp. 29–43). Guilford Press.

Barber, J. P., Muran, J. C., McCarthy, K. S., Keefe, J. R., & Zilcha-Mano, S. (2021). Research on dynamic therapies. In M. Barkham, W. Lutz, & L. G. Castonguay (Eds.), *Bergin and Garfield's handbook of psychotherapy and behavior change* (50th anniversary ed., pp. 387–419). John Wiley & Sons.

Barlow, D. H. (2010). Negative effects from psychological treatments: A perspective. *American Psychologist, 65*(1), 13–20. https://doi.org/10.1037/a0015643

Barth, F. D. (1997). Using daydreams in psychodynamic psychotherapy. *Clinical Social Work Journal*, 25, 265–280. https://doi.org/10.1023/A:1025730427420

Beebe, B., Lachmann, F., & Jaffe, J. (1997). Mother–infant interaction structures and presymbolic self- and object representations. *Psychoanalytic Dialogues*, 7(2), 133–182. https://doi.org/10.1080/10481889709539172

Bennett-Levy, J. (2019). Why therapists should walk the talk: The theoretical and empirical case for personal practice in therapist training and professional development. *Journal of Behavior Therapy and Experimental Psychiatry*, 62, 133–145. https://doi.org/10.1016/j.jbtep.2018.08.004

Bennett-Levy, J., & Finlay-Jones, A. (2018). The role of personal practice in therapist skill development: A model to guide therapists, educators, supervisors and researchers. *Cognitive Behaviour Therapy*, 47(3), 185–205. https://doi.org/10.1080/16506073.2018.1434678

Binder, J. L. (1999). Issues in teaching and learning time-limited psychodynamic psychotherapy. *Clinical Psychology Review*, 19(6), 705–719. https://doi.org/10.1016/S0272-7358(98)00078-6

Binder, J. L. (2004). *Key competencies in brief dynamic psychotherapy. Clinical practice beyond the manual*. Guilford Press.

Binder, J. L., & Betan, E. J. (2013). *Core competencies in brief dynamic psychotherapy. Becoming a highly effective and competent brief dynamic psychotherapist*. Routledge. https://doi.org/10.4324/9780203837412

Binder, J. L., & Betan, E. J. (2022). The cyclical maladaptive pattern. In T. D. Eells (Ed.), *Handbook of psychotherapy case formulation* (3rd ed., pp. 113–143). Guilford Press.

Binder, J. L., & Henry, W. P. (2010). Developing skills in managing negative process. In J. C. Muran & J. P. Barber (Eds.), *The therapeutic alliance: An evidence-based guide to practice* (pp. 285–303). Guilford Press.

Blagys, M. D., & Hilsenroth, M. J. (2000). Distinctive features of short-term psychodynamic-interpersonal psychotherapy: A review of the comparative psychotherapy process literature. *Clinical Psychology: Science and Practice*, 7(2), 167–188. https://doi.org/10.1093/clipsy.7.2.167

Blatt, S. J. (2008). *Polarities of experience: Relatedness and self-definition in personality development, psychopathology, and the therapeutic process*. American Psychological Association. https://doi.org/10.1037/11749-000

Bohart, A. C., & Wade, A. G. (2013). The client in psychotherapy. In M. J. Lambert (Ed.), *Bergin and Garfield's handbook of psychotherapy and behavior change* (6th ed., pp. 219–257). John Wiley & Sons.

Boterhoven De Haan, K. L., & Lee, C. W. (2014). Therapists' thoughts on therapy: Clinicians' perceptions of the therapy processes that distinguish schema, cognitive behavioural and psychodynamic approaches. *Psychotherapy Research*, 24(5), 538–549. https://doi.org/10.1080/10503307.2013.861092

Bowlby, J. (1982). *Attachment and loss: Vol. 1. Attachment*. Basic Books. (Original work published 1969)

Bowlby, J. (1985). The role of childhood experience in cognitive disturbance. In M. J. Mahoney and A. Freeman (Eds.), *Cognition and psychotherapy* (pp. 181–200). Plenum Press.

Bowlby, J. (1988). *A secure base*. Basic Books.

Brody, F., & Farber, B. (1996). The effects of therapist experience and diagnosis on countertransference. *Psychotherapy*, 33(3), 372–380. https://doi.org/10.1037/0033-3204.33.3.372

Brumbaugh, C. C., & Fraley, R. C. (2006). Transference and attachment: How do attachment patterns get carried forward from one relationship to the next? *Personality and Social Psychology Bulletin*, 32(4), 552–560. https://doi.org/10.1177/0146167205282740

Bugatti, M., & Boswell, J. F. (2016). Clinical errors as a lack of context responsiveness. *Psychotherapy*, 53(3), 262–267. https://doi.org/10.1037/pst0000080

Cabaniss, D. L., Cherry, S., Douglas, C. J., & Schwartz, A. (2011). *Psychodynamic psychotherapy: A clinical manual*. John Wiley & Sons.

Cartwright, C., Rhodes, P., King, R., & Shires, A. (2014). Experiences of countertransference: Reports of clinical psychology students. *Australian Psychologist*, 49(4), 232–240. https://doi.org/10.1111/ap.12062

Castonguay, L. G., Goldfried, M. R., Wiser, S., Raue, P. J., & Hayes, A. M. (1996). Predicting the effect of cognitive therapy for depression: A study of unique and common factors. *Journal of Consulting and Clinical Psychology, 64*(3), 497–504. https://doi.org/10.1037/0022-006X.64.3.497

Castonguay, L. G., & Hill, C. E. (Eds.). (2012). *Transformation in psychotherapy: Corrective experiences across cognitive behavioral, humanistic, and psychodynamic approaches.* American Psychological Association. https://doi.org/10.1037/13747-000

Christian, C., Safran, J. D., & Muran, J. C. (2012). The corrective emotional experience: A relational perspective and critique. In L. G. Castonguay & C. E. Hill (Eds.), *Transformation in psychotherapy: Corrective experiences across cognitive behavioral, humanistic, and psychodynamic approaches* (pp. 51–67). American Psychological Association. https://doi.org/10.1037/13747-004

Clarkin, J. F., Levy, K., Lenzenweger, M. F., & Kernberg, O. F. (2007). Evaluating three treatments for borderline personality disorder: A multiwave study. *American Journal of Psychiatry, 164*(6), 922–928. https://doi.org/10.1176/ajp.2007.164.6.922

Coker, J. (1990). *How to practice jazz.* Jamey Aebersold.

Cook, R. (2005). *It's about that time: Miles Davis on and off record.* Atlantic Books.

Cook, R. M., Welfare, L. E., & Jones, C. T. (2020). Incidence of intentional nondisclosure in clinical supervision by prelicensed counselors. *The Professional Counselor, 10*(1), 25–38. https://doi.org/10.15241/rmc.10.1.25

Csikszentmihalyi, M. (1997). *Finding flow: The psychology of engagement with everyday life.* HarperCollins.

Curtis, J. T., Silberschatz, G., Sampson, H., & Weiss, J. (1994). The Plan Formulation Method. *Psychotherapy Research, 4*(3–4), 197–207. https://doi.org/10.1080/10503309412331334032

Davis, D. E., DeBlaere, C., Owen, J., Hook, J. N., Rivera, D. P., Choe, E., Van Tongeren, D. R., Worthington, E. L., & Placeres, V. (2018). The multicultural orientation framework: A narrative review. *Psychotherapy, 55*(1), 89–100. https://doi.org/10.1037/pst0000160

Eagle, M. N. (2011). *From classical to contemporary psychoanalysis. A critique and integration.* Routledge. https://doi.org/10.4324/9780203868553

Ellis, M. V., Berger, L., Hanus, A. E., Ayala, E. E., Swords, B. A., & Siembor, M. (2014). Inadequate and harmful clinical supervision: Testing a revised framework and assessing occurrence. *The Counseling Psychologist, 42*(4), 434–472. https://doi.org/10.1177/0011000013508656

Ericsson, K. A. (2003). Development of elite performance and deliberate practice: An update from the perspective of the expert performance approach. In J. L. Starkes & K. A. Ericsson (Eds.), *Expert performance in sports: Advances in research on sport expertise* (pp. 49–83). Human Kinetics.

Ericsson, K. A. (2004). Deliberate practice and the acquisition and maintenance of expert performance in medicine and related domains. *Academic Medicine, 79*(Suppl. 10), S70–S81. https://doi.org/10.1097/00001888-200410001-00022

Ericsson, K. A. (2006). The influence of experience and deliberate practice on the development of superior expert performance. In K. A. Ericsson, N. Charness, P. J. Feltovich, & R. R. Hoffman (Eds.), *The Cambridge handbook of expertise and expert performance* (pp. 683–704). Cambridge University Press. https://doi.org/10.1017/CBO9780511816796.038

Ericsson, K. A., Hoffman, R. R., Kozbelt, A., & Williams, A. M. (Eds.). (2018). *The Cambridge handbook of expertise and expert performance* (2nd ed.). Cambridge University Press. https://doi.org/10.1017/9781316480748

Ericsson, K. A., Krampe, R. T., & Tesch-Römer, C. (1993). The role of deliberate practice in the acquisition of expert performance. *Psychological Review, 100*(3), 363–406. https://doi.org/10.1037/0033-295X.100.3.363

Ericsson, K. A., & Pool, R. (2016). *Peak: Secrets from the new science of expertise.* Houghton Mifflin Harcourt.

Eubanks, C. F., Muran, J. C., & Safran, J. D. (2018). Repairing alliance ruptures. In J. C. Norcross & B. E. Wampold (Eds.), *Psychotherapy relationships that work: Evidence-based responsiveness* (3rd ed., pp. 549–579). Oxford University Press.

Eubanks-Carter, C., Muran, J. C., & Safran, J. D. (2015). Alliance-focused training. *Psychotherapy, 52*(2), 169–173. https://doi.org/10.1037/a0037596

Fairbairn, W. R. D. (1952). *Psychoanalytic studies of the personality.* Tavistock.

Faulkner, W. (1951). *Requiem for a nun.* Random House.

Fauth, J., & Williams, E. N. (2005). The in-session self-awareness of therapist-trainees: Hindering or helpful? *Journal of Counseling Psychology, 52*(3), 443–447. https://doi.org/10.1037/0022-0167.52.3.443

Fisher, H., Atzil-Slonim, D., Bar-Kalifa, E., Rafaeli, E., & Peri, T. (2016). Emotional experience and alliance contribute to therapeutic change in psychodynamic therapy. *Psychotherapy, 53*(1), 105–116. https://doi.org/10.1037/pst0000041

Fisher, R. P., & Craik, F. I. M. (1977). Interaction between encoding and retrieval operations in cued recall. *Journal of Experimental Psychology: Human Learning and Memory, 3*(6), 701–711. https://doi.org/10.1037/0278-7393.3.6.701

Fonagy, P., & Bateman, A. W. (2006). Mechanisms of change in mentalization-based therapy of BPD. *Journal of Clinical Psychology, 62*(4), 411–430. https://doi.org/10.1002/jclp.20241

Freud, S. (1888). Hysteria. In J. Strachey (Ed.), *The standard edition of the complete psychological works of Sigmund Freud* (pp. 41–57). Hogarth Press, Inc.

Freud, S. (1937). Analysis terminable and interminable. In J. Strachey (Ed.), *The standard edition of the complete psychological works of Sigmund Freud* (Vol. 23, pp. 208–253). Hogarth Press.

Freud, S. (1957). Future prospects of psychoanalytic therapy. In J. Strachey (Ed.), *The standard edition of the complete works of Sigmund Freud* (Vol. 11, pp. 139–151). Hogarth Press. (Original work published 1910)

Freud, S. (1997). *The interpretation of dreams* (A. A. Brill, Trans.). Wordsworth Editions. (Original work published 1900)

Friedlander, M. L., Angus, L., Wright, S. T., Günther, C., Austin, C. L., Kangos, K., Barbaro, L., Macaulay, C., Carpenter, N., & Khattra, J. (2018). "If those tears could talk, what would they say?" Multi-method analysis of a corrective experience in brief dynamic therapy. *Psychotherapy Research, 28*(2), 217–234. https://doi.org/10.1080/10503307.2016.1184350

Friedlander, M. L., Angus, L. E., Xu, M., Wright, S. T., & Stark, N. M. (2020): A close look at therapist contributions to narrative-emotion shifting in a case illustration of brief dynamic therapy. *Psychotherapy Research, 30*(3), 402–416. https://doi.org/10.1080/10503307.2019.1609710

Furrow, J. L., Edwards, S. A., Choi, Y., & Bradley, B. (2012). Therapist presence in emotionally focused couple therapy blamer softening events: Promoting change through emotional experience. *Journal of Marital and Family Therapy, 38*(Suppl. 1), 39–49. https://doi.org/10.1111/j.1752-0606.2012.00293.x

Gabbard, G. O., & Wilkinson, S. M. (2000). *Management of countertransference with borderline patients.* Jason Aronson.

Geller, S. (2015). *Presence in psychotherapy* [Video]. https://www.youtube.com/watch?v=sShXDGjcjV0

Geller, S. (2017). *A practical guide to cultivating therapeutic presence.* American Psychological Association. https://doi.org/10.1037/0000025-000

Gelso, C., & Hayes, J. (2007). *Countertransference and the therapist's inner experience: Perils and possibilities.* Lawrence Erlbaum & Associates. https://doi.org/10.4324/9780203936979

Gelso, C. J., Kelley, F. A., Fuertes, J. N., Marmarosh, C., Holmes, S. E., Costa, C., & Hancock, G. R. (2005). Measuring the real relationship in psychotherapy: Initial validation of the therapist form. *Journal of Counseling Psychology, 52*(4), 640–649. https://doi.org/10.1037/0022-0167.52.4.640

Gill, M. M. (1954). Psychoanalysis and exploratory psychotherapy. *Journal of the American Psychoanalytic Association, 2*(4), 771–797. https://doi.org/10.1177/000306515400200413

Glausiusz, J. (2014). Living in an imaginary world. *Scientific American Mind, 23*(1). https://www.scientificamerican.com/article/living-in-an-imaginary-world/

Goldberg, S. B., Babins-Wagner, R., Rousmaniere, T., Berzins, S., Hoyt, W. T., Whipple, J. L., Miller, S. D., & Wampold, B. E. (2016). Creating a climate for therapist improvement: A case study of an agency focused on outcomes and deliberate practice. *Psychotherapy, 53*(3), 367–375. https://doi.org/10.1037/pst0000060

Goldberg, S. B., Rousmaniere, T., Miller, S. D., Whipple, J., Nielsen, S. L., Hoyt, W. T., & Wampold, B. E. (2016). Do psychotherapists improve with time and experience? A longitudinal analysis of outcomes in a clinical setting. *Journal of Counseling Psychology, 63*(1), 1–11. https://doi.org/10.1037/cou0000131

Goldman, R. N., Vaz, A., & Rousmaniere, T. (2021). *Deliberate practice in emotion-focused therapy.* American Psychological Association. https://doi.org/10.1037/0000227-000

Goodwin, B. J., Coyne, A. E., & Constantino, M. J. (2018). Extending the context-responsive psychotherapy integration framework to cultural processes in psychotherapy. *Psychotherapy, 55*(1), 3–8. https://doi.org/10.1037/pst0000143

Goodyear, R. K. (2015). Using accountability mechanisms more intentionally: A framework and its implications for training professional psychologists. *American Psychologist, 70*(8), 736–743. https://doi.org/10.1037/a0039828

Goodyear, R. K., & Nelson, M. L. (1997). The major formats of psychotherapy supervision. In C. E. Watkins, Jr. (Ed.), *Handbook of psychotherapy supervision* (pp. 328–344). John Wiley & Sons.

Goodyear, R. K., Wampold, B. E., Tracey, T. J., & Lichtenberg, J. W. (2017). Psychotherapy expertise should mean superior outcomes and demonstrable improvement over time. *The Counseling Psychologist, 45*(1), 54–65. https://doi.org/10.1177/0011000016652691

Greenberg, L. S., & Tomescu, L. R. (2017). *Supervision essentials for emotion-focused therapy.* American Psychological Association. https://doi.org/10.1037/15966-000

Greenberg, L. S., & Watson, J. (2006). *Emotion-focused therapy for depression.* Guilford Press. https://doi.org/10.1037/11286-000

Greenson, R. R. (1967). *The technique and practice of psychoanalysis* (Vol. 1). International Universities Press.

Haggerty, G., & Hilsenroth, M. J. (2011). The use of video in psychotherapy supervision. *British Journal of Psychotherapy, 27*(2), 193–210. https://doi.org/10.1111/j.1752-0118.2011.01232.x

Haig, M. (2020). *The midnight library.* Viking.

Harris, J., Jin, J., Hoffman, S., Phan, S., Prout, T. A., Rousmaniere, T., Vaz, A. (in press). *Deliberate practice in multicultural therapy.* American Psychological Association. https://doi.org/10.1037/0000357-000

Hatcher, R. L. (2015). Interpersonal competencies: Responsiveness, technique, and training in psychotherapy. *American Psychologist, 70*(8), 747–757. https://doi.org/10.1037/a0039803

Hayes, J. A., Gelso, C. J., Goldberg, S., & Kivlighan, D. M. (2018). Countertransference management and effective psychotherapy: Meta-analytic findings. *Psychotherapy, 55*(4), 496–507. https://doi.org/10.1037/pst0000189

Hayes, J. A., Gelso, C. J., & Hummel, A. M. (2011). Managing countertransference. In J. C. Norcross (Ed.), *Psychotherapy relationships that work: Evidence-based responsiveness* (2nd ed., pp. 239–258). Oxford University Press. https://doi.org/10.1093/acprof:oso/9780199737208.003.0012

Henry, W. P., Schacht, T. E., & Strupp, H. H. (1986). Structural analysis of social behavior: Application to a study of interpersonal process in differential psychotherapeutic outcome. *Journal of Consulting and Clinical Psychology, 54*(1), 27–31. https://doi.org/10.1037/0022-006X.54.1.27

Henry, W. P., Schacht, T. E., & Strupp, H. H. (1990). Patient and therapist introject, interpersonal process, and differential psychotherapy outcome. *Journal of Consulting and Clinical Psychology, 58*(6), 768–774. https://doi.org/10.1037/0022-006X.58.6.768

Henry, W. P., Strupp, H. H., Butler, S. F., Schacht, T. E., & Binder, J. L. (1993). Effects of training in time-limited dynamic psychotherapy: Changes in therapist behavior. *Journal of Consulting and Clinical Psychology, 61*(3), 434–440. https://doi.org/10.1037/0022-006X.61.3.434

Hill, C. E. (2020). *Helping skills: Facilitating exploration, insight, and action* (5th ed.). American Psychological Association. https://doi.org/10.1037/0000147-000

Hill, C. E., Gelso, C. J., Chui, H., Spangler, P. T., Hummel, A., Huang, T., Jackson, J., Jones, R. A., Palma, B., Bhatia, A., Gupta, S., Ain, S. C., Klingaman, B., Lim R. H., Liu, J., Hui, K., Jezzi, M. M., & Miles, J. R. (2014). To be or not to be immediate with clients: The use and perceived effects of immediacy in psychodynamic/interpersonal psychotherapy. *Psychotherapy Research, 24*(3), 299–315. https://doi.org/10.1080/10503307.2013.812262

Hill, C. E., Kivlighan, D. M. I. I. I., Rousmaniere, T., Kivlighan, D. M., Jr., Gerstenblith, J., & Hillman, J. (2020). Deliberate practice for the skill of immediacy: A multiple case study of doctoral student therapists and clients. *Psychotherapy, 57*(4), 587–597. https://doi.org/10.1037/pst0000247

Hill, C. E., & Knox, S. (2013). Training and supervision in psychotherapy: Evidence for effective practice. In M. J. Lambert (Ed.), *Handbook of psychotherapy and behavior change* (6th ed., pp. 775–811). Wiley.

Høglend, P., Amlo, S., Marble, A., Bøgwald, K.-P., Sørbye, O., Sjaastad, M. C., & Heyerdahl, O. (2006). Analysis of the patient–therapist relationship in dynamic psychotherapy: An experimental study of transference interpretations. *American Journal of Psychiatry, 163*(10), 1739–1746. https://doi.org/10.1176/ajp.2006.163.10.1739

Hook, J. N., Davis, D. D., Owen, J., & DeBlaere, C. (2017). *Cultural humility: Engaging diverse identities in therapy.* American Psychological Association. https://doi.org/10.1037/0000037-000

Horowitz, M. J. (1998). *Cognitive psychodynamics: From conflict to character.* John Wiley & Sons.

Howard, S. (2017). *Skills in psychodynamic counselling and psychotherapy* (2nd ed.). Sage Publications.

Inderbitzin, L. B., & Levy, S. T. (1990). Unconscious fantasy: A reconsideration of the concept. *Journal of the American Psychoanalytic Association, 38*(1), 113–130. https://doi.org/10.1177/000306519003800107

Kendall, P. C., & Beidas, R. S. (2007). Smoothing the trail for dissemination of evidence-based practices for youth: Flexibility within fidelity. *Professional Psychology, Research and Practice, 38*(1), 13–19. https://doi.org/10.1037/0735-7028.38.1.13

Kendall, P. C., & Frank, H. E. (2018). Implementing evidence-based treatment protocols: Flexibility within fidelity. *Clinical Psychology: Science and Practice, 25*(4), e12271. Advance online publication. https://doi.org/10.1111/cpsp.12271

Kiesler, D. J. (1988). *Therapeutic metacommunication: Therapist impact disclosure as feedback In psychotherapy.* Consulting Psychologists Press.

Kiesler, D. J., Schmidt, J. A., & Wagner, C. C. (1997). A circumplex inventory of impact messages. An operational bridge between emotion and interpersonal behavior. In R. Plutchik & H. R. Conte (Eds.), *Circumplex models of personality and emotions* (pp. 221–244). American Psychological Association. https://doi.org/10.1037/10261-010

Kohut, H. (1977). *The restoration of the self.* International Universities Press.

Koziol, L. F., & Budding, D. E. (2012). Procedural Learning. In N. M. Seel (Ed.), *Encyclopedia of the sciences of learning* (pp. 2694-2696). Springer. https://doi.org/10.1007/978-1-4419-1428-6_670

Kuhn, N., Andrews, S., Kaplan, A., Wolf, J., & Hurley, C. L. (2003). *Treating affect phobia: A manual for short-term dynamic psychotherapy.* Guilford Press.

Ladany, N., Hill, C. E., Corbett, M. M., & Nutt, E. A. (1996). Nature, extent, and importance of what psychotherapy trainees do not disclose to their supervisors. *Journal of Counseling Psychology, 43*(1), 10–24. https://doi.org/10.1037/0022-0167.43.1.10

Lambert, M. J. (2010). Yes, it is time for clinicians to monitor treatment outcome. In B. L. Duncan, S. C. Miller, B. E. Wampold, & M. A. Hubble (Eds.), *Heart and soul of change: Delivering what works in therapy* (2nd ed., pp. 239–266). American Psychological Association. https://doi.org/10.1037/12075-008

Lane, R. D., Ryan, L., Nadel, L., & Greenberg, L. (2015). Memory reconsolidation, emotional arousal, and the process of change in psychotherapy: New insights from brain science. *Behavioral and Brain Sciences, 38*, 1–64. https://doi.org/10.1017/S0140525X14000041

Levenson, H. (1995). *Time-limited dynamic psychotherapy: A guide to clinical practice*. Basic Books.

Levenson, H. (1999). *Time limited dynamic psychotherapy* [Film; educational DVD]. Pychotherapy. net. https://www.psychotherapy.net/video/time-limited-dynamic-psychotherapy

Levenson, H. (2003). Time-limited dynamic psychotherapy: An integrationist perspective. *Journal of Psychotherapy Integration, 13*(3–4), 300–333. https://doi.org/10.1037/1053-0479.13.3-4.300

Levenson, H. (2010). *Brief dynamic therapy over time* [Film; educational DVD]. American Psychological Association. https://www.apa.org/pubs/videos/4310871

Levenson, H. (2013). Time-limited dynamic psychotherapy: Working with reactions to chronically depressed clients. In A. W. Wolf, M. R. Goldfried, & J. C. Muran (Eds.), *Transforming negative reactions to clients: From frustration to compassion* (pp. 193–219). American Psychological Association. https://doi.org/10.1037/13940-009

Levenson, H. (2017). *Brief dynamic therapy* (2nd ed.). American Psychological Association. https://doi.org/10.1037/0000043-000

Levenson, H. (2018). *Time-limited dynamic psychotherapy: An integrative perspective* [includes video]. In M. J. Dewan, B. N. Steenbarger, & R. P. Greenberg (Eds.), *The art and science of brief psychotherapies: An illustrated guide* (3rd ed., Chapter 12). American Psychiatric Association Publishing. https://www.appi.org/Products/Psychotherapy/Art-and-Science-of-Brief-Psychotherapies-Third-Edi?SearchText=levenson,%20han&sku=37079

Levenson, H. (2020). Enlivening psychodynamic brief therapy with emotion-focused interventions: An integrative therapist's approach. *Clinical Social Work Journal, 48*(3), 267–278. https://doi.org/10.1007/s10615-020-00762-z

Levenson, H. (2021, March). *Enhancing responsiveness with deliberate practice*. Invited Address to the Responsive Therapist: Clinical, Conceptual, and Empirical Perspectives, Annual San Francisco Psychotherapy Research Group, San Francisco, CA, United States.

Levenson, H., Angus, L., & Pool, E. (2020). Viewing psychodynamic/interpersonal theory and practice through the lens of memory reconsolidation. In R. D. Lane & L. Nadel (Eds.), *Neuroscience of enduring change: Implications for psychotherapy* (pp. 296–323). Oxford University Press. https://doi.org/10.1093/oso/9780190881511.003.0012

Levenson, H., Butler, S., & Bein, E. (2002). Brief psychodynamic individual psychotherapy. In R. Hales, S. C. Yudofsky, & J. Talbot (Eds.), *American Psychiatric Press textbook of psychiatry* (pp. 11–17). American Psychiatric Press.

Levenson, H. (Guest Expert), & Carlson, J. (Host). (2008). *Brief dynamic therapy* [Film; educational DVD]. American Psychological Association. https://www.apa.org/pubs/videos/4310844

Levenson, H. (Guest Expert), & Carlson, J. (Host). (2010). *Brief dynamic therapy over time* [Film; educational DVD]. American Psychological Association. https://www.apa.org/pubs/videos/4310871

Levenson, H. (Guest Expert), & Friedlander, M. L. (Host). (in production). *Psychodynamic therapy skills* [Educational DVD]. American Psychological Association.

Levenson, H., & Strupp, H. H. (1999). Recommendations for the future of training in brief dynamic psychotherapy. *Journal of Clinical Psychology, 55*(4), 385–391. https://doi.org/10.1002/(SICI)1097-4679(199904)55:4<385::AID-JCLP2>3.0.CO;2-B

Levenson, H., & Strupp, H. H. (2007). Cyclical maladaptive patterns: Case formulation in time-limited dynamic psychotherapy. In T. D. Eells (Ed.), *Handbook of psychotherapy case formulation* (pp. 164–197). Guilford Press.

Levin, K. (1996). Unconscious phantasy in psychotherapy. *American Journal of Psychotherapy, 50*(2), 137–153.

Levy, K. N. (2009). Psychodynamic and psychoanalytic psychotherapies. In D. Richard & S. Huprich (Eds.), *Clinical psychology assessment, treatment, and research* (pp. 181–214). Elsevier Academic Press.

Levy, K. N., Keefe, J. R., & Ehrenthal, J. C. (2019). Research support for psychodynamic constructs. In D. Kealy & J. S. Ogrodniczuk (Eds.), *Evolving clinical practice* (pp. 89–106). Elsevier.

Levy, K. N., & Scala, J. W. (2012). Transference, transference interpretations, and transference-focused psychotherapies. *Psychotherapy, 49*(3), 391–403. https://doi.org/10.1037/a0029371

Lloyd, J. (2017). Therapeutic use of metaphor: Cultural connectivity. *Journal of Experiential Psychotherapy, 20*(2), 3–10.

Luo, X., Wang, J., Ng, T. (2022). *Delineating common microprocesses in psychodynamic psychotherapy using a dynamic systems approach* [Poster presentation]. 111th Annual Meeting of the American Psychoanalytic Association, New York, NY, United States.

Lyons-Ruth, K., Bruschweiler-Stern, N., Harrison, A. M., Morgan, A. C., Nahum, J. P., Sander, L., Stern, D. N., & Tronick, E. Z. (1999). Implicit relational knowing: Its role in development and psychoanalytic treatment. *Infant Mental Health Journal, 19*(3), 282–289.

MacDevitt, J. W. (1987). Therapists' personal therapy and professional self-awareness. *Psychotherapy, 24*(4), 693–703.

Malan, D. (1995). *Individual psychotherapy and the science of psychodynamics* (2nd ed.). Butterworth-Heinemann.

Malkomsen, A., Røssberg, J. I., Dammen, T., Wilberg, T., Løvgren, A., Ulberg, R., & Evensen, J. (2021). Digging down or scratching the surface: How patients use metaphors to describe their experiences of psychotherapy. *BMC Psychiatry, 21*, Article 533. https://doi.org/10.1186/s12888-021-03551-1

Markman, K. D., & Tetlock, P. E. (2000). Accountability and close-call counterfactuals: The loser who nearly won and the winner who nearly lost. *Personality and Social Psychology Bulletin, 26*(10), 1213–1224. https://doi.org/10.1177/0146167200262004

McCullough, L. (Guest Expert), & Carlson, J. (Host). (2005). *Affect-focused dynamic psychotherapy* [Film; educational DVD]. American Psychological Association. https://www.apa.org/pubs/videos/4310728

McCullough, L., Kuhn, N., Andrews, S., Kaplan, A., Wolf, J., & Hurley, C. L. (2003). *Treating affect phobia: A manual for short-term dynamic psychotherapy.* Guilford Press.

McGaghie, W. C., Issenberg, S. B., Barsuk, J. H., & Wayne, D. B. (2014). A critical review of simulation-based mastery learning with translational outcomes. *Medical Education, 48*(4), 375–385. https://doi.org/10.1111/medu.12391

McLeod, J. (2017). Qualitative methods for routine outcome measurement. In T. G. Rousmaniere, R. Goodyear, D. D. Miller, & B. E. Wampold (Eds.), *The cycle of excellence: Using deliberate practice to improve supervision and training* (pp. 99–122). John Wiley & Sons. https://doi.org/10.1002/9781119165590.ch5

McWilliams, N. (1999). *Psychoanalytic case formulation.* Guilford Press.

McWilliams, N. (2004). *Psychoanalytic psychotherapy: A practitioner's guide.* Guilford Press.

McWilliams, N. (2013). The impact of my own psychotherapy on my work as a therapist. *Psychoanalytic Psychology, 30*(4), 621–626. https://doi.org/10.1037/a0034582

McWilliams, N. (2021). *Psychoanalytic supervision.* Guilford Press.

McWilliams, N. (Guest Expert), & Carlson, J. (Host). (2008). *Psychoanalytic psychotherapy* [Film, educational DVD]. American Psychological Association. https://www.apa.org/pubs/videos/4310811

Messer, S. B., & Warren, C. S. (1995). *Models of brief psychodynamic therapy: A comparative approach.* Guilford Press.

Mitchell, S. A. (1988). *Relational concepts in psychoanalysis: An integration.* Harvard University Press. https://doi.org/10.4159/9780674041158

Muran, J. C., & Barber, J. P. (Eds.). (2010). *The therapeutic alliance: An evidence-based guide to practice.* Guilford Press.

Norcross, J. C., & Guy, J. D. (2005). The prevalence and parameters of personal therapy in the United States. In J. D. Geller, J. C. Norcross, & D. E. Orlinsky (Eds.), *The psychotherapist's own psychotherapy: Patient and clinician perspectives* (pp. 165–176). Oxford University Press.

Norcross, J. C., & Wampold, B. E. (Eds.). (2019). *Psychotherapy relationships that work* (Vols. 1–2, 3rd ed.). Oxford University Press.

Orlinsky, D. E., & Rønnestad, M. H., & Collaborative Research Network of the Society for Psychotherapy Research. (2005). *How psychotherapists develop: A study of therapeutic work and professional growth*. American Psychological Association. https://doi.org/10.1037/11157-000

Owen, J., & Hilsenroth, M. J. (2014). Treatment adherence: The importance of therapist flexibility in relation to therapy outcomes. *Journal of Counseling Psychology*, *61*(2), 280–288. https://doi.org/10.1037/a0035753

Peluso, P. R., & Freund, R. R. (2018). Therapist and client emotional expression and psychotherapy outcomes: A meta-analysis. *Psychotherapy*, *55*(4), 461–472. https://doi.org/10.1037/pst0000165

Pine, F. (1990). *Drive, ego, object, and self: A synthesis for clinical work*. Basic Books.

Prescott, D. S., Maeschalck, C. L., & Miller, S. D. (Eds.). (2017). *Feedback-informed treatment in clinical practice: Reaching for excellence*. American Psychological Association. https://doi.org/10.1037/0000039-000

Rousmaniere, T. G. (2016). *Deliberate practice for psychotherapists: A guide to improving clinical effectiveness*. Routledge Press. https://doi.org/10.4324/9781315472256

Rousmaniere, T. G. (2019). *Mastering the inner skills of psychotherapy: A deliberate practice manual*. Gold Lantern Press.

Rousmaniere, T. G., Goodyear, R., Miller, S. D., & Wampold, B. E. (Eds.). (2017). *The cycle of excellence: Using deliberate practice to improve supervision and training*. Wiley Publishers. https://doi.org/10.1002/9781119165590

Safran, J. D. (2012). *Psychoanalysis and psychoanalytic therapies*. American Psychological Association.

Safran, J. D. (Guest Expert), & Carlson, J. (Host). (2008). *Relational psychotherapy* [Film; educational DVD]. American Psychological Association. https://www.apa.org/pubs/videos/4310846

Safran, J. D. (Guest Expert), & Carlson, J. (Host) (2009). *Psychoanalytic psychotherapy over time* [Film; educational DVD]. American Psychological Association. https://www.apa.org/pubs/videos/4310864

Safran, J. D., & Kraus, J. (2014). Alliance ruptures, impasses, and enactments: A relational perspective. *Psychotherapy*, *51*(3), 381–387. https://doi.org/10.1037/a0036815

Safran, J. D., & Muran, J. C. (2000). *Negotiating the therapeutic alliance: A relational treatment guide*. Guilford Press.

Sandler, J., & Sandler, A. M. (1978). On the development of object relationships and affects. *The International Journal of Psycho-Analysis*, *59*(2–3), 285–296.

Sarnat, J. E. (2016). *Supervision essentials for psychodynamic psychotherapies*. American Psychological Association. https://doi.org/10.1037/14802-000

Schore, J. R., & Schore, A. N. (2008). Modern attachment theory: The central role of affect regulation in development and treatment. *Clinical Social Work Journal*, *36*(1), 9–20. https://doi.org/10.1007/s10615-007-0111-7

Sharpless, B. A., & Barber, J. P. (2012). Corrective emotional experiences from a psychodynamic perspective. In L. G. Castonguay & C. E. Hill (Eds.), *Transformation in psychotherapy: Corrective experiences across cognitive behavioral, humanistic, and psychodynamic approaches* (pp. 31–49). American Psychological Association. https://doi.org/10.1037/13747-003

Sharpless, B. A., Barber, J. P., & Summers, R. F. (2022). Psychodynamic psychotherapy. In G. Asmundson (Ed.), *Comprehensive clinical psychology* (2nd ed., Vol. 6, pp. 75–96). Elsevier.

Shedler, J. (2006). *That was then, this is now: Psychoanalytic psychotherapy for the rest of us*. https://jonathanshedler.com/wp-content/uploads/2020/07/Shedler-That-was-then-this-is-now-R10.pdf

Shedler, J. (2022). That was then, this is now: Psychoanalytic psychotherapy for the rest of us. *Contemporary Psychoanalysis*, *58*(2–3), 405–437. https://doi.org/10.1080/00107530.2022.2149038

Siegelman, E. Y. (1990). *Metaphor and meaning in psychotherapy.* Guilford Press.

Silberschatz, G. (2021). Responsiveness in control-mastery theory. In J. C. Watson & H. Wiseman (Eds.), *The responsive psychotherapist: Attuning to clients in the moment* (pp. 133–150). American Psychological Association.

Sims, P. A. (2003). Working with metaphor. *American Journal of Psychotherapy, 57*(4), 528–536. https://doi.org/10.1176/appi.psychotherapy.2003.57.4.528

Smith, S. M. (1979). Remembering in and out of context. *Journal of Experimental Psychology: Human Learning and Memory, 5*(5), 460–471. https://doi.org/10.1037/0278-7393.5.5.460

Squire, L. R. (2004). Memory systems of the brain: A brief history and current perspective. *Neurobiology of Learning and Memory, 82*(3), 171–177. https://doi.org/10.1016/j.nlm.2004.06.005

Stern, D., Sander, L., Nahum, J., Harrison, A., Lyons-Ruth, K., Morgan, B., & Tronick, E. (1998). Non-interpretative mechanisms in psychoanalytic therapy. The "something more" than interpretation. *International Journal of Psychoanalysis, 79,* 903–921.

Stiles, W. B., & Horvath, A. O. (2017). Appropriate responsiveness as a contribution to therapist effects. In L. G. Castonguay & C. E. Hill (Eds.), *How and why are some therapists better than others? Understanding therapist effects* (pp. 71–84). American Psychological Association. https://doi.org/10.1037/0000034-005

Stricker, G., & Gold, J. R. (1996). Psychotherapy integration: An assimilative, psychodynamic approach. *Clinical Psychology: Science and Practice, 3*(1), 47–58. https://doi.org/10.1111/j.1468-2850.1996.tb00057.x

Strupp, H. H., & Binder, J. L. (1984). *Psychotherapy in a new key: A guide to time-limited dynamic psychotherapy.* Basic Books.

Sullivan, H. S. (1954). *The interpersonal theory of psychiatry.* W. W. Norton & Company.

Taylor, J. M., & Neimeyer, G. J. (2017). Lifelong professional improvement: The evolution of continuing education. In T. G. Rousmaniere, R. Goodyear, S. D. Miller, & B. Wampold (Eds.), *The cycle of excellence: Using deliberate practice to improve supervision and training* (pp. 219–248). John Wiley & Sons.

Teyber, E., & Teyber F. M. (2014). Working with the process dimension in relational therapies: Guidelines for clinical training. *Psychotherapy, 51*(3), 334–341. https://doi.org/10.1037/a0036579

Tishby, O. (2021). Responsiveness in psychodynamic relational psychotherapy. In J. C. Watson & H. Wiseman (Eds.), *The responsive psychotherapist: Attuning to clients in the moment* (pp. 107–132). American Psychological Association. https://doi.org/10.1037/0000240-006

Tracey, T. J. G., Wampold, B. E., Goodyear, R. K., & Lichtenberg, J. W. (2015). Improving expertise in psychotherapy. *Psychotherapy Bulletin, 50*(1), 7–13.

Tracey, T. J. G., Wampold, B. E., Lichtenberg, J. W., & Goodyear, R. K. (2014). Expertise in psychotherapy: An elusive goal? *American Psychologist, 69*(3), 218–229. https://doi.org/10.1037/a0035099

Wachtel, P. L. (1993). *Therapeutic communication: Principles and effective practice.* Guilford Press.

Wachtel, P. L. (2008). *Relational theory and the practice of psychotherapy.* Guilford Press.

Wachtel, P. L. (2011). *Inside the session: What really happens in psychotherapy.* American Psychological Association. https://doi.org/10.1037/12321-000

Wachtel, P. L. (Guest Expert), & Carlson, J. (Host). (2007). *Integrative relational psychotherapy* [Film; educational DVD]. American Psychological Association.

Wampold, B. E., & Owen, J. (2021). Therapist effects. In L. G. Castonguay, M. Barkham, & W. Lutz (Eds.), *Handbook of psychotherapy and behavior change* (5th ed., pp. 297–326). John Wiley & Sons.

Wass, R., & Golding, C. (2014). Sharpening a tool for teaching: The zone of proximal development. *Teaching in Higher Education, 19*(6), 671–684. https://doi.org/10.1080/13562517.2014.901958

Westra, H. A., Norouzian, N., Poulin, L., Coyne, A. E., Constantino, M. J., Hara, K., Olson, D., & Antony, M. M. (2021). Testing a deliberate practice workshop for developing appropriate responsivity to resistance markers. *Psychotherapy, 58*(2), 175–185. https://doi.org/10.1037/pst0000311

Wiggins, J. S., & Broughton, R. (1985). The Interpersonal Circle: A structural model for the integration of personality research. In R. Hogan & W. H. Jones (Eds.), *Perspectives in personality* (Vol. 1, pp. 1–47). JAI Press.

Wolitzky, D. L. (2011). Psychoanalytic theories of psychotherapy. In J. C. Norcross, G. R. VanderBos, & D. K. Freedheim (Eds.), *History of psychotherapy: Continuity and change* (pp. 65–100). American Psychological Association. https://doi.org/10.1037/12353-003

Wrightsman, L. S., Jr. (1964). Measurement of philosophies of human nature. *Psychological Reports, 14*(3), 743–751. https://doi.org/10.2466/pr0.1964.14.3.743

Yalom, I. D. (1995). *The theory and practice of group psychotherapy.* Basic Books.

Yalom, I. D. (2002). *The gift of therapy: An open letter to a new generation of therapists and their patients.* Harper Perennial.

Zaretskii, V. (2009). The zone of proximal development: What Vygotsky did not have time to write. *Journal of Russian & East European Psychology, 47*(6), 70–93. https://doi.org/10.2753/RPO1061-0405470604

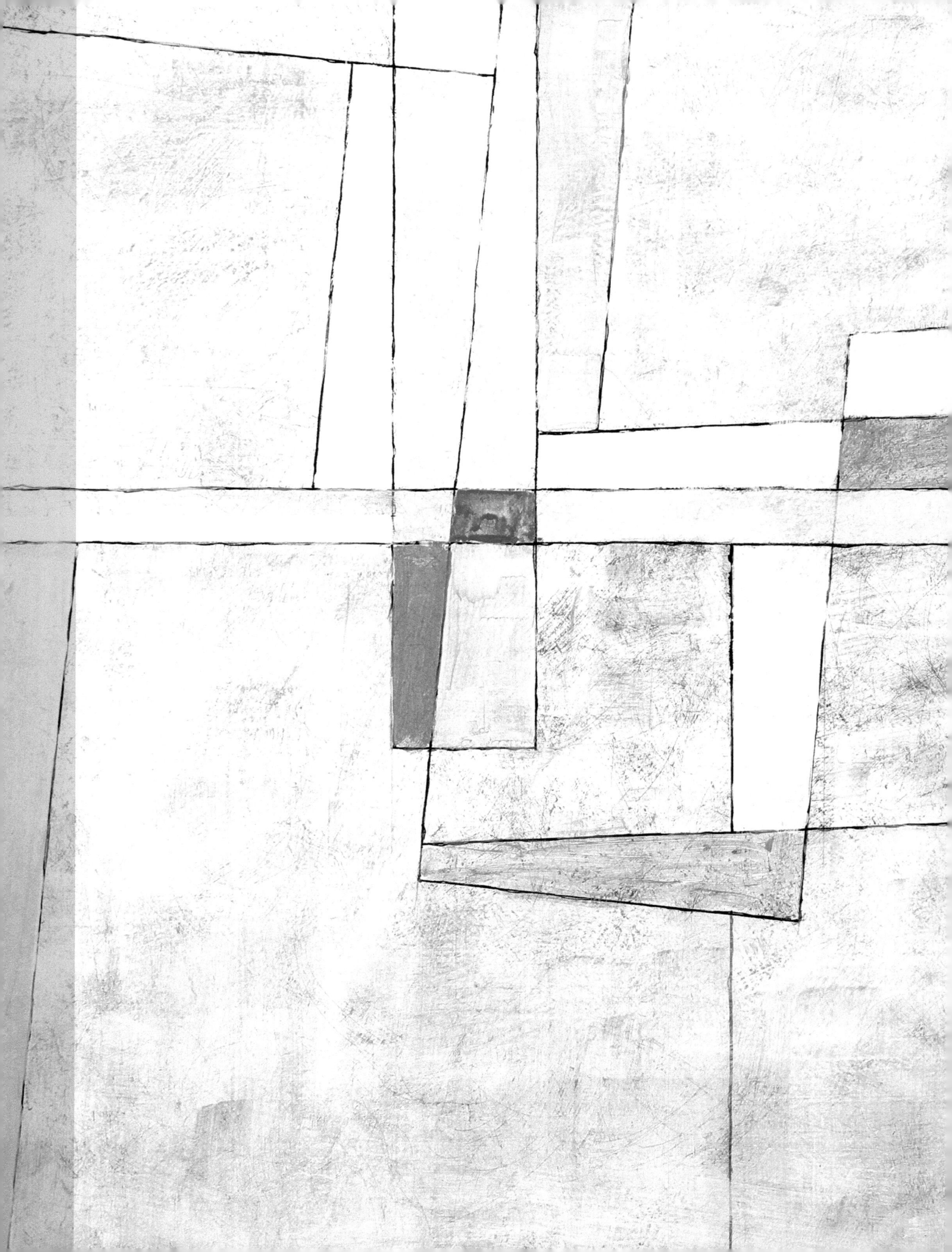

# Index

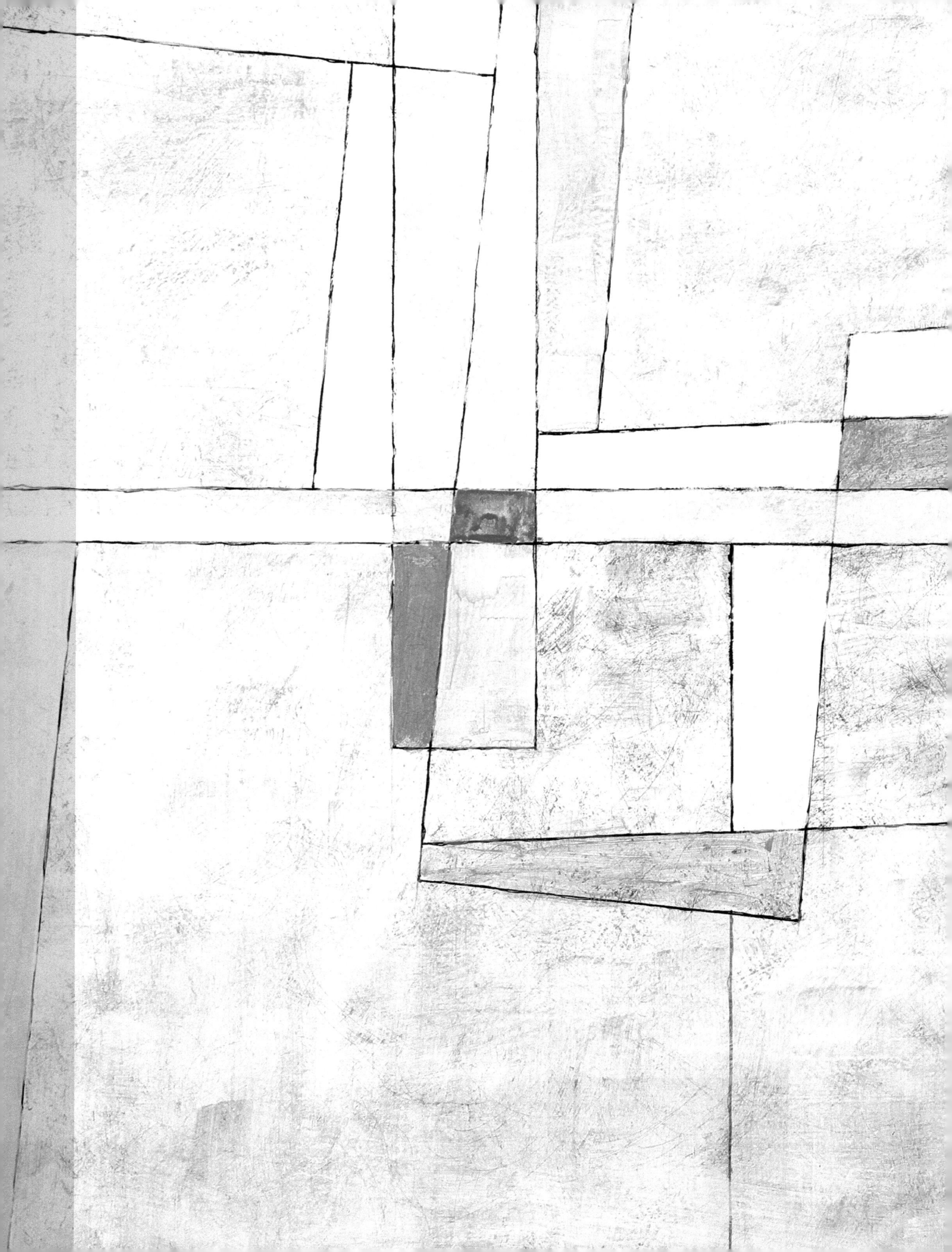

# About the Authors

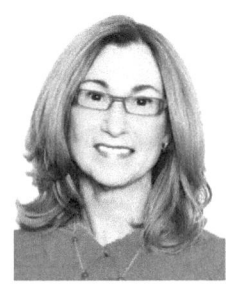

**Hanna Levenson, PhD,** is a professor at the Wright Institute in Berkeley, California, and a Fellow of the American Psychological Association (APA). In addition, she maintains a private practice in Oakland where she sees individuals and couples for therapy and professionals for consultation and supervision. For 20 years, Dr. Levenson was a clinical professor in the Department of Psychiatry, University of California Medical School, San Francisco (UCSF), and director of the Brief Therapy Program at the San Francisco VA Medical Center. She graduated from Vassar College (1967) with a BA in psychology and from Claremont University (1972) with a PhD in social psychology. After becoming an associate professor of psychology at Texas A&M University, she respecialized in clinical psychology, doing her internship training at Langley Porter Institute, UCSF (1976–1977). Dr. Levenson has been specializing in the areas of brief dynamic therapy and supervision for 40 years. She is the author of more than 85 professional papers and author or coauthor of three previous books (*Time-Limited Dynamic Psychotherapy: A Guide to Clinical Practice*, *Brief Dynamic and Interpersonal Therapy*, and *Brief Dynamic Therapy*). In her previous book (part of the APA Theories of Psychotherapy Series), Dr. Levenson integrates emotionally focused, experiential, and interpersonal approaches. She also has six professional videos illustrating her approach. Her most recent video is of two sessions highlighting psychodynamic skills and the use of deliberate practice as part of APA's Essentials of Deliberate Practice series. A recent project has been creating and hosting an 11 DVD and book series produced by APA on Essentials of Psychotherapy Supervision. Dr. Levenson has received the Distinguished Contribution to Psychology as a Profession Award given by the California Psychological Association.

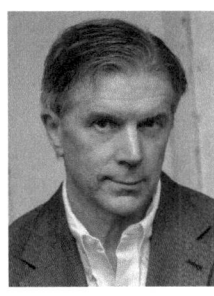

**Volney Gay, PhD,** is professor emeritus at Vanderbilt University. His degrees are BA, 1970, Reed College; MA, 1973, and PhD, 1976, the University of Chicago; he did his postdoctoral training at the St. Louis Psychoanalytic Institute. Dr. Volney retired in August 2018 as a professor of psychiatry, professor of religious studies, and professor of anthropology at Vanderbilt. At Vanderbilt, he was chair of religious studies, cofounder and director of the Center for the Study of Religion and Culture, and principal investigator, "Science and Religion," funded by the Templeton Foundation. He has directed 30 doctoral dissertations on psychology, religion, and anthropology. Dr. Volney is a training and supervising analyst at the St. Louis Psychoanalytic Institute, certified by the American Psychoanalytic Association, and a member of Section I, Division 39 (Society for Psychoanalysis and Psychoanalytic Psychology), of the American Psychological Association. He has published nine books on religion, psychiatry, and anthropology. He has won teaching awards from McMaster University and Vanderbilt University School of Medicine, the Heinz Hartmann Award given by the New York Psychoanalytic Institute, and the Outstanding Service Award from the American Psychoanalytic Association, and he was named Distinguished Psychoanalytic Educator by the International Forum for Psychoanalytic Education. His most recent book is *American Slavery: Privileges and Pleasures* (2021). In 1992, he founded the Nashville Psychoanalytic Study Group with Thomas Campbell, MD. In 2010, Dr. Volney endowed the Barbara Gay Lecture in Child Psychiatry at Vanderbilt University Medical Center.

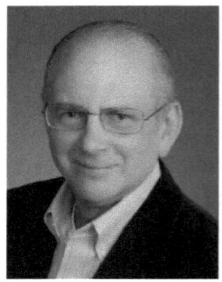

**Jeffrey L. Binder, PhD, ABPP,** is a clinical professor of psychiatry and behavioral science at Vanderbilt University, and a Fellow of the American Psychological Association, the Georgia Psychological Association, and the Academy of Clinical Psychology. He is also a diplomate in clinical psychology of the American Board of Professional Psychology. His professional career spans 51 years, during which he was at various times between 1991 and 2014 professor of psychology, program director, and dean at the Georgia School of Professional Psychology in Atlanta. Before that, Dr. Binder was clinical associate professor of psychology in psychiatry, Vanderbilt University (1980–1991); research associate professor of psychology, Vanderbilt University (1980–1983); clinical associate professor of psychiatry, University of Virginia (1976–1980); and assistant professor of psychiatry, University of Michigan (1972–1980). He also was director of outpatient services, Region Ten Community Mental Health Center, Charlottesville, Virginia (1976–1980), and director of adolescent and adult programs, Cumberland Hall Psychiatric Hospital, Nashville, Tennessee (1984–1989). Throughout his career, he has maintained a private practice in which he sees individuals and couples for therapy and trainees and professionals for consultation and supervision. Dr. Binder has authored or coauthored more than 45 articles and book chapters on psychotherapy practice, research, and supervision. Two of his papers ("Is It Time to Improve Psychotherapy Training?" and "Issues in Teaching and Learning Time-Limited Psychodynamic Psychotherapy," both published in the *Clinical Psychology Review*) were among the earliest proposals to improve psychotherapy training by applying instructional methods developed by cognitive scientists. Dr. Binder also has authored or coauthored four books, two of which present a model of time-limited psychodynamic–interpersonal therapy that incorporates principles derived from the findings of cognitive science research on the nature and development of expertise in complex performances.

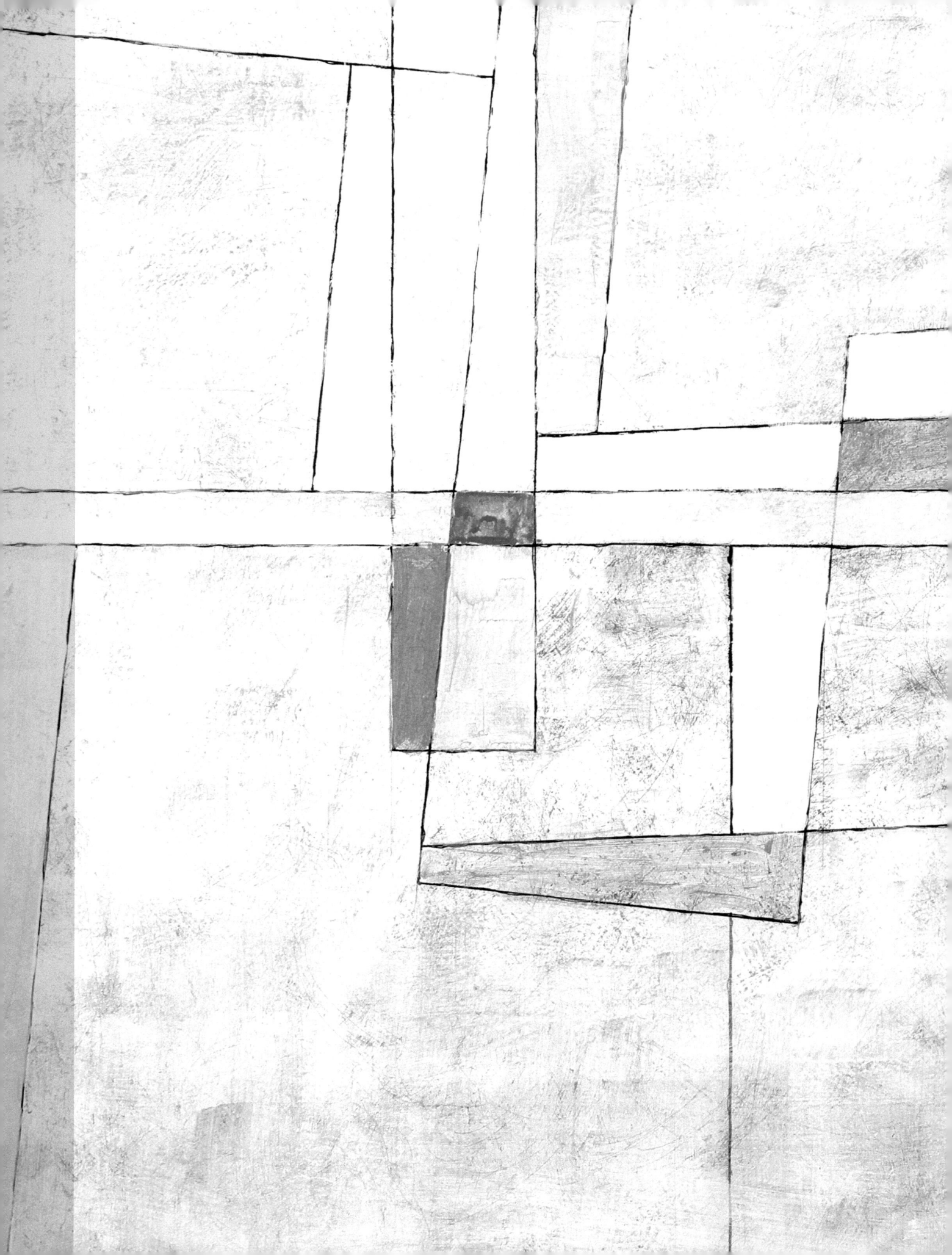

# About the Series Editors

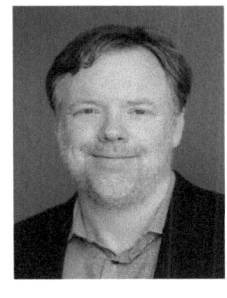

**Tony Rousmaniere, PsyD,** is cofounder and program director of Sentio University, Los Angeles, California. He provides workshops, webinars, and advanced clinical training and supervision to clinicians around the world. Dr. Rousmaniere is the author/coeditor of multiple books on deliberate practice and psychotherapy training and two series of clinical training books: The Essentials of Deliberate Practice (American Psychological Association) and Advanced Therapeutics, Clinical and Interpersonal Skills (Elsevier). In 2017, he published the widely cited article "What Your Therapist Doesn't Know" in *The Atlantic Monthly*. Dr. Rousmaniere supports the open-data movement and publishes his aggregated clinical outcome data, in deidentified form, on his website (https://drtonyr.com/). A Fellow of APA, he was awarded the Early Career Award by the Society for the Advancement of Psychotherapy (APA Division 29).

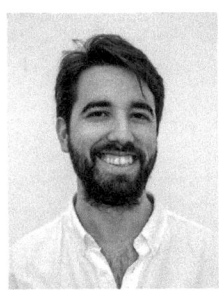

**Alexandre Vaz, PhD,** is cofounder and chief academic officer of Sentio University, Los Angeles, California. He provides deliberate practice workshops and advanced clinical training and supervision to clinicians around the world. Dr. Vaz is the author/coeditor of multiple books on deliberate practice and psychotherapy training and two series of clinical training books: The Essentials of Deliberate Practice (American Psychological Association) and Advanced Therapeutics, Clinical and Interpersonal Skills (Elsevier). He has held multiple committee roles for the Society for the Exploration of Psychotherapy Integration (SEPI) and the Society for Psychotherapy Research (SPR). Dr. Vaz is founder and host of "Psychotherapy Expert Talks," an acclaimed interview series with distinguished psychotherapists and therapy researchers.